Preface

The Directory of Private Medicine has be   /ith
information about private Consultants and   was
started in response to a demand by GPs fc   and
their clinics, so that they would have a mo   ıls.

As the demand for private medical services has increased, the public awareness of different treatment options has increased. In the past patients were quite content to allow GPs make all the decisions about their referrals. But with the increase in the choices available, patients now wish to play a greater role in the decision making process. This has led to a great demand amongst the public for more information about private medicine. We anticipate a great demand for information about quality standards in private medicine in the future.

We believe that patients have a right to be better informed. We also believe that our current referral system, with the GP referring patients to the Consultant, is the most appropriate. We welcome the GMC's stance on this and believe that protection of patients interests is paramount. We therefore advise patients to seek referral through their GP.

This edition of The Directory of Private Medicine provides details of private Consultants throughout the UK and details of GPs who offer private medical services. The Directory also provides a list of private hospitals in the UK.

Using The Directory of Private Medicine

Consultants and their clinics are organized according to specialty. Specialty sections are shown on the contents pages. Consultants are then subdivided according to the geographical area in which they practice. These geographical areas are represented by counties. The Directory covers the whole of the UK. Consultants are organized alphabetically within each area. There is an alphabetical list of the Consultants included in The Directory (see contents pages) enabling users to search for specific Consultants.

The Directory of Private Medicine includes an alphabetical list of Private GPs and Private Hospitals.

The Directory of Private Clinics
is published by QUIC Directory Limited.
20 Conway Road, Southgate, London N14 7BA

Tel: 0181 886 8888. Fax: 0181 351 4748
E-mail: admin@medicalnet.co.uk

Editor: Dr M F Kaleel

Copyright © 1999 QUIC Directory Limited.

All rights reserved. No part of this publication may be reproduced, stored in a retrieval system or transmitted in any form or by any means, electronic, mechanical, photocopying, recording or otherwise without the prior written permission of the publishers.

In accordance with General Medical Council Guidelines, it is strongly recommended that patients seeking referral to specialists do so via their General Practitioner. Inclusion in The Directory of Private Medicine does not constitute a recommendation as to the quality of services offered by practitioners or advertisers. Neither the proprietors, nor the publishers of The Directory of Private Medicine are liable in damages or otherwise for the quality or outcome of any treatment or services listed in The Directory of Private Medicine.

Qualifications, NHS Post and details of clinics have been entered as given by the Consultants. While every effort has been made to ensure the accuracy of entries in this Directory, neither the proprietors, the publishers, nor the printers of The Directory of Private Medicine, are liable in damages or otherwise for omission or incorrect insertion, whether as to wording, space or position of any entry or advertisement. The publishers reserve the right of acceptance or rejection of particulars submitted for insertion. Inclusion in The Directory of Private Medicine does not constitute a recommendation as to the quality of services offered by practitioners or advertisers.

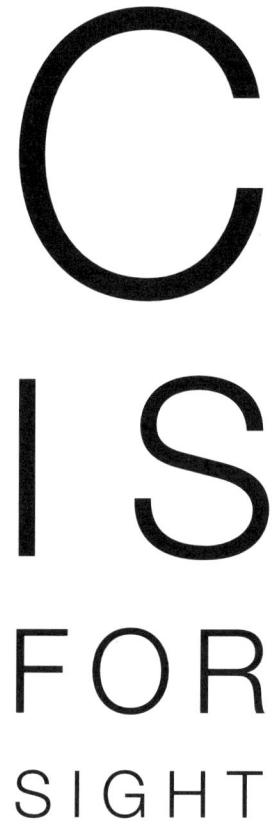

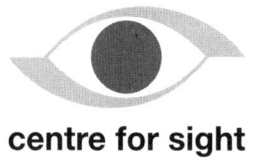

centre for sight

Laser and microsurgery for correction of shortsight, farsight and astigmatism. Consultants who specialise in medical and surgical diseases of the eye
For a brochure or details on a free seminar contact

07000 288 288

Offices in Harley Street London and Queen Victoria Hospital, NHS Trust, East Grinstead
www.centreforsight.com email lasik@compuserve.com

CONTENTS

Guide To Medical Qualifications	1
Royal Colleges	3
Allergy	4
London	4
West Yorkshire	4
Anaesthetics	5
(See also pain relief)	
Devon	5
London	5
West Sussex	5
Andrology	6
Cheshire	6
Essex	6
London	6
North Wales	7
Surrey	7
Audiological Medicine	8
Essex	8
London	8
Cardiology	9
Bath	9
Bristol	9
Buckinghamshire	9
Cheshire	9
Dumfries	10
Essex	10
Glasgow	10
Hertfordshire	10
Kent	11
Liverpool	11
London	12
Manchester	15
Middlesbrough	15
Surrey	15
Tyne & Wear	16
Dermatology	17
Berkshire	17
Cheshire	17
Enfield Middlesex	17
Essex	18
Glasgow	18
Hampshire	18
Hertfordshire	18
Kent	19
Leicestershire	19
London	19
Manchester	22
Middlesex	22
Norfolk	22
South Yorkshire	22
Warwickshire	23
West Midlands	23
West Sussex	23
ENT Surgery	24
Bedfordshire	24
Bristol	24
Buckinghamshire	24
Cheshire	24
Denbighshire	25
Devon	25
Enfield Middlesex	25
Essex	25
Hertfordshire	26

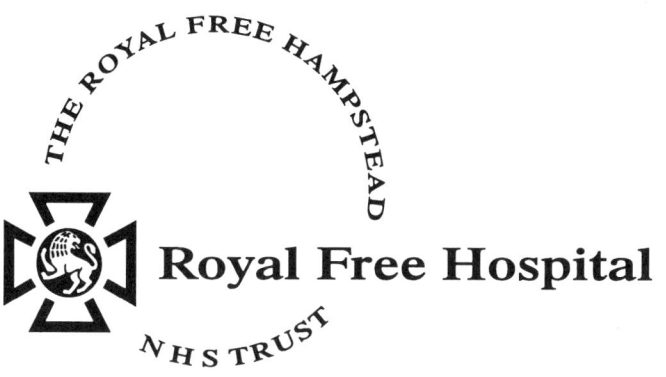

Royal Free Hospital

With panoramic views over London, the private unit has 53 single rooms, each with private bathroom, remote controlled television and private telephone.

Specialties include vascular surgery, general and orthopaedic surgery, medical oncology, dermatology and general medicine. Obstetric, gynaecology and paediatric services are also available.

The haematology department offers the most up-to-date treatment services to patients with all types of blood diseases.

The Royal Free founded one of the first liver units in the world established in the 1960's, the department has become a leading centre for liver medicine and transplantation.

The complete range of clinical support and diagnostic services available on site include: **Cardiac Catheter Laboratory, CT and MRI Scanner, Gamma and Renal Dialysis.**

24 hour medical cover is provided in all specialties. Special packages are available for bone marrow, liver and renal transplant as well as some of the more **common surgical procedures.**

The unit is fully recognised by all major UK medical insurers.

For further information please call on direct lines
In-patient services: 0171 830 2835
Out-patient services: 0171 830 2955

The Royal Free Hospital
Pond Street, Hampstead, London NW3 2QG

CONTENTS

Kent	26
London	28
Middlesex	33
Newcastle upon Tyne	33
Norfolk	33
North Hants	33
Nottinghamshire	34
Oxfordshire	34
South Yorkshire	34
Staffordshire	34
Surrey	35
Warwickshire	36
West Sussex	36

Endocrinology 37

Cheshire	37
Enfield Middlesex	37
Hertfordshire	37
London	38
Manchester	40
Middlesex	40
South Yorkshire	41

Gastroenterology 42

Birmingham	42
Devon	42
Essex	42
Glasgow	42
Herefordshire	43
London	43
Middlesex	46
Surrey	46
West Yorkshire	47

General Medicine 48

East Sussex	48
Enfield Middlesex	48
Hertfordshire	48
Kent	49
London	49
Middlesex	53
North Wales	53
South Yorkshire	53
Surrey	53
West Midlands	54
West Sussex	54

Genito-urinary Medicine 55

Berkshire	55
Buckinghamshire	55
Derbyshire	55
London	55

Geriatrics 57

Enfield Middlesex	57
Hertfordshire	57
London	57
Surrey	58

Haematology 59

Berkshire	59
Hampshire	59
Hertfordshire	59
London	59
Merseyside	60
Oxfordshire	60
Surrey	61
West Sussex	61

Hypertension 62

East Sussex	62

GORD Centre

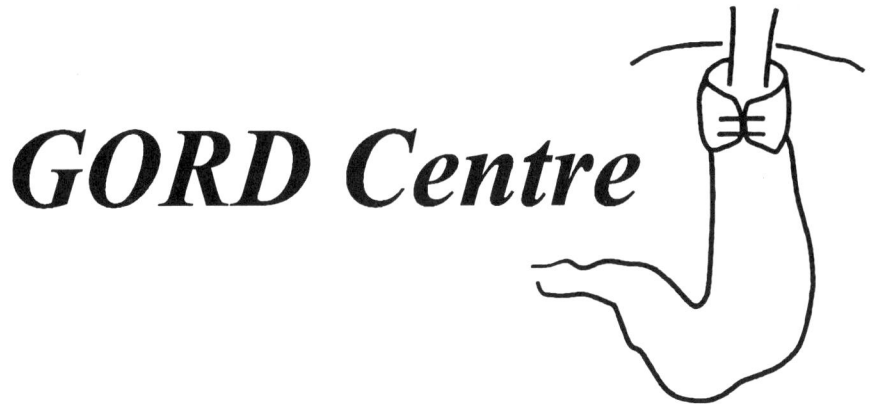

PPP/Colombia is pleased to announce its association with GORD Centre who have established Centres of Excellence for the investigation and management of Gastro-oesophageal reflux disease and anti-obesity surgery.

Specialists in:

- *Endoscopy*
- *24 hour oesophageal manometry and pH monitoring*
- *Laparoscopic anti-reflux surgery*
- *Laparoscopic anti-obesity surgery*

The Wellington Hospital
Wellington Place, London NW8 9LE

Secretary and Appointments
Tel: 0171 486 1515
Fax: 0171 935 4984

Website: www.gordcentre.org
E-mail: enquiries@gordcentre.org

CONTENTS

Infectious & Tropical Diseases	**63**
Leicestershire	63
London	63
Lipidology	**65**
Hertfordshire	65
London	65
Middlesex	66
West Sussex	66
Medical Genetics	**67**
London	67
Medico-Legal	**68**
Essex	68
London	68
Middlesex	69
Nottinghamshire	69
South Yorkshire	69
West Yorkshire	69
Metabolic Medicine	**70**
Cumbria	70
Hertfordshire	70
Kent	70
Liverpool	70
London	71
Middlesex	71
Nephrology	**72**
East Sussex	72
Hertfordshire	72
London	72
Middlesex	73
Neurology	**74**
Berkshire	74
Essex	74
Hampshire	75
Hertfordshire	75
London	75
Middlesex	79
Oxfordshire	79
Surrey	80
Neurophysiology (Clinical)	**81**
London	81
Staffordshire	81
Nuclear Medicine	**82**
London	82
Norfolk	82
Obstetrics & Gynaecology	**83**
Berkshire	83
Birmingham	83
Bristol	83
Buckinghamshire	84
Cambridgeshire	84
Cleveland	84
Derbyshire	84
Devon	85
Dorset	85
Down	85
Essex	85
Hampshire	87
Hertfordshire	87
Kent	88
Lancashire	88
Leeds	88
Lincolnshire	89
London	89
Middlesex	94

CONTENTS

Shropshire	94	Surrey	113
Surrey	94	West Glamorgan	114
Tyne & Wear	95	West Sussex	114
West Sussex	95	West Yorkshire	114

Oncology 96

East Sussex	96
Kent	96
London	96
Middlesex	98

Ophthalmology 99

Avon	99
Bedfordshire	99
Birmingham	99
Buckinghamshire	100
Cheshire	100
Devon	101
Dorset	101
Enfield Middlesex	101
Essex	101
Glamorgan	102
Gloucestershire	103
Hertfordshire	103
Kent	103
Lancashire	104
Leicestershire	104
London	104
Lothian	110
Manchester	110
Merseyside	111
Middlesex	111
North Yorkshire	112
Oxfordshire	112
Somerset	112

Orthopaedics 115

Avon	115
Berkshire	115
Bristol	115
Buckinghamshire	116
Cambridgeshire	116
Devonshire	116
East Sussex	116
Essex	117
Hertfordshire	118
Kent	118
Lancashire	119
London	120
Manchester	125
Merseyside	125
Middlesbrough	126
Middlesex	126
Norfolk	126
North Yorkshire	126
Oxfordshire	127
South Wales	127
Surrey	127
Tayside	129
West Sussex	129
West Yorkshire	129
Wirral	130
Worcestershire	130

CONTENTS

Orthopaedics - Hand Surgery   131
Berkshire · 131
Cheshire · 131
Glasgow · 131
London · 131

Orthopaedics - Knee Surgery   133
London · 133
Worcestershire · · · · · · · · · · · · · · · · 133

Orthopaedics - Spinal Surgery   134
London · 134
Suffolk · 134

Paediatric Surgery   135
Devon · 135
London · 135
Merseyside · · · · · · · · · · · · · · · · · · · 136
Surrey · 136

Paediatrics   137
Essex · 137
Hertfordshire · · · · · · · · · · · · · · · · · 137
Lancashire · · · · · · · · · · · · · · · · · · · 137
London · 138
Middlesex · 141
Surrey · 141

Pain Relief   143
(See also Anaesthetics)
Berkshire · 143
Essex · 143
Hertfordshire · · · · · · · · · · · · · · · · · 143
Kent · 144
London · 144
Middlesex · 144

Norfolk · 145
Oxfordshire · · · · · · · · · · · · · · · · · · 145
Surrey · 145
Warwickshire · · · · · · · · · · · · · · · · · 146

Pathology   147
Kent · 147
London · 147
West Midlands · · · · · · · · · · · · · · · · 147

Psychiatry   148
Berkshire · 148
Buckinghamshire · · · · · · · · · · · · · · 148
Cambridgeshire · · · · · · · · · · · · · · · 149
Cheshire · 149
Cleveland · 149
Dorset · 150
East Sussex · · · · · · · · · · · · · · · · · · 150
Essex · 150
Glasgow · 151
Greater Manchester · · · · · · · · · · · 151
Hampshire · · · · · · · · · · · · · · · · · · · 151
Hertfordshire · · · · · · · · · · · · · · · · · 152
Kent · 152
Lancashire · · · · · · · · · · · · · · · · · · · 152
London · 153
Merseyside · · · · · · · · · · · · · · · · · · · 159
Middlesex · 159
Nottinghamshire · · · · · · · · · · · · · · 160
Oxfordshire · · · · · · · · · · · · · · · · · · 160
Suffolk · 160
Surrey · 160
West Yorkshire · · · · · · · · · · · · · · · 161

Psychotherapy   162
Cleveland · 162

CONTENTS

Hertfordshire	162
Kent	162
London	162
Strathclyde	164
West Midlands	164

Radiology 165
Bedfordshire	165
Buckinghamshire	165
Durham	165
Hampshire	165
Hertfordshire	166
London	166
Norfolk	167

Renal Medicine 168
London	168

Respiratory Medicine 169
(See also Thoracic Medicine)
London	169

Rheumatology 170
Cheshire	170
Conwy	170
Essex	170
Hertfordshire	170
Kent	171
Lancashire	171
Leicestershire	171
London	171
Middlesex	174
Nottinghamshire	174
Surrey	175
Tyne & Wear	175

SURGERY - Breast 176
East Sussex	176
Essex	176
Hertfordshire	176
Kent	176
London	177
Manchester	178
Staffordshire	179
Surrey	179

SURGERY - Cardiothoracic 180
Cambridgeshire	180
London	180
Merseyside	181
Plymouth	181
Surrey	182

SURGERY - Colorectal & Gastrointestinal 183
Cheshire	183
Conwy	183
East Sussex	183
Enfield Middlesex	183
Essex	184
Hertfordshire	184
Kent	184
Lancashire	185
Liverpool	185
London	185
Middlesex	188
Oxfordshire	189
South Wales	189
Staffordshire	189
Surrey	189
West Midlands	190

CONTENTS

West Sussex · · · · · · · · · · · · · · · 190
Wrexham · · · · · · · · · · · · · · · · · 190

SURGERY - Endocrine 191
Devon · · · · · · · · · · · · · · · · · · · 191
Kent · 191
London · · · · · · · · · · · · · · · · · · 191
South Glamorgan · · · · · · · · · · · · 192

SURGERY - General 193
Bedfordshire · · · · · · · · · · · · · · · 193
Cheshire · · · · · · · · · · · · · · · · · 193
Devon · · · · · · · · · · · · · · · · · · · 193
East Sussex · · · · · · · · · · · · · · · 193
Enfield Middlesex · · · · · · · · · · · · 194
Essex · · · · · · · · · · · · · · · · · · · 194
Glasgow · · · · · · · · · · · · · · · · · 194
Hampshire · · · · · · · · · · · · · · · · 195
Hertfordshire · · · · · · · · · · · · · · · 195
Kent · 195
Liverpool · · · · · · · · · · · · · · · · · 196
London · · · · · · · · · · · · · · · · · · 197
Manchester · · · · · · · · · · · · · · · 200
Merseyside · · · · · · · · · · · · · · · 201
Middlesex · · · · · · · · · · · · · · · · 201
Oxfordshire · · · · · · · · · · · · · · · 201
Staffordshire · · · · · · · · · · · · · · · 202
Surrey · · · · · · · · · · · · · · · · · · · 202
West Sussex · · · · · · · · · · · · · · · 203

SURGERY - Hepatobiliary 204
Kent · 204

SURGERY - Neurology 205
Bristol · · · · · · · · · · · · · · · · · · · 205
Cleveland · · · · · · · · · · · · · · · · 205

Kent · 205
London · · · · · · · · · · · · · · · · · · 206
Nottinghamshire · · · · · · · · · · · · 207
South Yorkshire · · · · · · · · · · · · · 207
Tyne & Wear · · · · · · · · · · · · · · · 207
Warwickshire · · · · · · · · · · · · · · 207

SURGERY - Oncology 208
East Sussex · · · · · · · · · · · · · · · 208
Gwent · · · · · · · · · · · · · · · · · · · 208
Kent · 208
Liverpool · · · · · · · · · · · · · · · · · 208
London · · · · · · · · · · · · · · · · · · 209
Surrey · · · · · · · · · · · · · · · · · · · 209

SURGERY - Oral & Maxillofacial 210
Bedfordshire · · · · · · · · · · · · · · · 210
Bristol · · · · · · · · · · · · · · · · · · · 210
Buckinghamshire · · · · · · · · · · · · 210
Cambridgeshire · · · · · · · · · · · · · 211
Essex · · · · · · · · · · · · · · · · · · · 211
Hampshire · · · · · · · · · · · · · · · · 211
Hertfordshire · · · · · · · · · · · · · · · 212
London · · · · · · · · · · · · · · · · · · 212
Surrey · · · · · · · · · · · · · · · · · · · 213
Warwickshire · · · · · · · · · · · · · · 214
West Midlands · · · · · · · · · · · · · 214

SURGERY - Plastic 215
Avon · 215
Bedfordshire · · · · · · · · · · · · · · · 215
Berkshire · · · · · · · · · · · · · · · · · 215
Bristol · · · · · · · · · · · · · · · · · · · 216
Buckinghamshire · · · · · · · · · · · · 216
Cambridgeshire · · · · · · · · · · · · · 217
Cornwall · · · · · · · · · · · · · · · · · 217

CONTENTS

Devon	217
East Sussex	217
East Yorkshire	217
Enfield Middlesex	218
Essex	218
Gloucestershire	219
Hertfordshire	219
Kent	220
Leicestershire	220
London	220
Nottinghamshire	224
Oxfordshire	225
Surrey	225
Warwickshire	226
West Midlands	226
West Sussex	226
Wiltshire	227

SURGERY - Plastic - Hand Surgery   228

Bristol	228

SURGERY - Spinal   229

Buckinghamshire	229
London	229

SURGERY - Thoracic   230

London	230

SURGERY - Varicose Vein   231

Devon	231
East Sussex	231
Hampshire	231
Kent	231
Liverpool	232
London	232
South Glamorgan	233
Surrey	233
West Midlands	233

SURGERY - Vascular   234

Cheshire	234
County Durham	234
Devon	234
Essex	234
Glasgow	235
Hampshire	235
Kent	235
Lincolnshire	235
London	236
Merseyside	237
Surrey	237
West Midlands	237

Sexual Medicine   238

London	238
Suffolk	238

Sports Medicine & Surgery   239

Essex	239
London	239
Wiltshire	240

Thoracic Medicine   241

(See also Respiratory Medicine)

Berkshire	241
London	241
Surrey	242
West Sussex	242
Worcestershire	242

CONTENTS

Urology 243

Antrim · 243

Berkshire · · · · · · · · · · · · · · · · · · · 243

Buckinghamshire · · · · · · · · · · · · · · · 243

Enfield Middlesex · · · · · · · · · · · · · · · 244

Essex · 244

Gwent · 244

Hertfordshire · · · · · · · · · · · · · · · · · 244

Kent · 245

London · 245

Middlesex · · · · · · · · · · · · · · · · · · · 248

Norfolk · 248

North Wales · · · · · · · · · · · · · · · · · 249

Surrey · 249

West Sussex · · · · · · · · · · · · · · · · · · 249

West Yorkshire · · · · · · · · · · · · · · · · 250

Wrexham · 250

Consultant Index 251

General Practitioner List 260

Private Hospital List 265

Guide To Medical Qualifications

Basic Medical & Surgical Qualifications

In order to practice medicine General Practitioners need to hold one of the following basic medical and surgical qualifications.

BCh	Bachelor of Surgery. The basic surgical qualification awarded by the University of Oxford (where BCh is followed by Oxfd) or Queen's University of Belfast (where BCh is followed by Belf). Awarded with Bachelor of Medicine which is represented by the letters BM or MB.
BChir	Bachelor of Surgery. The basic surgical qualification awarded by the University of Cambridge, usually followed by the letters Camb. Awarded with Bachalor of Medicine which is represented by the letters MB.
BM	Bachelor of Medicine. Basic medical qualification.
ChB	Bachelor of Surgery. Equivalent to BCh and BChir.
MB	Bachelor of Medicine. Basic medical qualification.
LMSSA	Licenciate in Medicine and Surgery. Awarded by the Society of Apothecaries of London.
LRCP	Licenciate. LRCP Edin is awarded by the Royal College of Physicians of Edinborough. LRCP Lond is awarded by the Royal College of Physicians of London.
LRCS	Licenciate. LRCS Edin is awarded by the Royal College of Surgeons of Edinborough. LRCS Lond is awarded by the Royal College of Surgeons of London.
LRCPS	Licenciate. LRCPS Glas is awarded by the Royal College of Physicians and Surgeons of Glasgow.

Diplomas Obtained After Basic Degrees

The following diplomas can be obtained by medical practitoners after completion of their basic degrees.

DCH	Diploma in Child Health.
DLO	Diploma in Laryngology and Otology.
DMRT	Diploma in Medical Radio-Thrapy.
DRCOG	Diploma. Awarded by the Royal College of Obstetricians & Gynaecologists.

DTM&H   Diploma in Tropical Medicine and Hygene.
MRCGP   Member of the Royal College of General Practitioners. Additional qualification for general practice.

Consultant Qualifications

In order to practice as a Consultant, the relevant training has to be completed and exams passed.

FRCOG	Fellow of the Royal College of Obstetricians and Gynaecologists.
FRCOphth	Fellow of the Royal College of Ophthalmologists.
FRCP	Fellow of the Royal College of Physicians.
FRCPath	Fellow of the Royal College of Pathologists.
FRCPI	Fellow of the Royal College of Physicians of Ireland.
FRCPsych	Fellow of the Royal College of Psychiatrists.
FRCR	Fellow of the Royal College of Radiologists.
FRCS	Fellow of the Royal College of Surgeons of England. If FRCS Ed then Fellow of the Royal College of Surgeons of Edinborough.
MD	Doctor of Medicine.
MRCOG	Member of the Royal College of Obstetricians and Gynaecologists.
MRCP	Member of the Royal College of Physicians. If FRCP Ed then Member of the Royal College of Physicians of Edinborough.
MRCPsych	Member of the Royal College of Psychiatrists.
MS	Master of Surgery.

Royal Colleges

The Royal College of Anaesthetists.
48-49 Russel Square
London WC1B 4JY
Tel. 0171 813 1900

The Royal College of Obstetricians and Gynaecologists.
27 Sussex Place
London NW1 4RG
Tel: 0171 262 5425

The Royal College of Pathologists.
2 Carlton House Terrace
London SW1Y 5AF
Tel: 0171 930 5861

The Royal College of Radiologists.
38 Portland Place
London W1N 4JQ
Tel: 0171 636 4432

The Royal College of Surgeons of Edinborough.
18 Nicolson Street
Edinborough EH8 9DW
Tel. 0131 527 1600

The Royal College of Physicians of Edinborough.
9 Queen Street
Edinborough EH2 1JQ
Tel. 0131 225 7324

The Royal College of Paediatrics and Child Health.
5 St. Andrew's Place
London NW1 4LB
Tel. 0171 486 6151

The Faculty of Public Health Medicine of the Royal Colleges of Physicians.
4 St. Andrew's Place
London NW1 4LB
Tel. 0171 935 0243

The Royal College of General Practitioners.
14 Princes Gate
Hyde Park
London SW7 1PU
Tel. 0171 581 3232

The Royal College of Ophthalmologists.
17 Cornwall Terrace
London NW1 4QW
Tel. 0171 935 0702

The Royal College of Psychiatrists.
17 Belgrave Square
London SW1X 8PG
Tel. 0171 235 2351

The Royal College of Surgeons of England.
35/43 Lincoln's Inn Field
London WC2A 3PN

The Royal College of Physicians of London.
11 St. Andrew's Place
London NW1 4LE
Tel. 0171 935 1174

The Royal College of Physicians and Surgeons of Glasgow.
233-242 St. Vincent Street
Glasgow G2 5RJ
Tel. 0141 221 6072

The Faculty of Pharmaceutical Medicine of Royal Colleges of Physicians of the United Kingdom.
1 St. Andrew's Place
London NW1 4LB
Tel. 0171 224 0343

The Faculty of Occupational Medicine
6 St. Andrew's Place
London NW1 4LB
Tel. 0171

Allergy

London

Professor Jonathan Brostoff MA DM DSc FRCP FRCPath
- YEAR QUALIFIED: 1960
- NHS POST: Professor of Allergy and Environmental Health, Director of Centre for Allergy Research, University College London.
- SPECIAL INTEREST: Allergy and other hypersensitivity states including anaphylaxis, special interest in food allergy and food intolerance relating to IBS, ME/CFS, migraine, hyperactivity etc and the role of elimination diets.
- PRIVATE: 34 Fitzjohns Avenue, London NW3 5NB. Tel: 0171 435 1563 Fax: 0171 435 7648

Professor Tak Lee MBBChir MD ScD FRCPath FRCP
- NHS POST: Professor of Allergy and Respiratory Medicine Guy's & St. Thomas' Hospital
- SPECIAL INTEREST: Allergy and Asthma
- PRIVATE: The London Bridge Hospital, 27 Tooley Street, London, SE1 2PR.

West Yorkshire

Dr Jonathan Maberly MBBS FRCP FRACP
- YEAR QUALIFIED: 1962
- NHS POST: Airedale General Hospital.
- SPECIAL INTEREST: Investigating the association of environmental exposure to chemical inhalants and chronic conditions such as asthma, migraine and irritable bowel syndrome.
- PRIVATE: Airedale Allergy Centre, High Hall, St. Stephens Road, Steeton, Keighley, West Yorkshire BD20 6SB. Tel: 01535 656013 Fax: 01535 655456

Anaesthetics

Devon

Dr John C Pappin LRCP MRCS MBBS FRCA
- YEAR QUALIFIED: 1967
- NHS POST: Consultant Anaesthetist, Torbay Hospital, Lawes Bridge.
- SPECIAL INTEREST: Anaesthesia - general/regional/local for head and neck surgery, including craniofacial surgery; orthopaedics and general surgery.
- PRIVATE: Netherlee, Roundham Avenue, Paignton, Devon TQ4 6DE.
Tel: 01803 551430 Fax: 01803 654312

London

Dr Bhanu Mahendran FRCA
- YEAR QUALIFIED: 1978
- SPECIAL INTEREST: Anaesthetic services including pre and post operative management for elective and emergency surgery with particular emphasis on anaesthesia for neurosurgery; head and neck surgery and plastic surgery, as well as the management of acute post-operative pain.
- PRIVATE: 57 Redcliffe Gardens, London SW10 9JJ.
Tel: 0171 370 2120-Secretary. 01459 592250-Message Pager. 0831 689218-Mobile.

Dr David Nancekievill MBBS MRCS LRCP FFARCS FRCA DA
- NHS POST: Formerly - Clinical Director of Anaesthetic Services, St. Bartholomew's Hospital.
- SPECIAL INTEREST: Dental anaesthesia and sedation; ENT and facio-maxillary work; fully equipped to perform sedation in the dental surgery complete with all necessary monitoring equipment.
- PRIVATE: 50 Ormonde Terrace, Regents Park, London NW8 7LR.

West Sussex

Dr Peter John Venn MBBS FRCA
- NHS POST: Consultant Anaesthetist Queen Victoria Hospital
- SPECIAL INTEREST: Snoring and sleep apnoea
- PRIVATE: Victoria Hospital, Holtye Road, East Grinstead, West Sussex RH19 3DZ.
Tel: 01342 410 210 xt 256

Andrology

Cheshire

Miss Christine Mary Evans MD FRCS FRCSEd
- YEAR QUALIFIED: 1966
- NHS POST: Consultant Urologist, Glan Clwyd Hospital.
- SPECIAL INTEREST: Erectile dysfunction and penile deformity / implants; male to female gender reassignment; bladder reconstruction and surgery for stress incontinence.
- PRIVATE: Grosvenor Nuffield Hospital, Wrexham Road, Chester, Cheshire CH4 7QP. Tel: 01244 680444

Essex

Mr Henry Lewi FRCS
- YEAR QUALIFIED: 1974
- NHS POST: Consultant Urological Surgeon, Broomfield Hospital.
- SPECIAL INTEREST: Andrology and penile reconstructive surgery.
- PRIVATE: Dukes Priory Hospital, Stump Lane, Springfield Green, Springfield, Chelmsford Essex CM1 5SJ. Tel: 01245 345 345 Tel/Fax: 0245 462 151

London

Dr Malcolm Carruthers MD FRCPath MRCGP
- YEAR QUALIFIED: 1960
- SPECIAL INTEREST: Diagnosis and treatment of the male menopause or andropause, HRT for men and testosterone treatment of circulatory problems.
- PRIVATE: Gold Cross Medical Services, 82 Harley Street, London W1N 1AE. Tel: 0171 636 8283 Fax: 0171 636 8292 E-mail: carruthers@goldcrossmedical.com

Dr Louis Hughes MBBCh DObst RCOG
- SPECIAL INTEREST: Male infertility investigation; donor insemination; erectile dysfunction; sperm storage (pre-vasectomy and treatment); investigation of unexplained infertility; intra-uterine insemination.
- PRIVATE: 99 Harley Street, London W1N 1DF. Tel: 0171 935 9004 Fax: 0171 935 6494

North Wales

Miss Christine Mary Evans MD FRCS FRCSEd
- YEAR QUALIFIED: 1966
- NHS POST: Consultant Urologist, Glan Clwyd Hospital.
- SPECIAL INTEREST: Erectile dysfunction and penile deformity / implants; male to female gender reassignment; bladder reconstruction and surgery for stress incontinence.
- PRIVATE: North Wales Medical Centre, Queens Road, Llandudno, Conwy LL30 1UD. Tel: 01492 879031

Surrey

Mr Palaniappa Shanmugaraju FRCS FICS DUROL
- YEAR QUALIFIED: 1976
- NHS POST: Consultant Urologist, Mayday University Hospital.
- SPECIAL INTEREST: Andrology and male erectile dysfunction; renal and ureteric stones; uro-oncology.
- PRIVATE: Shirley Oaks Hospital, Poppy Lane, Shirley Oaks Village, Surrey, CR9 8AB.

Audiological Medicine

Essex

Mr Iynga Vanniasegaram MSc DLO FRCS(ENT)
- NHS POST: Consultant Audiological Physician St. George's & Great Ormond Street Hospitals
- SPECIAL INTEREST: Paediatric Audiology; Balance Disorders; Tinnitus Central Auditory Disorders; Noise Induced Hearing Loss (medico-legal). Glue Ear. Vertigo - Dizziness
- PRIVATE: Essex Nuffield Hospital, Shenfield Road, Brentwood, Essex, CM15 8EH. Tel: 01277 263263 ext 219 Fax: 01277 261924 E-mail: jx79@dial.pipex.com

London

Dr Mohamed Hariri MD DLO FRCS MSc
- NHS POST: Consultant Audiological Medicine, Charing Cross Hospital, Fulham Palace Road, London W6 8RF. Tel:0181 846 1004. Fax:0181 846 1070.
- SPECIAL INTEREST: Paediatric audiology; glue ear; congenital hearing loss; noise induced hearing loss; tinnitus; medico-legal cases.
- PRIVATE: Audiology Department, Portland Hospital for Women & Children, 234 Great Portland Street, London W1N 5PH. Tel: 0171 390 8060 Fax: 0171 390 8053

Dr Kusum S Sirimanna MBBS MS FRCS MSc DLO
- YEAR QUALIFIED: 1976
- NHS POST: Consultant Audiological Physician and Head of Department, Great Ormond Street Hospital for Children
- SPECIAL INTEREST: Paediatric audiology; hearing and balance disorders in children; tinnitus, noise and hearing loss; screening for hearing loss.
- PRIVATE: The Portland Hospital, 234 Great Portland Street, London W1N 5PA. Tel: 0171 390 8060 Fax: 0171 390 8053 E-mail: tsirimanna@baap.org.uk

Dr Sava O F Soucek MD PhD
- YEAR QUALIFIED: 1959
- NHS POST: Consultant Audiological Physician St Mary's Hospital
- SPECIAL INTEREST: Hearing loss in infants & young children. Adult and childhood ear problems including dizziness, balance, otalgia, deafness and tinnitus. Industrial hearing loss.
- PRIVATE: Department of Audiological Medicine, Portland Hospital for Women & Children, 234 Great Portland Street, London W1N 5PH. Tel: 0171 390 8060 Fax: 0171 390 8053 s.soucek@ic.ac.uk

Mr Iynga Vanniasegaram MSc DLO FRCS(ENT)
- NHS POST: Consultant Audiological Physician St. George's & Great Ormond Street Hospitals
- SPECIAL INTEREST: Paediatric Audiology; Balance Disorders; Tinnitus Central Auditory Disorders; Noise Induced Hearing Loss (medico-legal). Glue Ear. Vertigo - Dizziness
- PRIVATE: Depart. of Audiological Medicine, BMI Portland Hospital for Women & Children, 209 Great Portland Street, London, W1N 6AH. Tel: 0171 390 8060 Fax: 0171 390 8053 E-mail: jx79@dial.pipex.com

Cardiology

Bath

Dr William N Hubbard MA(Cantab) MBBS FRCP
YEAR QUALIFIED: 1980
NHS POST: Consultant Cardiologist, Royal United Hospital, Bath.
SPECIAL INTEREST: Coronary artery disease; cardiac failure; cardiac pacing.
PRIVATE: Longwood House, The Bath Clinic, Claverton Down Road, Combe Down, Bath BA2 7BR. Fax: 01225 835289

Bristol

Dr Timothy Cripps DM MRCP
YEAR QUALIFIED: 1980
NHS POST: Consultant Cardiologist, Bristol Royal Infirmary.
SPECIAL INTEREST: Angina coronary angioplasty; stents; arrhythmias; radiofrequency ablation; implantable defibrillators; general cardiology.
PRIVATE: Cardiology Department, Bristol Royal Infirmary, Bristol BS2 8HW.
Tel: 0117 928 2665 Fax: 0117 928 2666 E-mail: tim.cripps@bristol.ac.uk

Buckinghamshire

Dr Rodney A Foale MBBS FRCP FACC FESC
YEAR QUALIFIED: 1971
NHS POST: Director of Surgery and Cardiac Sciences and Consultant Cardiologist, St. Mary's Hospital.
SPECIAL INTEREST: Coronary artery disease treatment, medical / percutaneous balloon / stent / atherectomy. Hypertension and patient tailored therapy. All modalities of non invasive diagnosis.
PRIVATE: The Thames Valley Nuffield Hospital, Wexham Street, Slough, Buckinghamshire SL3 6NH.

Cheshire

Dr Jonathan Swan MBChB MD MRCP
YEAR QUALIFIED: 1983
NHS POST: Consultant Cardiologist, North Manchester General Hospital.
SPECIAL INTEREST: Ischaemic heart disease; coronary angiography; heart failure; echocardiography and cardiac pacing.
PRIVATE: Alexandra Hospital, Mill Lane, Cheadle, Cheshire SK8 2PX.
Tel: 0161 428 3656 Fax: 0161 654 9591

Dumfries

Dr Graeme W Tait MB ChB MD FRCP
YEAR QUALIFIED: 1982
NHS POST: Consultant Cardiologist and Physician, Dumfries and Galloway Royal Infirmary.
SPECIAL INTEREST: Coronary atherosclerosis; management of hyperlipidaemia in ischaemic heart disease; pre-hospital thrombolysis; patient education in coronary disease; atrial dysrhythmias.
PRIVATE: Lochthorn Private Clinic, Edinburgh Road, Dumfries, DG1 1TR.
Tel: 01387 252882 Fax: 01387 264932

Essex

Dr John Stephens MD FRCP
NHS POST: Consultant Cardiologist Havering Hospitals & Royal Hospitals NHS Trust
SPECIAL INTEREST: General cardiology; non-invasive and invasive investigations.
PRIVATE: 29 Crossways, Shenfield, Essex CM15 8QY.
Tel: 01277 221254 Fax: 01277 234518
Oaks Hospital, Mile End Road, Colchester, Essex CO4 5XR.

Glasgow

Dr Graeme W Tait MB ChB MD FRCP
YEAR QUALIFIED: 1982
NHS POST: Consultant Cardiologist and Physician, Dumfries and Galloway Royal Infirmary.
SPECIAL INTEREST: Coronary atherosclerosis; management of hyperlipidaemia in ischaemic heart disease; pre-hospital thrombolysis; patient education in coronary disease; atrial dysrhythmias.
PRIVATE: Ross Hall Hospital, 221 Crookston Road, Glasgow G52 3NQ.
Tel: 0141 810 3151

Hertfordshire

Dr David Hackett MD FRCP
NHS POST: Consultant Cardiologist, St. Albans & Hemel Hempstead Hospital, and St. Mary's Hospital, London.
SPECIAL INTEREST: Coronary artery disease
PRIVATE: BUPA Hospital Harpenden, Ambrose Lane, Harpenden, Herts, AL5 4BP.
Tel: 01582 760 290 Fax: 01582 462 301

Dr Peter Keir MA MB BChir FRCP
NHS POST: Consultant Physician, Queen Elizabeth II Hospital.
SPECIAL INTEREST:
PRIVATE: BUPA Hospital Harpenden, Ambrose Lane, Harpenden, Herts, AL5 4BP.
Tel: 0800 585 112/01582 763191/769067 Fax: 01582 761 358
Queen Elizabeth II Hospital, Howlands, Welwyn Garden City, Hertfordshire, AL7 4HQ.
Tel: 01707 365 036 Fax: 01707 365 058

Dr David P Lipkin BSc MD FRCP
- NHS POST: Consultant, Royal Free Hospital.
- SPECIAL INTEREST: Angina; coronary angiography; interventional cardiology including coronary angioplasty and coronary artery stenting.
- PRIVATE: BUPA Hospital Bushey, Heathbourne Rd, Bushey, Watford, Hertfordshire WD2 1RD. Tel: 0171 586 5959 Appointments & Fax: 0181 202 8495

Kent

Dr Cliff Bucknall MD FRCP
- NHS POST: Consultant Cardiologist, Guy's & St. Thomas' Hospital.
- SPECIAL INTEREST: Complex coronary angioplasty; stenting; pacing.
- PRIVATE: BMI Sloane Hospital, 125 Albermarle Road, Beckenham, Kent, BR3 2HS. Tel: 0181 460 6998

Dr John Chambers MA MD FRCP FESC FACC
- NHS POST: Consultant, Guy's and St. Thomas' Hospital, London and Maidstone Hospital, Kent.
- SPECIAL INTEREST: Echocardiography; valve disease; chest pain.
- PRIVATE: BUPA Alexandra Hospital, Impton Lane, Walderslade, Chatham, Kent ME5 9PG. Tel: 01634 687 166

Dr Paul V L Curry MD FRCP
- YEAR QUALIFIED: 1969
- NHS POST: Honorary Consultant Cardiologist Guy's & St. Thomas' Hospitals.
- SPECIAL INTEREST: General cardiology; coronary angioplasty & stents; cardiac arrhythmias; pacemakers.
- PRIVATE: BUPA Tunbridge Wells Hospital, Fordcombe Road, Fordcombe, Tunbridge Wells, Kents TN3 0RD. Tel: 0171 403 0824 Fax: 0171 403 2306
  E-mail: DRPAULCURRY@COMPUSERVE.COM

Liverpool

Dr Raphael Adam Perry FRCP DM FACC BSc
- YEAR QUALIFIED: 1980
- NHS POST: Consultant Cardiologist, CTC - Liverpool NHS Trust.
- SPECIAL INTEREST: Coronary intervention/angioplasty; also balloon vacuotomy; echocardiography including toe and stress echo.
- PRIVATE: 45 Rodney Street, Liverpool, L1. Tel: 0151 228 1616 Fax: 0151 428 2146

London

Dr Stephen J D Brecker BSc MB BS MRCP MD FACC
- YEAR QUALIFIED: 1984
- NHS POST: Consultant Cardiologist, St. George's Hospital.
- SPECIAL INTEREST: The interventional management of coronary artery disease, angioplasty and coronary stenting, echocardiography and general cardiology.
- PRIVATE: The Heart Hospital, 50 Wimpole Street, London W1M 7DG.
  Tel: 0181 725 1390 Fax: 0181 725 0211
  Parkside Hospital, 53 Parkside, Wimbledon, London, SW19 5NX.
  Tel: 0181 725 1390 Fax: 0181 725 0211

Dr Cliff Bucknall MD FRCP
- NHS POST: Consultant Cardiologist, Guy's & St. Thomas' Hospital.
- SPECIAL INTEREST: Complex coronary angioplasty; stenting; pacing.
- PRIVATE: Suite 302, Emblem House London Bridge Hospital, 27 Tooley Street, London, SE1 2PR.
  Tel: 0171 407 0292 Fax: 0171 357 0994

Dr John Chambers MA MD FRCP FESC FACC
- NHS POST: Consultant, Guy's and St. Thomas' Hospital, London and Maidstone Hospital, Kent.
- SPECIAL INTEREST: Echocardiography; valve disease; chest pain.
- PRIVATE: Guy's Nuffield House, Newcomen Street, London, SE1 1YR.
  Tel: 0171 955 4752

Dr Paul V L Curry MD FRCP
- YEAR QUALIFIED: 1969
- NHS POST: Honorary Consultant Cardiologist Guy's & St. Thomas' Hospitals.
- SPECIAL INTEREST: General cardiology; coronary angioplasty & stents; cardiac arrhythmias; pacemakers.
- PRIVATE: Heart Hospital, 50 Wimpole Street, London W1M 7DG.
  Tel: 0171 403 0824 Fax: 0171 403 2306
  E-mail: DRPAULCURRY@COMPUSERVE.COM
  Emblem House London Bridge Hospital, 27 Tooley Street, London, SE1 2PR.
  Tel: 0171 403 0824 Fax: 0171 403 2306
  E-mail: DRPAULCURRY@COMPUSERVE.COM
  Parkside Hospital, 53 Parkside, Wimbledon, London, SW19 5NX.
  Tel: 0171 403 0824 Fax: 0171 403 2306
  E-mail: DRPAULCURRY@COMPUSERVE.COM
  Lister Hospital, Chelsea Bridge Road, London, SW1W 8RH.
  Tel: 0171 403 0824 Fax: 0171 403 2306
  E-mail: DRPAULCURRY@COMPUSERVE.COM

Dr Wyn Davies MD FRCP
- YEAR QUALIFIED: 1976
- NHS POST: Consultant Cardiologist, St. Mary's Hospital, Praed Street, London W2 1NY.
- SPECIAL INTEREST: Interventional Management of Arrhythmias by Ablation Techniques and of Coronary Disease by means of Angioplasty.
- PRIVATE: 66 Harley Street, London W1N 1AE.
  Tel: 0171 636 6340 Fax: 0171 631 1306

Cardiology. London

Professor John Deanfield MA MB BChir FRCP
- NHS POST: Consultant Cardiologist, Great Ormond Street Hospital for Children NHS Trust and University College London Hospitals.
- SPECIAL INTEREST: Paediatric cardiology; coronary disease and coronary risk factor management.
- PRIVATE: Harley Street Clinic, 35 Weymouth Street, London, W1N 4BJ.
  Tel: 0171 404 5094   Fax: 0171 813 8263

Dr Duncan S Dymond MD FRCP FACC FESC
- NHS POST: Consultant Cardiologist St. Bartholomew's Hospital
- SPECIAL INTEREST: Clinical Cardiology with special interest in Coronary Artery Disease. Angioplasty and Stenting. Prognostic Assessments.
- PRIVATE: 50 Wimpole Street, London W1M 7DG.
  Tel: 0171 486 8963   Fax: 0171 486 7918

Dr Rodney A Foale MBBS FRCP FACC FESC
- YEAR QUALIFIED: 1971
- NHS POST: Director of Surgery and Cardiac Sciences and Consultant Cardiologist, St. Mary's Hospital.
- SPECIAL INTEREST: Coronary artery disease treatment, medical / percutaneous balloon / stent / atherectomy. Hypertension and patient tailored therapy. All modalities of non invasive diagnosis.
- PRIVATE: 66 Harley Street, London W1N 1AE.
  Tel: 0171 323 4687   Fax: 0171 631 5341   E-mail: info@smht-foale.co.uk
  The Lindo Wing, St. Mary's Hospital, South Wharf Road, Paddington, London W2 1NY.

  The Heart Hospital, 16-18 Westmoreland Street, London W1M 8PH.

Dr David E Jewitt BSc MB FRCP FESC
- NHS POST: Director of Cardiac Department & Consultant Cardiologist, King's College Hospital
- SPECIAL INTEREST: Clinical and interventional cardiology.
- PRIVATE: Cromwell Hospital, Cromwell Road, London SW5 0TU.
  Tel: 0171 370 4233   Fax: 0171 244 6678
  Emblem House London Bridge Hospital, 27 Tooley Street, London, SE1 2PR.
  Tel: 0171 403 4884   Fax: 0171 407 3162
  The Guthrie Clinic, King's College Hospital, Denmark Hill, London, SE5 9RS.
  Tel: 0171 346 3379   Fax: 0171 346 3489

Dr David P Lipkin BSc MD FRCP
- NHS POST: Consultant, Royal Free Hospital.
- SPECIAL INTEREST: Angina; coronary angiography; interventional cardiology including coronary angioplasty and coronary artery stenting.
- PRIVATE: Wellington Hospital South, Wellington Place, London NW8 9LE.
  Tel: 0171 586 5959 Appointments &   Fax: 0181 202 8495

Dr John R Muir DM(Oxon) FRCP MA
- NHS POST: Formerly Professor of Cardiology- University Hospital of Wales.
- SPECIAL INTEREST: Coronary artery disease; hypertension; valvular heart disease.
- PRIVATE: Flat 1, 21 Devonshire Place, London W1N 1PD.
  Tel: 0171 486 8738   Fax: 0171 580 9988

Cardiology. London

Dr Anthony Rickards FRCP FACC FESC
- **YEAR QUALIFIED:** 1968
- **NHS POST:** Consultant Cardiologist, Royal Brompton Hospital
- **SPECIAL INTEREST:** Clinical cardiology; coronary artery disease; coronary intervention; cardiac pacing and arrhythmias.
- **PRIVATE:** The Heart Hospital, 47 Wimpole Street, London W1M 7DG.
  Tel: 0171 573 8899 Fax: 0171 573 8898

Dr Michael Rigby MD FRCP
- **NHS POST:** Consultant Paediatric Cardiologist Royal Brompton Hospital
- **SPECIAL INTEREST:** Paediatric cardiology.
- **PRIVATE:** Private Outpatient Clinic, Royal Brompton Hospital, Sydney Street, London SW3 6NP.
  Tel: 0171 351 8542 Fax: 0171 351 8547 E-mail: m.rigby@rbh.nthames.nhs.uk

Dr Elliot Shinebourne MD FRCP FRCPCH
- **NHS POST:** Consultant Paediatric Cardiologist Royal Brompton Hospital/National Heart & Lung Institute
- **SPECIAL INTEREST:** Congenital heart disease - diagnosis, investigation and management in infants, children, adolescents and young adults. Cardiac arrhythmias in children.
- **PRIVATE:** Private Consulting Rooms, Royal Brompton Hospital, Sydney Street, London SW3 6NP.
  Tel: 0171 351 8541 Fax: 0171 351 8544

Dr Ulrich Sigwart MD FRCP FACC FACA FESC
- **YEAR QUALIFIED:** 1967
- **NHS POST:** Consultant Cardiologist, Royal Brompton National Heart & Lung Hospital
- **SPECIAL INTEREST:** Invasive cardiology; interventional cardiology; cardiomyopathy; coronary heart disease; valvular heart disease.
- **PRIVATE:** 47 Wimpole Street, London W1M 7DG.
  Tel: 0171 573 8899 Fax: 0171 573 8898 E-mail: u.sigwart@rbh.nthames.nhs.uk

Dr John Stephens MD FRCP
- **NHS POST:** Consultant Cardiologist Havering Hospitals & Royal Hospitals NHS Trust
- **SPECIAL INTEREST:** General cardiology; non-invasive and invasive investigations.
- **PRIVATE:** 93 Harley Street, London W1N 1DF.
  Tel: 0121 632 5881

Dr Robert Howard Swanton MA MD FRCP FESC
- **YEAR QUALIFIED:** 1969
- **NHS POST:** Consultant Cardiologist, Middlesex Hospital.
- **SPECIAL INTEREST:** All general adult cardiology with a special interest in interventional cardiology (angioplasty), pacing and valve disease.
- **PRIVATE:** 42 Wimpole Street, London W1M 7AF.
  Tel: 0171 486 7416 Fax: 0171 487 2569

Dr Robert M R Tulloh BM BCh MA MRCP FRCPCH
- **NHS POST:** Consultant Paediatric Cardiologist Guy's & St. Thomas' NHS Trust
- **SPECIAL INTEREST:** Paediatric cardiology; diagnosis and interventional treatment of children's heart disease.
- **PRIVATE:** Guy's Hospital, St Thomas Street, London, SE1 9RT.
  Tel: 0171 955 4616 Fax: 0171 955 4614 E-mail:r.tulloh@umds.ac.uk

Cardiology. London

Dr John Malcolm Walker BSc MD FRCP
- YEAR QUALIFIED: 1975
- NHS POST: Consultant Cardiologist, University College and Middlesex Hospitals.
- SPECIAL INTEREST: Adult general cardiology including intervention and pacemaker therapy. Ischaemic preconditioning; thalassaemia cardiac care clinic.
- PRIVATE: Private Rooms Department, Cardiology University College Hospital, Cecil Fleming House, Gower Street, London WC1E 6AU.
  Tel: 0171 380 9756 Fax: 0181 388 5095

Dr Michael Murray Webb-Peploe MB FRCP
- YEAR QUALIFIED: 1960
- NHS POST: Consultant Cardiologist, St. Thomas' Hospital, London.
- SPECIAL INTEREST: Adult cardiology; interventional cardiology.
- PRIVATE: 199 Westminster Bridge Road, London SE1 7UT.
  Tel: 0171 261 9877 Fax: 0171 922 8301

Manchester

Dr Jonathan Swan MBChB MD MRCP
- YEAR QUALIFIED: 1983
- NHS POST: Consultant Cardiologist, North Manchester General Hospital.
- SPECIAL INTEREST: Ischaemic heart disease; coronary angiography; heart failure; echocardiography and cardiac pacing.
- PRIVATE: Roselands, 4 Middleton Road, Prestwich, Manchester M8 5DS.
  Tel: 0161 795 9111 Fax: 0161 654 9591

Middlesbrough

Dr Mark Andrew de Belder MA MD FRCP
- YEAR QUALIFIED: 1980
- NHS POST: Consultant Cardiologist, South Cleveland Hospital.
- SPECIAL INTEREST: Interventional cardiology; ischaemic heart disease.
- PRIVATE: South Cleveland Hospital, Marton Road, Middlesbrough TS4 3BW.
  Tel: 01642 854620 Fax: 01642 282408

Surrey

Dr Stephen J D Brecker BSc MB BS MRCP MD FACC
- YEAR QUALIFIED: 1984
- NHS POST: Consultant Cardiologist, St. George's Hospital.
- SPECIAL INTEREST: The interventional management of coronary artery disease, angioplasty and coronary stenting, echocardiography and general cardiology.
- PRIVATE: St. Anthony's Hospital, London Road, North Cheam, Surrey, SM3 9DW.
  Tel: 0181 725 1390 Fax: 0181 725 0211

Dr Olusola Odemuyiwa MD MRCP(UK)
YEAR QUALIFIED: 1978
NHS POST: Consultant Cardiologist, Epsom Generals Hospital, London.
SPECIAL INTEREST: Myocardial infarction: diagnosis and management of acute and chronic coronary syndromes.
PRIVATE: Ashtead Hospital, The Warren, Ashtead, Surrey KT21 2SB.
Tel: 01372 276161 Fax: 01372 278704
St. Anthony's Hospital, London Road, North Cheam, Surrey, SM3 9DW.
Tel: 0181 337 6691 Fax: 0181 337 0816; 330 1037

Tyne & Wear

Dr Stephen Furniss MA MBBS FRCP
YEAR QUALIFIED: 1979
NHS POST: Consultant Cardiologist, Freeman Hospital
SPECIAL INTEREST: Electrophysiology - catheter ablation of arrhythmias; coronary intervention - PTCA / stents / valvuloplasty.
PRIVATE: BUPA Hospital Washington, Picktree Lane, Rickleton, Washington, Tyne & Wear NE38 9JZ. Tel: 0191 415 1272 E-mail: s.s.furniss@ncl.ac.uk

Dr Mark Andrew de Belder MA MD FRCP
YEAR QUALIFIED: 1980
NHS POST: Consultant Cardiologist, South Cleveland Hospital.
SPECIAL INTEREST: Interventional cardiology; ischaemic heart disease.
PRIVATE: BUPA Hospital Washington, Picktree Lane, Rickleton, Washington, Tyne & Wear NE38 9JZ. Tel: 0191 415 1272 Fax: 0191 415 5541

Dermatology

Berkshire

Professor John L M Hawk BSc MD FRCP
YEAR QUALIFIED: 1969
NHS POST: Consultant Dermatologist, St. Thomas' Hospital, London SE1 7EH.
SPECIAL INTEREST: Sunlight-induced skin disease; psoralen photochemotherapy (PUVA).
PRIVATE: 47 Alma Road, Windsor, Berkshire SL4 3HH.
Tel: 01753 831 254 Fax: 01753 858 569

Dr Martin James MB BSc FRCP
YEAR QUALIFIED: 1972
NHS POST: Consultant Dermatologist, Royal Berkshire Hospital.
SPECIAL INTEREST: Dermatological surgery and treatment of skin cancer; laser resurfacing for acne and actinic damage; sclerotherapy of superficial leg telangiectasia; laser treatment of vascular and pigmented lesions.
PRIVATE: Consulting Rooms, BUPA Dunedin Hospital, 72 Berkeley Avenue, Reading, Berkshire RG1 6HY. Tel: 01734 584 711 Fax: 01734 588 110
Berkshire Independent Hospital, Wensley Road, Coley Park, Reading, Berkshire RG1 6UZ. Tel: 01734 560 056 Fax: 01734 566 333

Cheshire

Dr Paul J August FRCP
YEAR QUALIFIED: 1967
NHS POST: Consultant Dermatologist, Selfend Royal Hospital Trust, Central Manchester Trust.
SPECIAL INTEREST: General dermatology; laser surgery; atopic dermatitis.
PRIVATE: South Cheshire Private Hospital, Crewe, Cheshire
Tel: 01606 889179 Fax: 01606 301134

Enfield Middlesex

Dr John James Ryan Almeyda MBBS FRCP(Lond)
YEAR QUALIFIED: 1960
NHS POST: Consultant Dermatologist, Enfield & Harringay.
SPECIAL INTEREST: All skin diseases: Acne; eczema; psoriasis; moles; skin cancers.
PRIVATE: North London Nuffield Hospital, Cavell Drive, Uplands Park Road, Enfield, EN2 7PR.
Tel: 0181 366 2122
Kings Oak Hospital, Chase Farm (North side), The Ridgeway, Enfield, Middlesex EN2 8SD. Tel: 0181 370 9505

Essex

Dr Sarah Vijayasingam-Henderson MBBS MRCP MMED(int med)
- YEAR QUALIFIED: 1982
- NHS POST: Consultant Dermatologist Southend Healthcare Trust
- SPECIAL INTEREST: Wound-healing; atopic eczema; skin problems associated with internal diseases; psoriasis; paediatric dermatology; skin cancer.
- PRIVATE: BUPA Wellesley Hospital, Eastern Avenue, Southend on Sea SS2 4XH.

Glasgow

Dr John Thomson MD FRCP(Glas, Edin) FChS D.Obst RCOG
- YEAR QUALIFIED: 1965
- NHS POST: Consultant Dermatologist, Glasgow Royal Infirmary, Glasgow.
- SPECIAL INTEREST: Dermatological surgery; medico-legal work.
- PRIVATE: Ross Hall Hospital, 221 Crookston Road, Glasgow G52 3NQ. Tel: 0141 810 3151 Fax: 0141 882 7439

Hampshire

Dr Richard Eric Ashton MA MD FRCP
- YEAR QUALIFIED: 1974
- NHS POST: Consultant Dermatologist, Royal Hospital Haslar, Gosport, Hampshire.
- SPECIAL INTEREST: Dermatological surgery; MOH's surgery; dermatological lasers.
- PRIVATE: BUPA Hospital Portsmouth, Bartons Road, Havant, Hampshire PO9 5NP. Tel: 01705 454511
  BUPA Chalybeate Hospital, Chalybeate Close, Tremona Road, Southampton, Hampshire SO16 6UY. Tel: 01703 775544

Hertfordshire

Dr Paul Maurice MA MD FRCP
- YEAR QUALIFIED: 1977
- NHS POST: Consultant Dermatologist, St. Albans & Hemel Hempstead NHS Trust.
- SPECIAL INTEREST: Skin cancer; psoriasis; dermatological surgery and acne.
- PRIVATE: BUPA Hospital Harpenden, Ambrose Lane, Harpenden, Herts, AL5 4BP. Tel: 01582 763 191/0800 585 112 Fax: 01582 761 358

Kent

Dr Alastair Barkley MB BS FRCP (Lond)
- YEAR QUALIFIED: 1978
- NHS POST: Consultant Dermatologist, The Whittington Hospital.
- SPECIAL INTEREST: Skin cancer, PUVA photochemotherapy.
- PRIVATE: Fawkham Manor Hospital, Manor Lane, Fawkham, Longfield, Kent DA3 8ND.
  Tel: 01474 879900 Fax: 01474 879827

Leicestershire

Dr John Berth-Jones MB BS FRCP
- YEAR QUALIFIED: 1979
- NHS POST: Consultant Dermatologist, Walsgrave Hospital Coventry and George Eliot Hospital, Nuneaton.
- SPECIAL INTEREST: Psoriasis, atopic dermatitis, cutaneous neoplasia, dermatological therapeutics.
- PRIVATE: Leicester Nuffield Hospital, Scraptoft Lane, Leicester, Leicestershire LE5 1HY.
  Tel: 0116 276 9401 Fax: 0116 246 1076

London

Dr John James Ryan Almeyda MBBS FRCP(Lond)
- YEAR QUALIFIED: 1960
- NHS POST: Consultant Dermatologist, Enfield & Harringay.
- SPECIAL INTEREST: All skin diseases: Acne; eczema; psoriasis; moles; skin cancers.
- PRIVATE: 111 Harley Street, London W1N 1DG.
  Tel: 0171 935 4013

Dr Harvey Baker MD FRCP (Lond)
- YEAR QUALIFIED: 1954
- SPECIAL INTEREST: Psoriasis; eczema; hair disorders.
- PRIVATE: 152 Harley Street, London W1N 1HH.
  Tel: 0171 935 8868/2477 Fax: 0171 224 2574

Dr Alastair Barkley MB BS FRCP (Lond)
- YEAR QUALIFIED: 1978
- NHS POST: Consultant Dermatologist, The Whittington Hospital.
- SPECIAL INTEREST: Skin cancer, PUVA photochemotherapy.
- PRIVATE: The London Bridge Hospital, 27 Tooley Street, London, SE1 2PR.
  Tel: 0171 815 3653 Fax: 0171 815 3654

Dermatology. London

Dr Veronique Bataille MD MRCP PhD
- YEAR QUALIFIED: 1985
- NHS POST: Consultant Dermatologist, Royal London Hospital.
- SPECIAL INTEREST: Melanoma; familial melanoma; atypical mole syndrome; atypical naevi and family cancer syndromes; skin cancer.
- PRIVATE: Newark Dermatology Clinic, 2 Newark Street, Whitechapel, London E1 2AT.
Tel: 0171 295 7169 Fax: 0171 295 7171 E-mail: bataille@icrf.icnet.uk

Dr Martin M Black MD FRCP FRCPath
- YEAR QUALIFIED: 1963
- NHS POST: Consultant Dermatologist, St John's Institute of Dermatology.
- SPECIAL INTEREST: Clinical dermatology; bullous diseases; cutaneous amyloidosis; panniculitis; skin pathology; cutaneous immunofluorescence.
- PRIVATE: York House Consulting Rooms, 199 Westminster Bridge Road, London SE1 7UT.
Tel: 0171 928 5485

Dr Christopher Bunker MA MD FRCP
- YEAR QUALIFIED: 1981
- NHS POST: Consultant Dermatologist Chelsea & Westminster, Charing Cross and Royal Marsden Hospitals.
- SPECIAL INTEREST: HIV / Penis disorders.
- PRIVATE: 152 Harley Street, London W1N 1HH.
Tel: 0171 935 0444 Fax: 0171 224 2574

Dr David A Fenton MBChB MRCP MRCS
- NHS POST: Consultant Dermatologist, St Thomas' Hospital, London SE1 and St Andrew's Hospital, London E3.
- SPECIAL INTEREST: Disorders of hair, scalp and nails.
- PRIVATE: Consulting Rooms, 80 Harley Street, London W1N 1AE.
Tel: 0171 580 8356 Fax: 0171 637 0242

Dr David Harris FRCP
- NHS POST: Consultant Dermatologist, The Whittington Hospital NHS Trust.
- SPECIAL INTEREST: Skin cancer therapy including micrographic (Mohs) surgery. Cosmetic and laser dermatology for scarring and treatment of birthmarks.
- PRIVATE: Consulting Rooms, The Wellington Hospital, Wellington Place, London, NW8 9LE.
Tel: 0171 586 3213/5959 ext 6022
Hospital of St. John & St. Elizabeth, 60 Grove End Road, St Johns Wood, London, NW8 9NH. Tel: 0171 286 5126, Practice Manager- 0171 431 2714

Dr Anne Kobza Black MD FRCP
- YEAR QUALIFIED: 1963
- NHS POST: Consultant Dermatologist, St John's Institute of Dermatology & St. Thomas' Hospital.
- SPECIAL INTEREST: General, female dermatological problems; urticaria; vulval problems.
- PRIVATE: York House Consulting Rooms, 199 Westminster Bridge Road, London SE1 7UT.
Tel: 0171 928 5485 Fax: 0171 928 3748

Dermatology. London

Professor Irene M Leigh MD FRCP
- **NHS POST:** Consultant Dermatologist (Honorary), Royal Hospitals Trust, St. Bartholomew's And The Royal London School Of Medicine & Dentistry.
- **SPECIAL INTEREST:** Skin Cancer - non melanoma/melanoma; vulval disease; pigmented lesion clinic; dermatological surgery; erythema multiforme; photobiology; wound healing; paediatric dermatology.
- **PRIVATE:** Newark Dermatology Clinic, 2 Newark Street, Whitechapel, London E1 2AT.
  Tel: 0171 295 7169 Fax: 0171 295 7171 E-mail: brame@icrf.icnet.uk

Dr Andrew C Markey MD FRCP
- **YEAR QUALIFIED:** 1980
- **NHS POST:** Consultant Dermatologist, St. John's Institute of Dermatology, St. Thomas' Hospital.
- **SPECIAL INTEREST:** Cosmetic dermatology; laser skin surgery; skin tumours; dermatological surgery.
- **PRIVATE:** Lister Hospital, Chelsea Bridge Road, London, SW1W 8RH.
  Tel: 0171 730 1219 Fax: 0171 730 1368

Dr Trevor W E Robinson MA MB BChir FRCP
- **YEAR QUALIFIED:** 1968
- **NHS POST:** Emeritus Consultant Dermatologist, University College (London) Hospitals.
- **SPECIAL INTEREST:** Virus infections; solar skin damage with/without premalignant and malignant change.
- **PRIVATE:** 99 Harley Street, London W1N 1DF.
  Tel: 0171 637 7325 Fax: 0171 637 5383

Dr Christopher Rowland Payne MBBS MRCP
- **NHS POST:** Honorary Consultant Dermatologist, Royal Marsden Hospital.
- **SPECIAL INTEREST:** Medical and surgical treatment of skin malignancies, benign tumours and cosmetic problems.
- **PRIVATE:** Cromwell Hospital, Cromwell Road, London SW5 0TU.
  Tel: 0171 460 2000 Fax: 0171 233 7393
  The London Clinic, 149 Harley Street, London, W1N 2DE.
  Tel: 0171 935 4444 Fax: 0171 233 7393

Dr Robin Russell Jones MA FRCP
- **NHS POST:** Director, Skin Tumour Unit - St. John's Institute of Dermatology St Thomas' Hospital. Consultant Dermatologist Ealing & Hammersmith Hospitals
- **SPECIAL INTEREST:** Skin tumours, skin pathology, acne, eczema
- **PRIVATE:** Cromwell Hospital, Cromwell Road, London SW5 0TU.
  Tel: 0171 460 2000

Dr Malcolm Rustin BSc MD FRCP
- **NHS POST:** Consultant Dermatologist Royal Free Hospital
- **SPECIAL INTEREST:** General dermatology; atopic eczema; connective tissue diseases.
- **PRIVATE:** 53 Wimpole Street, London W1M 7DF.
  Tel: 0171 935 9266 Fax: 0171 935 3060

Dr Sean Whittaker MB MD FRCP
- YEAR QUALIFIED: 1981
- NHS POST: Consultant in Dermatology, Royal Free Hospital, London.
- SPECIAL INTEREST: Skin cancer; melanoma.
- PRIVATE: The Wellington Hospital, Wellington Place, London, NW8 9LE.
Tel: 0171 586 3213 Fax: 0171 483 0297

Manchester

Dr Paul J August FRCP
- YEAR QUALIFIED: 1967
- NHS POST: Consultant Dermatologist, Selfend Royal Hospital Trust, Central Manchester Trust.
- SPECIAL INTEREST: General dermatology; laser surgery; atopic dermatitis.
- PRIVATE: 23 St. John Street, Manchester M3 4DT.
Tel: 0161 834 0363 Fax: 0161 834 4205

Middlesex

Dr Robin Russell Jones MA FRCP
- NHS POST: Director, Skin Tumour Unit - St. John's Institute of Dermatology St Thomas' Hospital. Consultant Dermatologist Ealing & Hammersmith Hospitals
- SPECIAL INTEREST: Skin tumours, skin pathology, acne, eczema
- PRIVATE: Ealing Hospital, Uxbridge Road, Southall, Middlx, UB1 3EW.
Tel: 0181 967 5435

Norfolk

Dr Robert Graham MB BS FRCP
- YEAR QUALIFIED: 1977
- NHS POST: Consultant Dermatologist at the James Paget NHS Trust, Great Yarmouth, Norfolk.
- SPECIAL INTEREST: Skin signs of systemic disease; skin tumours; paediatric dermatology; contact dermatitis Reiter's disease.
- PRIVATE: Hill House Consulting Rooms, BUPA Hospital, Old Watton Road, Norwich, Norfolk NR4 7TD. Tel: 01603 255507 Fax: 01603 505851

The Coastal Clinic, 4 Park Road, Gorleston, Great Yarmouth, Norfolk NR31 6EJ.
Tel: 01493 601770 Fax: 01493 442430

South Yorkshire

Dr Christine I Harrington MB ChB(Hons) MD(Cam) FRCP(UK)
- YEAR QUALIFIED: 1971
- NHS POST: Consultant Dermatologist, Royal Hallmshire Hospital, Sheffield.
- SPECIAL INTEREST: Vulval disease, skin and systemic disease, skin malignancy, eczema, psoriasis, acne, psycho-dermatology.
- PRIVATE: Somersby, 3 Endcliffe Grove Avenue, Sheffield, South Yorkshire S10 3EJ.
Tel: 0114 266 7201 Fax: 0114 267 1210

Warwickshire

Dr John Berth-Jones MB BS FRCP
- YEAR QUALIFIED: 1979
- NHS POST: Consultant Dermatologist, Walsgrave Hospital Coventry and George Eliot Hospital, Nuneaton.
- SPECIAL INTEREST: Psoriasis, atopic dermatitis, cutaneous neoplasia, dermatological therapeutics.
- PRIVATE: Nuneaton Private Hospital, 132 Coventry Road, Nuneaton, Warwickshire CV10 7AD.
Tel: 01203 353000 Fax: 01203 346645

West Midlands

Dr John Berth-Jones MB BS FRCP
- YEAR QUALIFIED: 1979
- NHS POST: Consultant Dermatologist, Walsgrave Hospital Coventry and George Eliot Hospital, Nuneaton.
- SPECIAL INTEREST: Psoriasis, atopic dermatitis, cutaneous neoplasia, dermatological therapeutics.
- PRIVATE: Coventry Consulting Rooms, 11 Dalton Road, Earlesdon, Coventry, West Midlands CV5 6PD. Tel: 01203 677444 Fax: 01203 691436

West Sussex

Dr Peter R Coburn MB FRCP
- NHS POST: Consultant Dermatologist, Worthing & Chichester Hospitals.
- SPECIAL INTEREST: Skin tumours and photo-dermatology.
- PRIVATE: 116 Heene Road, Worthing, West Sussex BN11 4PN.
Tel: 01903 200 938 Fax: 01903 232 532
24 West Street, Chichester, West Sussex PO19 1QP.
Tel: 01243 789 630 Fax: 01243 536 591

Dr Ashley V Levantine MBBS MRCS LRCP FRCP
- NHS POST: Consultant Dermatologist, Chichester and Worthing Trusts.
- SPECIAL INTEREST: PUVA, Psoriasis
- PRIVATE: King Edward VII Hospital, Midhurst, West Sussex, GU29 0BL.
Tel: 01730 812 341 Fax: 01730 816 333
Sherburne Hospital, 78 Broyle Road, Chichester, West Sussex PO19 4BE.
Tel: 01243 530 600 Fax: 01243 532 244
116 Heene Road, Worthing, West Sussex BN11 4PN.
Tel: 01903 200 938 Fax: 01903 232 532

ENT Surgery

Bedfordshire

Mr David Johnston BSc MB ChB FRCS(Ed) FRCS(Eng)(ORL)
- NHS POST: ENT Consultant, St. Albans Hospital, Hemel Hempstead NHS Trust.
- SPECIAL INTEREST: Paediatric ENT; otology; rhinology.
- PRIVATE: Cobham Clinic, Luton and Dunstable Hospital, Lewsey Road, Luton, Bedfordshire, LU4 0DZ. Tel: Secretary-01582 760274 Fax: 01582 760274

Bristol

Mr Philip G Bicknell MB BCh FRCS FRCSE
- YEAR QUALIFIED: 1962
- NHS POST: Consultant Surgeon, St Michaels Hospital, Bristol.
- SPECIAL INTEREST: Nasal and sinus disorders; paediatric ENT.
- PRIVATE: Litfield House Medical Centre, 1 Litfield Place, Clifton Down, Bristol BS8 3LS. Tel: 0117 973 1323 Fax: 0117 973 3303

Buckinghamshire

Mr Peter M Brown FRCS (Eng) FRCS (Ed)
- YEAR QUALIFIED: 1969
- NHS POST: Consultant ENT Surgeon, Milton Keynes General NHS Trust.
- SPECIAL INTEREST: Rhinology including endoscopic sinus surgery; functional and cosmetic rhinoplasty; laryngology, including voice clinic; general ENT.
- PRIVATE: Saxon Clinic, Saxon Street, Eaglestone, Milton Keynes, Buckinghamshire MK6 5LR. Tel: 01908 665 533 ext 221 Fax: 01908 608 112
  E-mail: susanbrown@uk_consultants.co.uk

Cheshire

Mr Philip Hodgson Jones MA MB BChir FRCS
- YEAR QUALIFIED: 1973
- NHS POST: Consultant ENT Surgeon and Clinical Director, Wythenshawe Hospital.
- SPECIAL INTEREST: Phonosurgery; rhinitis; middle ear surgery.
- PRIVATE: The Croft, 161 Brooklands Road, Cheshire M33 3PD. Tel: 0161 976 3355 Fax: 0161 969 3547

Denbighshire

Mr Jonathan Osborne MB BS FRCS(Ed) FRCS(Eng) DLO
- YEAR QUALIFIED: 1978
- NHS POST: Consultant Otolaryngologist, Glan Clwyd Hospital.
- SPECIAL INTEREST: Paediatric otology and cochlear implants; voice and phonosurgery; sleep disorders and their surgery.
- PRIVATE: ENT Department, Glan Clwyd Hospital, Bodelwyddan, Denbighshire, LL18 5UY. Tel: 01745 534233 Fax: 01745 534160
E-mail: caroline.jones@glanclwyd-tr.wales.nhs.uk

Devon

Mr Paul C Windle-Taylor MA MB BChir FRCS MBA
- YEAR QUALIFIED: 1972
- NHS POST: Consultant Otolaryngologist, Plymouth Hospitals NHS Trust.
- SPECIAL INTEREST: Disorders of hearing and balance; tinnitus; otological and neuro-otological surgery; bone anchored; hearing aids and cochlear implantation.
- PRIVATE: Nuffield Hospital, Derriford Road, Plymouth, Devon PL6 8BG. Tel: 01752 775861 Fax: 01752 768969

Enfield Middlesex

Mr Dennis I Choa MA(Cantab) MA BM BCh(Oxon) FRCS
- NHS POST: Consultant ENT Surgeon, Royal National Throat Nose & Ear Hospital, Whittington Hospital and Middlesex (UCL) Hospital.
- SPECIAL INTEREST: Stapedectomy and other middle ear/mastoid surgery including paediatric; FESS: surgery for chronic sinus disease; surgery for snoring; rhinoplasty; general adult and paediatric ENT.
- PRIVATE: Kings Oak Hospital, Chase Farm (North side), The Ridgeway, Enfield, Middlesex EN2 8SD. Tel: 0181 366 0036 Fax: 0181 364 6779

Essex

Mr Chitta Ranjan Chowdhury MBBS FRCS FICS FCSHK
- YEAR QUALIFIED: 1970
- NHS POST: Consultant ENT Surgeon, Haroldwood / Oldchurch Hospital, Romford, Essex.
- SPECIAL INTEREST: Paediatric ENT; microsurgery; endoscopic sinus surgery.
- PRIVATE: BUPA Hartswood Hospital, Eagle Way, Brentwood, Essex, CM13 3LE. Tel: 0850 944614; 01708 442268 Fax: 01277 232525; 01708 708275

ENT Surgery. Essex

Mr Bhik Kotecha MBBCh, FRCS(Ed & Eng) FRCS(Orl) MPhil DLO
- NHS POST: Consultant Otolaryngologist, Royal National Throat, Nose And Ear Hospital and Havering Hospitals NHS Trust.
- SPECIAL INTEREST: Snoring and sleep disorders; otology; functional endoscopic sinus surgery; nasal allergy.
- PRIVATE: BUPA Roding Hospital, Roding Lane South, Redbridge, Ilford, Essex IG4 5PZ.
  Tel: 0181 551 1100 Fax: 0181 551 6415
  Essex Nuffield Hospital, Shenfield Road, Brentwood, Essex, CM15 8EH.
  Tel: 01277 263263
  BUPA Hartswood Hospital, Eagle Way, Brentwood, Essex, CM13 3LE.
  Tel: 01277 232525

Mr Chandra B Singh MB BS FRCS DLO
- YEAR QUALIFIED: 1961
- NHS POST: Consultant ENT Surgeon Mid Essex Hospital Trust
- SPECIAL INTEREST: Septo-rhinoplasty.
- PRIVATE: Springfield Hospital, Lawn Lane, Springfield, Chelmsford, Essex CM1 7GU.
  Tel: 01245 461777

Hertfordshire

Mr David Johnston BSc MB ChB FRCS(Ed) FRCS(Eng)(ORL)
- NHS POST: ENT Consultant, St. Albans Hospital, Hemel Hempstead NHS Trust.
- SPECIAL INTEREST: Paediatric ENT; otology; rhinology.
- PRIVATE: BUPA Hospital Bushey, Heathbourne Rd, Bushey, Watford, Hertfordshire WD2 1RD.
  Tel: 0181 950 8550. Secretary-01442 287042. Fax: 0181 950 7556
  BUPA Hospital Harpenden, Ambrose Lane, Harpenden, Herts, AL5 4BP.
  Tel: 01582 763191. Secretary-01582 760274 Fax: 01582 760 274

Mr Kalpesh S Patel BSc(Hons) MBBS FRCS(orl)
- YEAR QUALIFIED: 1984
- NHS POST: Consultant ENT / Head and Neck Surgeon, St Mary's Hospital
- SPECIAL INTEREST: Sinus problems; nasal allergy; endoscopic sinus surgery; head and neck surgical oncology; facial dermatological surgery.
- PRIVATE: North London Nuffield Hospital, Cavell Drive, Uplands Park Road, Enfield, EN2 7PR.
  Tel: 0181 366 2122 Fax: 0181 362 3629

Kent

Mr David Anthony Bowdler MBBS FRCS (Gen Surg) FRCS (OTOL)
- NHS POST: Consultant ENT Surgeon, Lewisham Hospital, Memorial Hospital and Queén Mary's Hospital, Sidcup.
- SPECIAL INTEREST: General ENT with a special interest in paediatric ENT and otology.
- PRIVATE: Fawkham Manor Hospital, Manor Lane, Fawkham, Longfield, Kent DA3 8ND.
  Tel: Appointments-01474 879900, Secretary-0181 2954802. Fax: 0181 295 4803
  E-mail: dbowdler@uk-consultants.co.uk
  Chelsfield Park Hospital, Bucks Cross Road, Chelsfield, Kent, BR6 7RG.
  Tel: Appoinments-01689 877855, Secretary-0181 2954802. Fax: 0181 295 4803
  E-mail: dbowdler@uk-consultants.co.uk

ENT Surgery. Kent

Mr David Golding-Wood BSc FRCS FRCS Ed
- YEAR QUALIFIED: 1980
- NHS POST: Consultant ENT and Head and Neck Surgeon, Bromley Hospitals NHS Trust.
- SPECIAL INTEREST: Rhinology; otology, particularly tympanomastoid disease and paediatric ENT.
- PRIVATE: Chelsfield Park Hospital, Bucks Cross Road, Chelsfield, Kent, BR6 7RG.
  Tel: 01689 877 855 Fax: 01689 837 439
  The Sloane Hospital, 125 Albemarle Road, Beckenham, Kent BR3 2HS.
  Tel: 0181 460 6998 Fax: 0181 313 9547

Mr Andrew N Johns MA FRCS
- NHS POST: Consultant ENT Surgeon, Kent and Sussex Weald Trust
- SPECIAL INTEREST: E.N.T.
- PRIVATE: Somerfield Hospital, 63-77 London Road, Maidstone, Kent, ME16 0DU.
  Tel: 01622 208000
  BUPA Alexandra Hospital, Impton Lane, Walderslade, Chatham, Kent ME5 9PG.
  Tel: 01634 687166
  Private Consulting Rooms, 16 Bower Mount Road, Maidstone, Kent ME16 8AU.
  Tel: 01622 692154

Miss Catherine Milton BSc FRCS
- NHS POST: Consultant Otorhinolaryngologist, Kent and Sussex Hospital.
- SPECIAL INTEREST: Paediatrics, Parotid and salivary gland surgery.
- PRIVATE: BUPA Hospital Tunbridge Wells, Fordcombe Road, Fordcombe, Tunbridge Wells, Kent TN3 0RD. Tel: 01892 740 047 Fax: 01892 740 046
  Nuffield Hospital Tunbridge Wells, Kingswood Road, Tunbridge Wells, Kent TN2 4UL.
  Tel: 01892 531 111 Fax: 01892 515 689
  2 Kingswood Close, Tunbridge Wells, Kent
  Tel: 01892 537 430 Fax: 01892 517 873

Mr Padman Ratnesar FRCS FACS DLO
- YEAR QUALIFIED: 1961
- NHS POST: Consultant Otolaryngologist - part time Farnborough Hospital.
- SPECIAL INTEREST: Paediatric otolaryngology; early detection of deafness and rehabilitation; otology.
- PRIVATE: BMI Sloane Hospital, 125 Albermarle Road, Beckenham, Kent BR3 2HS.
  Tel: 0181 466 6911 Fax: 0181 464 1443
  Chelsfield Park Hospital, Bucks Cross Road, Chelsfield, Kent, BR6 7RG.
  Tel: 01689 877855 Fax: 01689 837539

Miss Patricia Robinson DCH FRCS FRCSI
- YEAR QUALIFIED: 1978
- NHS POST: Consultant ENT Surgeon William Harvey Hospital
- SPECIAL INTEREST: Paediatric otolaryngology; endoscopic sinus surgery.
- PRIVATE: St. Saviour's Hospital (BUPA), 73 Seabrook, Hythe, Kent, CT21 5QW.
  Tel: 01303 265 581
  The Chaucer Hospital, Nackington Road, Canterbury, Kent CT4 7AR.
  Tel: 01227 825100

Mr Roland Mark Terry MBBS FRCS
NHS POST: Consultant ENT Surgeon Farnborough Hospital
SPECIAL INTEREST: Paediatric otolaryngology; endoscopic nasal surgery; salivary gland surgery and thyroid.
PRIVATE: Ravensbourne House, Sloane Hospital, 125 Albermarle Road, Beckenham, Kent BR3 5HS. Tel: 0181 466 6911
Chelsfield Park Hospital, Bucks Cross Road, Chelsfield, Kent, BR6 7RG.
Tel: 01689 877855 Fax: 01689 837439

London

Mr Solomon Abramovich MSc FRCS
NHS POST: Consultant, St. Mary's Hospital and Central Middlesex Hospital.
SPECIAL INTEREST: ENT surgery.
PRIVATE: 152 Harley Street, London W1N 1HH.
Tel: 0171 935 3834 Fax: 0171 224 2574
Consulting Rooms, 5th Floor, The Wellington Hospital, Wellington Place, London, NW8 9LE. Tel: 0171 586 3213 Fax: 0171 483 0297

Mr David M Albert MB BS FRCS
YEAR QUALIFIED: 1979
NHS POST: Consultant Paediatric Otolaryngologist, Great Ormond Street Hospital for Sick Children.
SPECIAL INTEREST: Paediatric otolaryngology; paediatric airway obstruction; cochlear implants; laryngeal reconstruction; paediatric ear disease; otitis media; glue ear; tonsils adenoids.
PRIVATE: BMI Portland Hospital for Women & Children, 234 Great Portland Street, London W1N 6AH. Tel: 0171 390 8300 Fax: 0171 383 4269 E-mail: albert@easynet.co.uk

Mr C Martin Bailey BSc FRCS
YEAR QUALIFIED: 1973
NHS POST: Consultant E.N.T. Surgeon, Great Ormond Street Hospital For Children.
SPECIAL INTEREST: Paediatric otolaryngology.
PRIVATE: 55 Harley Street, London W1N 1DD.
Tel: 0171 580 2426 Fax: 0171 436 1645

Mr David Anthony Bowdler MBBS FRCS (Gen Surg) FRCS (OTOL)
NHS POST: Consultant ENT Surgeon, Lewisham Hospital, Memorial Hospital and Queen Mary's Hospital, Sidcup.
SPECIAL INTEREST: General ENT with a special interest in paediatric ENT and otology.
PRIVATE: BMI Blackheath Hospital, 40-42 Lee Terrace, London, SE3 9UD.
Tel: Appointments-0181 318 7722, Secretary-0181 2954802 Fax: 0181 295 4803
E-mail: dbowdler@uk-consultants.co.uk

Miss Elfy B Chevretton BSc MS FRCS
YEAR QUALIFIED: 1978
NHS POST: Consultant ENT Surgeon, Guy's & St Thomas' Hospital Trust.
SPECIAL INTEREST: General ENT surgery with a special interest in head & neck surgery, salivary gland surgery, endoscopic sinus surgery and phonosurgery.
PRIVATE: Suite 305, Emblem House London Bridge Hospital, 27 Tooley Street, London, SE1 2PR.
Tel: 0171 403 4501 Fax: 0171 357 6172

ENT Surgery. London

Mr Dennis I Choa MA(Cantab) MA BM BCh(Oxon) FRCS
- NHS POST: Consultant ENT Surgeon, Royal National Throat Nose & Ear Hospital, Whittington Hospital and Middlesex (UCL) Hospital.
- SPECIAL INTEREST: Stapedectomy and other middle ear/mastoid surgery including paediatric; FESS: surgery for chronic sinus disease; surgery for snoring; rhinoplasty; general adult and paediatric ENT.
- PRIVATE: (Wednesday Afternoon), The London Clinic, 149 Harley Street, London, W1N 2DE.
  Tel: 0171 935 4444 Fax: 0171 616 7533
  (Thursday Morning), 66 New Cavendish Street, London W1M 7LD.
  Tel: 0171 637 5111 Fax: 0171 580 9749

Mr Charles B Croft FRCS FRCS(Ed)
- YEAR QUALIFIED: 1965
- NHS POST: Consultant ENT Surgeon and Clinical Director, The Royal National Throat, Nose & Ear Hospital
- SPECIAL INTEREST: Head and neck surgery; snoring/sleep apnoea.
- PRIVATE: 55 Harley Street, London, W1N 1DD.
  Tel: 0171 580 2426 Fax: 0171 436 1645

Mr Charles A East MB FRCS
- YEAR QUALIFIED: 1981
- NHS POST: Consultant Otolaryngology, Head and Neck Surgery, Royal National Throat Nose and Ear Hospital and The Royal Free Hospital NHS Trust.
- SPECIAL INTEREST: General ENT; rhinoplasty and sinus disease.
- PRIVATE: 150 Harley Street, London W1N 1AH.
  Tel: 0171 935 7435 Fax: 0171 935 3635

Mr Ian Fraser BSc MBBS FRCS
- YEAR QUALIFIED: 1966
- NHS POST: Consultant - ENT, Head & Neck Cancer Unit, Charing Cross Hospital.
- SPECIAL INTEREST: General ENT including rhinosinusitis, tinnitus and noise induced hearing loss.
- PRIVATE: 126 Harley Street, London W1N 1AH.
  Tel: 0171 935 8735 / 2030 Fax: 0171 224 2520
  Cromwell Hospital, Cromwell Road, London SW5 OTU.
  Tel: Appointments-0171 935 8735. Hospital-0171 460 2000 Fax: 0171 460 5555

Mr David Garfield Davies MBBS FRCS HON. FRAM
- NHS POST: Consultant in Otolaryngology, The Royal National Throat, Nose & Ear Hospital.
- SPECIAL INTEREST: Vocal problems; hearing loss; nasal problems; snoring.
- PRIVATE: The London Clinic, 149 Harley Street, London, W1N 2DE.
  Tel: 0171 935 4444 Fax: 0171 333 0340

Professor Michael Gleeson FRCS
- YEAR QUALIFIED: 1976
- NHS POST: Guy's Hospital
- SPECIAL INTEREST: E.N.T. - Salivary gland and skull base surgery.
- PRIVATE: Guy's Hospital, St Thomas Street, London, SE1 9RT.
  Tel: 0171 955 4474, 0171 955 4350

ENT Surgery. London

Mr Henry R Grant MB BS FRCS
- YEAR QUALIFIED: 1964
- NHS POST: Consultant Otolaryngologist, Royal National Throat Nose And Ear Hospital.
- SPECIAL INTEREST: General ENT; head and neck oncology; sleep apnoea and snoring; middle ear surgery and voice problems.
- PRIVATE: 31 Wimpole Street, London W1M 7AE.
  Tel: 0171 935 3593 Fax: 0171 224 1957

Dr Mohamed Hariri MD DLO FRCS MSc
- NHS POST: Consultant Audiological Medicine, Charing Cross Hospital, Fulham Palace Road, London W6 8RF. Tel:0181 846 1004. Fax:0181 846 1070.
- SPECIAL INTEREST: Paediatric audiology; glue ear; congenital hearing loss; noise induced hearing loss; tinnitus; medico-legal cases.
- PRIVATE: Audiology Department, Portland Hospital for Women & Children, 234 Great Portland Street, London W1N 5PH. Tel: 0171 390 8060 Fax: 0171 390 8053

Mr Thomas Martin Harris MA FRCS
- YEAR QUALIFIED: 1973
- NHS POST: Consultant ENT Surgeon, University Hospital Lewisham, London
- SPECIAL INTEREST: Especially voice disorders; microsurgery of the larynx; multi-disciplinary voice care.
- PRIVATE: The Blackheath Hospital, 40-42 Lee Terrace, Blackheath, London, SE3 9UD.
  Tel: 0181 318 7722 Fax: 0181 318 2542

Mr Anthony C John MBBS FRCS
- YEAR QUALIFIED: 1970
- NHS POST: Consultant ENT Surgeon, St. Helier Hospital, Carshalton (P/T) and St. George's Hospital
- SPECIAL INTEREST: Treatment of rhinitis and sinusitis; otology especially children.
- PRIVATE: Parkside Hospital, 53 Parkside, Wimbledon, London, SW19 5NX.
  Tel: 0181 946 4202 Fax: 0181 944 8461

Mr Jamsheed Khan BSc MB BS FICS DLO PhD
- SPECIAL INTEREST: Sinus surgery; nasalplastics; otology and head & neck surgery.
- PRIVATE: Private Health Centre, Green Street, East Ham, London E7 8DA.
  Tel: 0181 472 0170
  26 Preston Drive, Wanstead E11 2SB.
  Tel: 0181 989 8133

Mr Bhik Kotecha MBBCh, FRCS(Ed & Eng) FRCS(Orl) MPhil DLO
- NHS POST: Consultant Otolaryngologist, Royal National Throat, Nose And Ear Hospital and Havering Hospitals NHS Trust.
- SPECIAL INTEREST: Snoring and sleep disorders; otology; functional endoscopic sinus surgery; nasal allergy.
- PRIVATE: Royal National Throat, Nose & Ear Hospital, 330 Grays Inn Road, London, WC1X 8DA. Tel: 0171 915 1434

ENT Surgery. London

Mrs Susanna Leighton Consultant Paediatric Otolaryngologist
- YEAR QUALIFIED: 1983
- NHS POST: Consultant Paediatric Otolaryngologist, Great Ormond Street Hospital For Children NHS Trust.
- SPECIAL INTEREST: All areas of paediatric otolaryngology including glue ear, acute and chronic infection, upper and lower airway disease and cochlear implantation.
- PRIVATE: 234 Great Portland Street, London W1N 5PH.
Tel: 0171 390 8301 Fax: 0171 383 4269

Mr Harold Ludman MA MB FRCS
- YEAR QUALIFIED: 1957
- NHS POST: Consultant Otolaryngologist (Emeritus), National Hospital for Neurology & Neurosurgery, London
- SPECIAL INTEREST: Otology and neuro-otology
- PRIVATE: The London Clinic, 149 Harley Street, London, W1N 2DE.
Tel: 0171 935 4444

Mr Gavin A J Morrison MA MBBS FRCS
- NHS POST: Consultant Ear Nose & Throat Surgeon, Guy's & St. Thomas' Hospitals And King's College Hospital.
- SPECIAL INTEREST: Neonatal and paediatric otolaryngology; otology and neuro otology; vertigo and otology; endoscopic sinus surgery.
- PRIVATE: The Lister Hospital, Chelsea Bridge Road, London, SW1W 8RH.
150 Harley Street, London W1N 1AH.
Tel: 0171 928 7315 Fax: 0171 935 3635
Consulting Rooms,, York House,, 199 Westminster Bridge Road, London SE1 7UT.
Tel: 0171 928 7315 Fax: 0171 928 3748
BMI Blackheath Hospital, 40-42 Lee Terrace, London, SE3 9UD.
Tel: 0181 318 7722 Fax: 0181 318 2542

Mr Terence Mugliston MRCP FRCS
- NHS POST: Consultant, Queen Mary's University Hospital
- SPECIAL INTEREST: Paediatrics; sinus surgery; rhinoplasty head and neck.
- PRIVATE: Parkside Hospital, 53 Parkside, Wimbledon, London, SW19 5NX.
Tel: 0181 946 4202 Secretary Tel: 0181 947 1841
Lister Hospital, Chelsea Bridge Road, London, SW1W 8RH.
Tel: 0171 730 3417 Secretary Tel: 0181 947 1841

Mr Paul O'Flynn MBBS FRCS
- NHS POST: Consultant Royal National Throat, Nose, Ear NHS Trust
- SPECIAL INTEREST: General otolaryngology; head and neck surgery.
- PRIVATE: 55 Harley Street, London W1N 1DD.
Tel: 0171 580 4111-appts. 0171 436 3902-office Fax: 0171 436 4901

ENT Surgery. London

Mr Kalpesh S Patel BSc(Hons) MBBS FRCS(orl)
- YEAR QUALIFIED: 1984
- NHS POST: Consultant ENT / Head and Neck Surgeon, St Mary's Hospital
- SPECIAL INTEREST: Sinus problems; nasal allergy; endoscopic sinus surgery; head and neck surgical oncology; facial dermatological surgery.
- PRIVATE: Cromwell Hospital, Cromwell Road, London SW5 OTU.
  Tel: 0171 460 2000 Fax: 0171 460 5555
  Clementine Churchill Hospital, Sudbury Hill, Harrow, Middlesex, HA1 3RX.
  Tel: 0181 872 3939 Fax: 0181 872 3871
  149 Harley Street, London W1N 2DE.
  Tel: 0171 262 0297 Fax: 0171 886 1390

Mr Robert E Quiney FRCS FRCS(Ed) MBBS
- YEAR QUALIFIED: 1980
- NHS POST: Consultant ENT Surgeon, Royal Free Hospital, London NW3
- SPECIAL INTEREST: All aspects of both adult and paediatric otolaryngology but with a special interest in otology, neuro-otology and skull base surgery.
- PRIVATE: 55 Harley Street, London, W1N 1DD.
  Tel: 0171 580 2426 Fax: 0171 436 1645

Mr David Roberts MBBS BSc FRCS FRCS(Orl)
- YEAR QUALIFIED: 1987
- NHS POST: Consultant ENT and Facial Plastic Surgeon, Guys and St Thomas NHS Trust.
- SPECIAL INTEREST: Rhinology; sinus disease; endoscopic nasal surgery; rhinoplasty; facial plastic surgery.
- PRIVATE: 55 Harley Street, London, W1N 1DD.
  Tel: 0171 580 4111 Fax: 0181 785 7515 E-mail: dr@easynet.co.uk
  The London Bridge Hospital, 27 Tooley Street, London, SE1 2PR.
  Tel: 0171 815 3648 Fax: 0181 785 7515 E-mail: dr@easynet.co.uk

Dr Kusum S Sirimanna MBBS MS FRCS MSc DLO
- YEAR QUALIFIED: 1976
- NHS POST: Consultant Audiological Physician and Head of Department, Great Ormond Street Hospital for Children
- SPECIAL INTEREST: Paediatric audiology; hearing and balance disorders in children; tinnitus, noise and hearing loss; screening for hearing loss.
- PRIVATE: The Portland Hospital, 234 Great Portland Street, London W1N 5PA.
  Tel: 0171 390 8060 Fax: 0171 390 8053 E-mail: tsirimanna@baap.org.uk

Mr Iynga Vanniasegaram MSc DLO FRCS(ENT)
- NHS POST: Consultant Audiological Physician St. George's & Great Ormond Street Hospitals
- SPECIAL INTEREST: Paediatric Audiology; Balance Disorders; Tinnitus Central Auditory Disorders; Noise Induced Hearing Loss (medico-legal). Glue Ear. Vertigo - Dizziness
- PRIVATE: Depart. of Audiological Medicine, BMI Portland Hospital for Women & Children, 209 Great Portland Street, London, W1N 6AH.
  Tel: 0171 390 8060 Fax: 0171 390 8053 E-mail: jx79@dial.pipex.com

Mr Colin E Wallace MBBS FRCS T(s)
- YEAR QUALIFIED: 1963
- SPECIAL INTEREST: General adult and paediatric ENT; surgery for snoring and nocturnal apnoea; nasal and sinus surgery; voice disorders and microlaryngeal surgery; ENT allergy.
- PRIVATE: Cromwell Hospital, Cromwell Road, London SW5 OTU.
  Tel: 0171 460 5700 / 460 2000 - appointments Fax: 0171 460 5555
  148 Harley Street, London W1N 1AH.
  Tel: 0171 935 1207/1900 - appointments

Middlesex

Mr Solomon Abramovich MSc FRCS
- NHS POST: Consultant, St. Mary's Hospital and Central Middlesex Hospital.
- SPECIAL INTEREST: ENT surgery.
- PRIVATE: The Clementine Churchill Hospital, Sudbury Hill, Harrow, Middlesex, HA1 3RX.
  Tel: 0181 422 3464 Fax: 0181 864 1747

Newcastle upon Tyne

Mr John Hill MBBS FRCS FRCSEd
- YEAR QUALIFIED: 1984
- NHS POST: Consultant Otolaryngologist, Freeman Hospital, Newcastle upon Tyne.
- SPECIAL INTEREST: Otology and rhinology; general adult and paediatric otolaryngology.
- PRIVATE: Newcastle Nuffield Hospital, Clayton Road, Newcastle upon Tyne NE2 1JP.
  Tel: 0191 281 6131 E-mail: johnhillfrcs@compuserve.com

Norfolk

Mr Anthony J Innes MB BS FRCS
- YEAR QUALIFIED: 1972
- NHS POST: Consultant Otolaryngologist, Norfolk and Norwich NHS Healthcare Trust.
- SPECIAL INTEREST: Paediatric ear, nose and throat disease; surgical treatment of pharyngeal pouch; snoring. General ear, nose and throat problems.
- PRIVATE: Hill House Consulting Rooms, BUPA Hospital, Old Watton Road, Norwich, Norfolk NR4 7TD. Tel: 01603 504622 Fax: 01603 504622 E-mail: AInnes441@aol.com

North Hants

Mr Robin John Lee MB BCh BAO MA MD FRCSI
- YEAR QUALIFIED: 1978
- NHS POST: Consultant ENT Surgeon, Kettering General Hospital.
- SPECIAL INTEREST: Otology and rhinology.
- PRIVATE: The Woodland Hospital, Rothwell Road, Kettering, North Hants NN16 8XF.
  Tel: 01536 414515 Fax: 01536 412155

Nottinghamshire

Mr S Ali FRCS DLO
- YEAR QUALIFIED: 1972
- NHS POST: Consultant ENT Surgeon, The King's Mill Centre.
- SPECIAL INTEREST: Rhinology; paediatric ENT surgery and noise induced hearing loss.
- PRIVATE: The Park Hospital Sherwood Lodge Drive, Arnold, Nottingham NG5 8RX.
  Tel: 0115 967 0670 Fax: 0115 967 0381
  The Private Clinic, 14 Woodhouse Road, Mansfield, Nottingham NG1 8 2AD.
  Tel: 01623 624137 Fax: 01623 422137

Oxfordshire

Mr Grant James Bates BSc BmBch FRCS
- NHS POST: Consultant Otolaryngologist, Radcliffe Infirmary Oxford and Senior Lecturer, Oxford University.
- SPECIAL INTEREST: All aspects of rhinology including endoscopic sinus surgery, orbital decompression for thyroid eye disease and rhinoplasty. Pharyngeal pouch stapling - endoscopic. Monthly voice clinic with speech therapists.
- PRIVATE: Felstead House, 23 Banbury Road, Oxford, Oxon OX2 6NX.
  Tel: 01865 311105 Fax: 01865 310342 E-mail: grant.bates@nds.ox.ac.uk

South Yorkshire

Mr Jack Michael Lancer MB ChB(Sheff) FRCS(Eng)
- YEAR QUALIFIED: 1978
- NHS POST: Consultant ENT Surgeon, Rotherham District General Hospital (R.D.G.H.).
- SPECIAL INTEREST: Ear surgery; all aspects especially stapedectomy; rhinoplasty; general and paediatric; facial plastics.
- PRIVATE: Parkfield Hospital, Parkfield Road, Rotherham, South Yorkshire S65 2AJ.
  Tel: 01709 828928 Fax: 01777 817158

Staffordshire

Mr James Timothy Little MB ChB(Sheffield) FRCS(England)
- YEAR QUALIFIED: 1965
- NHS POST: Consultant ENT Surgeon, North Staffordshire Hospital, Stoke-on-Trent.
- SPECIAL INTEREST: Paediatric ENT; middle ear surgery.
- PRIVATE: S.T. Little Parklands, 9 Second Avenue, Porthill, Newcastle-under-Lyme, Staffordshire ST5 8NU. Tel: 01782 639866 Fax: 01782 639866

Surrey

Mr Kemal Bevan MB BS ChM FRCS
- NHS POST: Consultant ENT Surgeon, Crawley Hospital, East Surrey Hospital, Horsham Hospital, Dorking Hospital.
- SPECIAL INTEREST: Aesthetic surgery to nose, rhinology, functional endoscopic sinus surgery, otology, assessment of hearing in children, laser surgery to larynx/snoring; laser-assisted uvulopalatoplasty.
- PRIVATE: BUPA Gatwick Park Hospital, Povey Cross Road, Horley, Surrey RH6 0BB.
  Tel: 01293 785511 Fax: 01293 774883
  North Downs Hospital, 46 Tupwood Lane, Caterham, Surrey CR3 6DP.
  Tel: 01883 348 981 Fax: 01883 341 163
  BUPA Redwood Hospital East Surrey, Canada Drive, Redhill, Surrey RH1 5BY.
  Tel: 01737 277277 Fax: 01737 277288

Mr Patrick Chapman LRCP MRCS MBBS FRCS
- YEAR QUALIFIED: 1968
- NHS POST: Consultant Otololaryngologist / Head & Neck Surgeon, St. Peter's Hospital, Chertsey and Ashford Hospital Middlesex and Royal Surrey County Hospital, Guilford.
- SPECIAL INTEREST: General otolaryngology; paediatric otolaryngology; endoscopic sinus surgery and rhinoplasty surgery; head & neck surgery and laser surgery.
- PRIVATE: Lee Farm, New Lane, Sutton Green, Guildford, Surrey GU4 7QF.
  Tel: 01483 714991 Fax: 01483 723805
  Woking Nuffield Hospital, Shores Road, Woking, Surrey, GU21 4BY.
  Tel: 01483 763 511 Fax: 01483 722 966

Mr Ian Fraser BSc MBBS FRCS
- YEAR QUALIFIED: 1966
- NHS POST: Consultant - ENT, Head & Neck Cancer Unit, Charing Cross Hospital.
- SPECIAL INTEREST: General ENT including rhinosinusitis, tinnitus and noise induced hearing loss.
- PRIVATE: New Victoria Hospital, 184 Coombe Lane West, Kingston Upon Thames, Surrey, KT2 7EG. Tel: Appointments-0171 935 8735. Hospital-0181 949 9000 Fax: 0181 949 9099

Mr Anthony C John MBBS FRCS
- YEAR QUALIFIED: 1970
- NHS POST: Consultant ENT Surgeon, St. Helier Hospital, Carshalton (P/T) and St. George's Hospital
- SPECIAL INTEREST: Treatment of rhinitis and sinusitis; otology especially children.
- PRIVATE: St. Anthony's Hospital, London Road, North Cheam, Surrey, SM3 9DW.
  Tel: 0181 337 6691 Fax: 0181 335 3325

Mr Jeffrey R Knight FRCS (otolaryngol) MB ChB
- NHS POST: Consultant ENT Surgeon Mayday University Hospital and St. George's Hospital.
- SPECIAL INTEREST: Otology & Otoneurology
- PRIVATE: Shirley Oaks Hospital, Poppy Lane, Shirley Oaks Village, Surrey, CR9 8AB.
  Tel: 0181 655 2255 xt 301/317/360 appts. Fax: 0181 656 2868

Mr Peter J Robb BSc(Hons) MBBS FRCS FRCS(Ed)
- NHS POST: Consultant ENT Surgeon, Epsom General Hospital, KT18 7EG.
- SPECIAL INTEREST: Paediatric ENT; allergy, salivary gland diseases; laser surgery; voice; laryngology.
- PRIVATE: Ashtead Hospital, The Warren, Ashtead, Surrey KT21 2SB.
  Tel: Appts-01372 276 161. Sec-01372 275 161 Fax: 01372 278 704

Warwickshire

Mr David Esmond Phillips MB BS FRCS
- YEAR QUALIFIED: 1982
- NHS POST: Consultant Otorhinolaryngologist/Head and Neck Surgeon, Warwick Hospital.
- SPECIAL INTEREST: Perennial rhinitis; chronic rhinosinusitis; rhinoplasty and medico-legal aspects of occupational rhinitis and nasal injuries; thyroid surgery.
- PRIVATE: The Warwickshire Nuffield Hospital, Old Milverton Lane, Leamington Spa, Warwickshire CV32 6RW. Tel: 01926 427971 Fax: 01926 428791

West Sussex

Mr Kemal Bevan MB BS ChM FRCS
- NHS POST: Consultant ENT Surgeon, Crawley Hospital, East Surrey Hospital, Horsham Hospital, Dorking Hospital.
- SPECIAL INTEREST: Aesthetic surgery to nose, rhinology, functional endoscopic sinus surgery, otology, assessment of hearing in children, laser surgery to larynx/snoring; laser-assisted uvulopalatoplasty.
- PRIVATE: Ashdown Hospital, Burrell Road, Haywards Heath, West Sussex RH16 1UD.
  Tel: 01444 456999 Fax: 01444 454111

Endocrinology

Cheshire

Dr David Ewins BM(Hons) DM MRCP
  YEAR QUALIFIED: 1983
  NHS POST: Consultant Physician, Countess of Chester Hospital.
  SPECIAL INTEREST: General medicine specialising in endocrinology and diabetes, including lipids and metabolic bone disease.
  PRIVATE: Grosvenor Nuffield Hospital, Wrexham Road, Chester, Cheshire CH4 7QP. Tel: 01244 684318 Fax: 01244 680812

Enfield Middlesex

Dr Rodwin Jackson FCP(SA) MD FRCP
  NHS POST: Consultant Physician, Chase Farm Hospital.
  SPECIAL INTEREST: Diabetes and endocrinology.
  PRIVATE: Kings Oak Hospital, Chase Farm (North side), The Ridgeway, Enfield, Middlesex EN2 8SD. Tel: 0181 364 5520
  North London Nuffield Hospital, Cavell Drive, Uplands Park Road, Enfield, EN2 7PR. Tel: 0181 366 2122

Dr Ian Ramsay MD FRCP FRCPE
  SPECIAL INTEREST: Thyroid; radioactive iodine; osteoporosis; endocrine hair disorders.
  PRIVATE: Kings Oak Hospital, Chase Farm (North side), The Ridgeway, Enfield, Middlesex EN2 8SD. Tel: 0181 370 9505 Fax: 0181 370 9551

Hertfordshire

Dr Michael R Clements MD FRCP
  YEAR QUALIFIED: 1976
  NHS POST: Consultant Physician & Endocrinologist, Watford General Hospital.
  SPECIAL INTEREST: Endocrinology and metabolism including diabetes; thyroid; pituitary and adrenal disease; lipids; reproductive endocrinology and metabolic bone disease; osteoporosis and HRT.
  PRIVATE: BUPA Hospital Bushey, Heathbourne Rd, Bushey, Watford, Hertfordshire WD2 1RD. Tel: 0181 901 5555 Fax: 01923 217455

Dr Colin Johnston MA MB BCh MD FRCP
  NHS POST: Consultant Physician & Endocrinologist, St. Albans & Hemel Hempstead NHS Trust.
  SPECIAL INTEREST: All aspects of medicine and endocrinology including diabetes, thyroid disease and impotence.
  PRIVATE: Hemel Hempstead General Hospital Hillfield Road, Hemel Hempstead, Herts, HP2 4AD. Tel: 01582 460 129

London

Dr Ralph Abraham MA PhD BM BCh MRCP
- YEAR QUALIFIED: 1971
- SPECIAL INTEREST: Diabetes; endocrinology; lipid disorders; obesity; hypertension; impotence.
- PRIVATE: The London Diabetes & Lipid Centre, 14 Wimpole Street, London W1M 7AB. Tel: 0171 636 9901 Fax: 0171 636 9902

Professor Charles G D Brook MA MD FRCP FRCPCH
- YEAR QUALIFIED: 1964
- NHS POST: Consultant Paediatric Endocrinologist, Great Ormond Street Hospital For Children and Middlesex Hospital.
- SPECIAL INTEREST: Growth disorders; endocrine problems; physical development; puberty disorders.
- PRIVATE: Middlesex Hospital, Mortimer Street, London, W1N 8AA. Tel: 0171 380 9221

Dr Desmond N Croft MA DM FRCP
- NHS POST: Consultant Physician, St. Thomas' Hospital.
- SPECIAL INTEREST: Thyroid disease.
- PRIVATE: York House Consulting Rooms, 199 Westminster Bridge Road, London SE1 7UT. Tel: 0171 928 5485 Fax: 0171 928 3748

Dr Rodwin Jackson FCP(SA) MD FRCP
- NHS POST: Consultant Physician, Chase Farm Hospital.
- SPECIAL INTEREST: Diabetes and endocrinology.
- PRIVATE: Hospital of St. John & St. Elizabeth, 60 Grove End Road, St Johns Wood, London, NW8 9NH. Tel: 0171 286 5126
  Garden Hospital, 46-50 Sunny Gardens Road, Hendon, London, NW4 1RX. Tel: 0181 203 6832

Professor Howard S Jacobs MD FRCP FRCOG
- YEAR QUALIFIED: 1962
- NHS POST: Emeritus Professor of Reproductive Endocrinology & Honorary Consultant, The Middlesex Hospital
- SPECIAL INTEREST: Reproductive endocrinology; ovulation and menstrual disturbances; hirsutism; acne; menopause.
- PRIVATE: The London Diabetes & Lipid Centre, 14 Wimpole Street, London W1M 7AB. Tel: 0171 636 9901 Fax: 0171 636 9902 E-mail: HSJacobs1@aol.com

Dr Maurice Katz FCP(SA) FRCP
- YEAR QUALIFIED: 1963
- NHS POST: Consultant Endocrinologist, University College London Hospitals.
- SPECIAL INTEREST: Reproductive endocrinology; menstrual disorders; androgenised females; PCO.; premenstrual syndrome; menopause; osteoporosis; male and female infertility; psychosexual problems and endocrinology of ageing; pituitary; thyroid; adrenal.
- PRIVATE: 148 Harley Street, London W1N 1AH. Tel: 0171 383 7911 Fax: 0171 380 9816

Endocrinology. London

Dr Geoffrey J Lloyd BSc LLB MB BS FRCP
- PRIVATE: Flat C, 21 Devonshire Place, London W1N 1PD.
  Tel: 0171 935 8071 Fax: 0171 935 4913

Dr Karim Meeran MBBS BSc MRCP MD
- YEAR QUALIFIED: 1988
- NHS POST: Consultant Endocrinologist, Hammersmith Hospital.
- SPECIAL INTEREST: Pituitary disease; Cushing's disease; Addison's disease; thyroid disorders.
- PRIVATE: Robert & Lisa Sainsbury Wing, Hammersmith Hospital, Du Cane Road, London, W12 OHS. Tel: 0181 383 3113 Fax: 0181 383 3142

Dr Nigel Oakley MD FRCP
- YEAR QUALIFIED: 1958
- NHS POST: Consultant Physician St. George's Hospital
- SPECIAL INTEREST: Diabetes mellitus.
- PRIVATE: 44 Wimpole Street, London W1M 7DG.
  Tel: 0171 935 0552 Fax: 0171 224 0629

Dr Ian Ramsay MD FRCP FRCPE
- SPECIAL INTEREST: Thyroid; radioactive iodine; osteoporosis; endocrine hair disorders.
- PRIVATE: Cromwell Hospital, Cromwell Road, London SW5 OTU.
  Tel: 0171 460 5700 Fax: 0171 460 5555
  The Lister Hospital, Chelsea Bridge Road, London, SW1W 8RH.
  Tel: 0171 730 8298 Fax: 0171 259 9218

Dr Edmund Peter Shephard BA MA(Oxon) MB BS MRCP MD
- YEAR QUALIFIED: 1970
- SPECIAL INTEREST: Diabetes thyroid; hypertension; diagnostic problems.
- PRIVATE: 80 Harley Street, London W1N 1AE.
  Tel: 0171 637 4962 Fax: 0171 637 4963

Dr Richard Stanhope BSc MD DCH FRCP
- NHS POST: Consultant Paediatric Endocrinologist Great Ormond Street Hospital for Children NHS Trust & The Middlesex Hospital (UCLH)
- SPECIAL INTEREST: Adolescent and Paediatric Endocrinology especially disorders of puberty and growth
- PRIVATE: The Portland Hospital, 205-209 Great Portland Street, London W1N 6AH.
  Tel: Appts - 0181 670 1957 Fax: 0181 670 1957
  Great Ormond Street Hospital for Children NHS Trust, Great Ormond Street, London WC1N 3JH. Tel: (44) 171 9052139, 0181 6701957-appts. Fax: (44) 171 8138496, 0181 6701957-private appts.

Professor John Vallance-Owen MA MD FRCP FRCPI FRCPath FHKCP
- SPECIAL INTEREST: General (internal) medicine; diabetes; endocrinology.
- PRIVATE: London Independent Hospital, 1 Beaumont Square, Stepney Green, London E1 4NL.
  Tel: 0171 790 0990 Fax: 0171 265 9032

Endocrinology. London

Dr Richard W E Watts MD DSc PhD FRCP
- NHS POST: Honorary Consultant Physician Hammersmith Hospital
- SPECIAL INTEREST: Endocrinology; metabolism; diabetes; renal medicine; general medicine.
- PRIVATE: Harley Street Clinic, 35 Weymouth Street, London, W1N 4BJ.
  Tel: 0171 935 7700, Appointments: 0171 586 5959 ext 2572
  Wellington Hospital,, Wellington Place, St John's Wood, London NW8 9LE.
  Tel: 0171 586 5959 xt 2572 Fax: 0171 483 0297 Aircall- 01459 126538
  Highgate Private Clinic, 17-19 View Road, Highgate, London, N6.
  Tel: Appts.-0171 586 5959 xt 2572. 0181 341 4182 Fax: 0181 342 8347 Aircall- 01459 126538
  Sainsbury Wing, Hammersmith Hospital, Du Cane Road, London, W12 OHS.
  Tel: Appts: 0171 586 5959 ext.2572. Fax: 0171 483 0297
  E-mail: info@wellingtonchc.demon.co.uk

Manchester

Dr Frederick C W Wu BSc(Hon) MD FRCP FRCP(Edin)
- YEAR QUALIFIED: 1972
- NHS POST: Honorary Consultant Endocrinologist, Machester Royal Infirmatry.
- SPECIAL INTEREST: Reproductive endocrinology; andrology; androgen replacement; hormone replacement therapy; pubertal disorders; hypogonadism.
- PRIVATE: Department of Endocrinology, Manchester Royal Infirmary, Oxford Road, Manchester M13 9WL. Tel: 0161 276 4256 Fax: 0161 276 8019

Middlesex

Dr Christopher Baynes DM MRCP
- YEAR QUALIFIED: 1982
- NHS POST: Consultant Physician, Chase Farm.
- SPECIAL INTEREST: General clinical endocrinology and diabetes.
- PRIVATE: Kings Oak Hospital, Chase Farm (North side), The Ridgeway, Enfield, Middlesex EN2 8SD. Tel: 0181 370 9500 Fax: 0181 370 9501

Dr Michael R Clements MD FRCP
- YEAR QUALIFIED: 1976
- NHS POST: Consultant Physician & Endocrinologist, Watford General Hospital.
- SPECIAL INTEREST: Endocrinology and metabolism including diabetes; thyroid; pituitary and adrenal disease; lipids; reproductive endocrinology and metabolic bone disease; osteoporosis and HRT.
- PRIVATE: Bishops Wood Hospital, Rickmansworth Road, Northwood, Middlesex HA6 2JW.
  Tel: 01923 835 814 Fax: 01923 217455

South Yorkshire

Dr Jonathan Webster MA MD(Cantab) MRCP(UK)
- YEAR QUALIFIED: 1983
- NHS POST: Consultant Physician and Endocrinologist, Northern General Hospital, Sheffield.
- SPECIAL INTEREST: General endocrinology; particular interest in pituitary disease; hyperprolactinaemia; medical therapy of pituitary tumours; thyroid; adrenal.
- PRIVATE: Claremont Hospital, 401 Sandygate Road, Sheffield, South Yorkshire S10 5UB. Tel: 0114 263 0330 Fax: 0114 263 2119

Gastroenterology

Birmingham

Dr Carol Anne Cobb MBBS BSc MRCP
- YEAR QUALIFIED: 1982
- NHS POST: Consultant Physician and Gastroenterologist, Sandwell Healthcare NHS Trust.
- SPECIAL INTEREST: Endoscopy including therapeutic colonoscopy and ERCP, inflammatory bowel disease and liver diseases.
- PRIVATE: BMI Priory Hospital, Priory Road, Edgbaston, Birmingham B5 7UG.
  Tel: 0121 440 2323

Devon

Dr Simon Travis DPhil FRCP
- YEAR QUALIFIED: 1981
- NHS POST: Consultant Gastroenterologist, Derriford Hospital, Plymouth.
- SPECIAL INTEREST: All gastrointestinal and hepatobiliary disorders; inflammatory bowel disease; endoscopy (including upper GI, colonoscopy and ERCP).
- PRIVATE: Nuffield Hospital, Derriford Road, Plymouth, Devon PL6 8BG.
  Tel: 01752 761835 Fax: 01752 768969

Essex

Dr Waseem Ashraf BSc MRCP FACG
- YEAR QUALIFIED: 1982
- NHS POST: Consultant Gastroenterologist, King George Hospital, Essex.
- SPECIAL INTEREST: Interventional/therapeutic endoscopy and colonoscopy; therapeutic ERCP; gastrointestinal motility.
- PRIVATE: BUPA Roding Hospital, Roding Lane South, Redbridge, Ilford, Essex IG4 5PZ.
  Tel: 0181 551 1100 Fax: 0181 551 9452
  Holly House Hospital, High Road, Buckhurst Hill, Essex, IG9 5HX.
  Tel: 0181 505 3311 Fax: 0181 502 9735

Glasgow

Dr William Stuart Hislop MB ChB FRCP FACG
- YEAR QUALIFIED: 1973
- NHS POST: Consultant Physician, Royal Alexandra Hospital.
- SPECIAL INTEREST: Liver disease.
- PRIVATE: Ross Hall Hospital, 221 Crookston Road, Glasgow G52 3NQ.
  Tel: 0141 810 3151

Gastroenterology. Glasgow

Dr Peter R Mills MD FRCP FACP
- YEAR QUALIFIED: 1972
- NHS POST: Consultant Physician and Gastroenterologist, Western Infirmary, Glasgow.
- SPECIAL INTEREST: Diagnostic and therapeutic endoscopy; gastroenterology; liver disease; general internal medicine.
- PRIVATE: Glasgow Nuffield Hospital, Beaconsfield Road, Glasgow G12 0PJ.
  Tel: 0141 334 9441 Fax: 0141 339 1352

Herefordshire

Dr Michael J Hall MD MSc FRCP
- YEAR QUALIFIED: 1972
- NHS POST: Consultant Physician and Gastroenterologist, County Hospital, Hereford.
- SPECIAL INTEREST: Upper and lower gastrointestinal endoscopy and ERCP; investigating and management of patients with dyspepsia, IBS, inflammatory bowel disease, malabsorption and liver disease; interest in iron deficiency anaemia and coeliac disease.
- PRIVATE: Wye Valley Nuffield Hospital, Venns Lane, Hereford, Herefordshire HR1 1DF.
  Tel: 01432 364064 Fax: 01432 364054

London

Dr Andrew K Burroughs MBChB Hons, FRCP
- YEAR QUALIFIED: 1976
- NHS POST: Consultant Physician and Hepatologist, Royal Free Hospital.
- SPECIAL INTEREST: Liver disease and liver transplantation.
- PRIVATE: Lyndhurst Rooms, Royal Free Hospital, Pond Street, Hampstead, London, NW3 2QG.
  Tel: 0171 794 0500 xt 3978 Fax: 0171 794 4688
  E-mail: andrew.burroughs@talk21.com

Professor Paul J Ciclitira MD PhD FRCP
- NHS POST: Professor of Gastroenterology, St. Thomas' Hospital, Guy's & St. Thomas' NHS Trust.
- SPECIAL INTEREST: Coeliac disease/malabsorption; gastroenterology; general internal medicine.
- PRIVATE: Albert Embankment Consulting Rooms, St. Thomas' Hospital, Lambeth Palace Road, London, SE1 7EH.
  Tel: 0171 928 5485-ap 0171 928 9292 xt 2354-sec. Fax: 0171 620 2597

Dr John Croker MA BM BCh FRCP
- YEAR QUALIFIED: 1970
- NHS POST: Consultant, Middlesex Hospital.
- SPECIAL INTEREST: Geriatrics; general medicine; gastroenterology.
- PRIVATE: The London Clinic, 20 Devonshire Place, London, W1N 2DH.
  Tel: 0171 616 7781 Fax: 0171 486 1755

Gastroenterology. London

Dr Michael J Glynn MA MD FRCP
- YEAR QUALIFIED: 1977
- NHS POST: Consultant Physician & Gastroenterologist, Royal London Hospital and St. Bartholomew's Hospital.
- SPECIAL INTEREST: Hepatobiliary disease and endoscopy.
- PRIVATE: The London Independent Hospital, 1 Beaumont Square, Stepney Green, London E1 4NL. Tel: 0171 790 0990-appointments Fax: 0171 702 8495 Secretary: 07071 780743

Dr Geoffrey J Lloyd BSc LLB MB BS FRCP
- PRIVATE: Flat C, 21 Devonshire Place, London W1N 1PD.
  Tel: 0171 935 8071 Fax: 0171 935 4913

Dr Neil Ian McNeil MA MD FRCP
- NHS POST: Consultant Gastroenterologist and Physician, Ealing Hospital.
- SPECIAL INTEREST: Dyspepsia and Helicobacter pylori; diarrhoea and constipation; acid-peptic disease and functional and inflammatory intestinal problems
- PRIVATE: Clementine Churchill Hospital, Sudbury Hill, Harrow, Middlesex, HA1 3RX.
  Tel: 0181 872 3872
  Cromwell Hospital, Cromwell Road, London SW5 OTU.
  Tel: 0171 460 5700

Dr J J Misiewicz BSc MBBS FRCP (Lond, Edin)
- NHS POST: Honorary Consultant Physician, Central Middlesex Hospital.
- SPECIAL INTEREST: Peptic ulcer; irritable bowel syndrome; inflammatory bowel disease; ulcerative colitis; Crohn's disease; gastro-oesophageal reflux.
- PRIVATE: Princess Grace Hospital, 42-52 Nottingham Place, London, W1M 3FD.
  Tel: 0171 486 1234 Fax: 0171 487 4476

Dr Iain M Murray-Lyon BSc MD FRCP FRCP(Ed)
- YEAR QUALIFIED: 1964
- NHS POST: Consultant Gastroenterologist, Charing Cross Hospital and Chelsea & Westminster Hospital.
- SPECIAL INTEREST: Gastroenterology; liver disease.
- PRIVATE: 149 Harley Street, London W1N 2DE.
  Tel: 0171 935 6747 Fax: 0171 935 7017

Gastroenterology. London

Dr Ana H. Raimundo MD PhD
- NHS POST: Consultant Gastroenterologist Central Middlesex Hospital
- SPECIAL INTEREST: GI motility investigations (24 hour ambulatory techniques); functional bowel (IBS, pseudo-obstruction syndromes); gastro-oesophageal reflux disease; oesophageal motor disorders; non-cardiac chest pain; ambulatory oesophageal motility and pH monitoring; inflammatory bowel disease (U.C./Crohn's).
- PRIVATE: 80 Harley Street, London W1N 1AE.
Tel: 0171 636 8248 Fax: 0171 935 4984 E-mail: ahraimundo@dial.pipex.com
The Lister Hospital, Chelsea Bridge Road, London, SW1W 8RH.
Tel: 0171 7303417. appts.-0171 7308298 sec-0171 6368248 Fax: 0171 935 4984
E-mail: ahraimundo@dial.pipex.com
The Princess Grace Hospital, 42-52 Nottingham Place, London W1M 3FD.
Tel: appts: 0171 636 8248 Fax: 0171 935 4984 E-mail: ahraimundo@dial.pipex.com
The Wellington Hospital, Wellington Place, London, NW8 9LE.
Tel: 0171 636 8248 Fax: 0171 935 4984 E-mail: ahraimundo@dial.pipex.com
Cromwell Hospital, Cromwell Road, London SW5 0TU.
Tel: 0171 460 2000. Secretary - 0171 636 8248 Fax: 0171 935 4984
E-mail: ahraimundo@dial.pipex.com

Dr Jeremy Sanderson MB BS MD FRCP
- YEAR QUALIFIED: 1984
- NHS POST: Consultant Gastroenterologist Guy's & St Thomas' Hospitals
- SPECIAL INTEREST: Inflammatory bowel disease; colonoscopy; colorectal cancer screening.
- PRIVATE: Suite 406, Emblem House London Bridge Hospital, 27 Tooley Street, London, SE1 2PR.
Tel: 0171 403 3814

Dr Martin Sarner MD FRCP
- NHS POST: University College Hospital
- SPECIAL INTEREST: Gastroenterology; pancreatic and inflammatory bowel disease.
- PRIVATE: Private Patients Wing, University College Hospital, Gower Street, London WC1E 6AU.
Tel: 0171 388 3894 Fax: 0171 380 9816

Dr Brian Paul Saunders MB BS MD MRCP
- YEAR QUALIFIED: 1988
- NHS POST: Senior Lecturer in Endoscopy, Consultant Physician, St. Mark's Hospital and Northwick Park Hospital.
- SPECIAL INTEREST: Gastrointestinal endoscopy, particularly colonoscopy; colorectal cancer prevention/detection; inflammatory bowel disease.
- PRIVATE: The London Clinic, 20 Devonshire Place, London, W1N 2DH.
Tel: 0171 616 7782 Fax: 0171 486 1755 E-mail: wolfsonendoscopy@btinternet.com

Dr Allan D Thomson Bsc MB ChB PhD FRCP (Ed) FRCP
- YEAR QUALIFIED: 1963
- NHS POST: Consultant Physician/ Gastroenterologist Greenwich District Hospital
- SPECIAL INTEREST: Gastroenterology; liver disease.
- PRIVATE: BMI Blackheath Hospital, 40-42 Lee Terrace, London, SE3 9UD.
Tel: 0181 318 7722 Fax: 0181 318 2542

Gastroenterology. London

Dr Robin Vicary FRCP
- YEAR QUALIFIED: 1969
- NHS POST: Consultant Gastroenterologist and Physician, Whittington Hospital.
- SPECIAL INTEREST: Abdominal pain.
- PRIVATE: Highgate Private Hospital, 17-19 View Road, Highgate, London N6 4DJ.
Tel: 0181 341 6989 Fax: 0181 348 7205 E-mail: robin@flossy.demon.co.uk

Dr Mark L Wilkinson BSc MD FRCP
- YEAR QUALIFIED: 1974
- NHS POST: Consultant in Gastroenterology Guy's Hospital, Guy's & St. Thomas' Hospital Trust.
- SPECIAL INTEREST: Hepato-biliary and pancreatic disease; endoscopy, especially ERCP; general hepatology and gastroenterology. Director of specialist medicine, Guy's & St. Thomas' Hospital Trust. Education Secretary, Endoscopy Committee, British Society of Gastroenterology.
- PRIVATE: Emblem House London Bridge Hospital, 27 Tooley Street, London, SE1 2PR.
Tel: 0171 403 3814

Middlesex

Dr J J Misiewicz BSc MBBS FRCP (Lond, Edin)
- NHS POST: Honorary Consultant Physician, Central Middlesex Hospital.
- SPECIAL INTEREST: Peptic ulcer; irritable bowel syndrome; inflammatory bowel disease; ulcerative colitis; Crohn's disease; gastro-oesophageal reflux.
- PRIVATE: Clementine Churchill Hospital, Sudbury Hill, Harrow, Middlesex, HA1 3RX.
Tel: 0181 872 3872 Fax: 0181 872 3836

Dr Brian Paul Saunders MB BS MD MRCP
- YEAR QUALIFIED: 1988
- NHS POST: Senior Lecturer in Endoscopy, Consultant Physician, St. Mark's Hospital and Northwick Park Hospital.
- SPECIAL INTEREST: Gastrointestinal endoscopy, particularly colonoscopy; colorectal cancer prevention/detection; inflammatory bowel disease.
- PRIVATE: Wolfson Unit for Endoscopy, St. Mark's Hospital, Watford Road, Harrow, Middlesex HA1 3UJ. Tel: 0181 235 4225 Fax: 0181 423 3588
E-mail: wolfsonendoscopy@btinternet.com

Surrey

Dr Peter Finch MD FRCP
- YEAR QUALIFIED: 1980
- NHS POST: Consultant Gastroenterologist, St Peter's Hospital NHS Trust.
- SPECIAL INTEREST: Endoscopy; oesophageal motility; ERCP.
- PRIVATE: Runnymede Hospital, Guildford Road, Ottershaw, Surrey, KT16 0RQ.
Tel: 01483 721 812 Fax: 0870 0567897 E-mail: finchpj@dsk.co.uk
Woking Nuffield Hospital, Shores Road, Woking, Surrey, GU21 4BY.
Tel: 01483 721812 Fax: 0870 0567897 E-mail: finchpj@dsk.co.uk

Gastroenterology. Surrey

Dr Ian Strickland FRCP
NHS POST: Consultant Physician Kingston Hospital
SPECIAL INTEREST: Gastroenterology
PRIVATE: New Victoria Hospital, 184 Coombe Lane West, Kingston Upon Thames, Surrey, KT2 7EG. Tel: 0181 949 9020 Fax: 0181 949 9099

West Yorkshire

Professor Anthony Axon MD FRCP
YEAR QUALIFIED: 1965
NHS POST: Consultant Physician, The General Infirmary at Leeds.
SPECIAL INTEREST: Gastroenterology, dyspepsia, inflammatory bowel disease, pancreatico-biliary disease, endoscopy, diagnosis of gastro-intestinal malignancy, helicobacter pylori.
PRIVATE: BUPA Hospital Leeds, Roundhay Hall, Jackson Avenue, Leeds, West Yorkshire LS8 1NT. Tel: 0113 269 3939 Fax: 0113 268 1340
The Mid Yorkshire Nuffield Hospital, Outwood Lane, Horsforth, West Yorkshire LS18 4HP. Tel: 0113 258 8756 Fax: 0113 258 3108

General Medicine

East Sussex

Dr John C Kingswood FRCP
- NHS POST: Consultant Physician, Royal Sussex County Hospital.
- SPECIAL INTEREST: Nephrology & Hypertension
- PRIVATE: Sussex Diagnostic Centre, 13 New Church Road, Hove, East Sussex BN3 4AA. Tel: 01273 770044 / 724174 Fax: 01273 726931

Enfield Middlesex

Dr Rodwin Jackson FCP(SA) MD FRCP
- NHS POST: Consultant Physician, Chase Farm Hospital.
- SPECIAL INTEREST: Diabetes and endocrinology.
- PRIVATE: Kings Oak Hospital, Chase Farm (North side), The Ridgeway, Enfield, Middlesex EN2 8SD. Tel: 0181 364 5520
  North London Nuffield Hospital, Cavell Drive, Uplands Park Road, Enfield, EN2 7PR. Tel: 0181 366 2122

Hertfordshire

Dr Michael R Clements MD FRCP
- YEAR QUALIFIED: 1976
- NHS POST: Consultant Physician & Endocrinologist, Watford General Hospital.
- SPECIAL INTEREST: Endocrinology and metabolism including diabetes; thyroid; pituitary and adrenal disease; lipids; reproductive endocrinology and metabolic bone disease; osteoporosis and HRT.
- PRIVATE: BUPA Hospital Bushey, Heathbourne Rd, Bushey, Watford, Hertfordshire WD2 1RD. Tel: 0181 901 5555 Fax: 01923 217455

Dr Colin Johnston MA MB BCh MD FRCP
- NHS POST: Consultant Physician & Endocrinologist, St. Albans & Hemel Hempstead NHS Trust
- SPECIAL INTEREST: All aspects of medicine and endocrinology including diabetes, thyroid disease and impotence.
- PRIVATE: Hemel Hempstead General Hospital Hillfield Road, Hemel Hempstead, Herts, HP2 4AD. Tel: 01582 460 129

Dr Alfa Sa' adu BSc MSc PhD MBBS MRCP DTM & H
- NHS POST: Consultant Physician Watford General Hospital
- PRIVATE: BUPA Hospital Bushey, Heathbourne Rd, Bushey, Watford, Hertfordshire WD2 1RD. Tel: 0181 950 8550/01923 217 741 Fax: 0181 444 0919

Kent

Dr D S Jonathan Maw MB FRCP
YEAR QUALIFIED: 1962
NHS POST: Consultant Physician
SPECIAL INTEREST: Wide experience in acute general medicine, diabetes and endocrinology, including out-patient & inpatient investigation and management. Senior examiner for insurance companies. Expert medical reports for medico-legal purposes.
PRIVATE: 53 Madeira Park, Tunbridge Wells, Kent TN2 5SY.
Tel: 01892 534815 Fax: 01892 534815
Chelsfield Park Hospital, Bucks Cross Road, Chelsfield, Kent, BR6 7RG.
Tel: 01689 877855 Fax: 01689 827544

Dr Christopher F P Wharton MA DM FRCP
NHS POST: Consultant Physician, Bromley Acute Trust Farnborough Hospital, Farnborough, Kent BR6 8ND
SPECIAL INTEREST: Cardiology, especially hypertension and coronary disease; heart failure.
PRIVATE: Chelsfield Park Hospital, Bucks Cross Road, Chelsfield, Kent, BR6 7RG.
Tel: 01689 877 855
BMI Sloane Hospital, 125 Albermarle Road, Beckenham, Kent, BR3 2HS.
Tel: 0181 466 6911

London

Dr Ralph Abraham MA PhD BM BCh MRCP
YEAR QUALIFIED: 1971
SPECIAL INTEREST: Diabetes; endocrinology; lipid disorders; obesity; hypertension; impotence.
PRIVATE: The London Diabetes & Lipid Centre, 14 Wimpole Street, London W1M 7AB.
Tel: 0171 636 9901 Fax: 0171 636 9902

Dr Laurence R I Baker MA MD FRCP FRCPE
YEAR QUALIFIED: 1963
NHS POST: Consultant Physician and Nephrologist, St. Bartholomew's Hospital / Royal London Hospital, London.
SPECIAL INTEREST: Nephrology
PRIVATE: The London Clinic, 20 Devonshire Place, London, W1N 2DH.
Tel: 0171 224 5234 Fax: 0171 486 8706

Professor Paul J Ciclitira MD PhD FRCP
NHS POST: Professor of Gastroenterology, St. Thomas' Hospital, Guy's & St. Thomas' NHS Trust.
SPECIAL INTEREST: Coeliac disease/malabsorption; gastroenterology; general internal medicine.
PRIVATE: Albert Embankment Consulting Rooms, St. Thomas' Hospital, Lambeth Palace Road, London, SE1 7EH. Tel: 071 928 5485-ap 071 928 9292 xt 2354-sec. Fax: 0171 620 2597

General Medicine. London

Dr Simon L Cohen MB FRCP
- NHS POST: Consultant Physician, University College London Hospitals, including Middlesex & the St Peter's Group of Hospitals.
- SPECIAL INTEREST: General medicine; nephrology; intensive care; hypertension; medical ethics.
- PRIVATE: Private Consulting Room, University College Hospital, Gower Street, London, WC1E 6BD. Tel: 0171 388 3894 Fax: 0171 380 9816

Dr Desmond N Croft MA DM FRCP
- NHS POST: Consultant Physician, St. Thomas' Hospital.
- SPECIAL INTEREST: Thyroid disease.
- PRIVATE: York House Consulting Rooms, 199 Westminster Bridge Road, London SE1 7UT. Tel: 0171 928 5485 Fax: 0171 928 3748

Dr P Bruce S Fowler DM FRCP
- NHS POST: Honorary Reader and Honorary Consultant, Charing Cross Hospital.
- SPECIAL INTEREST: Impaired thyroid function; treatable cause of coronary artery disease in women. (Last Article Nov/Dec. JRCP 1996).
- PRIVATE: 152 Harley Street, London W1N 1HH. Tel: 0171 935 8868 Fax: 0171 224 2574

Dr Stewart Goodwin MB BChir MD FRCPath FRCPA
- YEAR QUALIFIED: 1958
- SPECIAL INTEREST: Chronic fatigue syndrome (myalgic encephalo-myelitis); diet treatment that relieves 60% of symptoms in 60% of patients within 8 weeks, while recognising other aetiological factors.
- PRIVATE: P O Box 13683, Wimbledon, London SW19 7ZL. Tel: 0410 416430 Fax: 0181 879 1611

Dr Barry I Hoffbrand MA DM FRCP
- YEAR QUALIFIED: 1958
- NHS POST: Consultant Physician and Nephrologist, Whittington Hospital (Retired).
- SPECIAL INTEREST: Nephrology; hypertension; cerebrovascular disease.
- PRIVATE: Highgate Private Hospital, 17-19 View Road, Highgate, London N6 4DJ. Tel: 0181 341 4182 Fax: 0181 342 8347 Secretary & Appointments: 0181 348 6990 Fax: 0181 340 1376
  Wellington Hospital South, Wellington Place, London NW8 9LE. Tel: 0171 586 3213 Fax: 0171 483 0297

Dr Rodwin Jackson FCP(SA) MD FRCP
- NHS POST: Consultant Physician, Chase Farm Hospital.
- SPECIAL INTEREST: Diabetes and endocrinology.
- PRIVATE: Hospital of St. John & St. Elizabeth, 60 Grove End Road, St John's Wood, London, NW8 9NH. Tel: 0171 286 5126
  Garden Hospital, 46-50 Sunny Gardens Road, Hendon, London, NW4 1RX. Tel: 0181 203 6832

General Medicine. London

Dr John P D Keet MBBS MRCP
- YEAR QUALIFIED: 1968
- NHS POST: Consultant Physician since 1977, Mayday University Hospital, Croydon, CR7 7YE. Tel: 0181 401 3618. Fax: 0181 401 3620.
- SPECIAL INTEREST: Cognitive disorders; memory clinics; neurology; cardiology; nutrition medicine, primary prevention and rehabilitation in older people. General geriatrics and general medicine in older people. Medico-legal work. Telemedicine.
- PRIVATE: Cromwell Hospital, Cromwell Road, London SW5 OTU. Tel: 0171 460 2000. 0171 486 2729. 0171 486 9259 Fax: 0171 460 5555. 0171 486 9259 Mobile: 0956 855 157. 0410 306 065(GSM). Web site:www.medicalnet.co.uk/Dr_John_Keet

Dr Geoffrey K Knowles MD FRCP
- YEAR QUALIFIED: 1970
- NHS POST: Consultant Physician, Kingston Hospital.
- SPECIAL INTEREST: All aspects of respiratory medicine including asthma, allergy, infections and cancer.
- PRIVATE: Parkside Hospital, 53 Parkside, Wimbledon, London, SW19 5NX. Tel: 0181 946 4202 Fax: 0181 946 7775

Dr Felix I D Konotey-Ahulu MD(Lond) FRCP(Lond) DTMH(L'Pool)
- YEAR QUALIFIED: 1959
- SPECIAL INTEREST: Tropical medicine and haemoglobinopathy.
- PRIVATE: Consulting Rooms, 10 Harley Street, London, W1N 1AA. Tel: 0171 467 8300 Fax: 0171 467 8312
  Cromwell Hospital, Cromwell Road, London SW5 OTU. Tel: 0171 460 2000 Fax: 0171 460 5601

Professor James Malone-Lee MD, FRCP
- YEAR QUALIFIED: 1974
- NHS POST: Consultant Physician, St. Pancras Hospital.
- SPECIAL INTEREST: Urodynamics and incontinence.
- PRIVATE: St. Pancras Hospital, 4 St. Pancras Way, London, NW1 OPE. Tel: 0171 530 3320 Fax: 0171 388 4364 E-mail: james.malone-lee@ucl.ac.uk

Dr Milton B Maltz MBBS MPhil(Cardiology)
- YEAR QUALIFIED: 1980
- NHS POST: Clinical Assistant Cardiology Whipps Cross Hospital And Royal Free Hospital
- SPECIAL INTEREST: Exercise test in patients with arrhythmias and coronary artery disease
- PRIVATE: Medical Centre for Cardiac Research Ltd, 48 Harley Street, London W1N 1AD. Tel: 0171 580 3145 Fax: 0171 323 3484

Dr Frank Marsh MA FRCP MB B Chir
- YEAR QUALIFIED: 1960
- NHS POST: Consultant Physician & Nephrologist, Royal London Hospital, Whitechapel, London E1 1BB. Tel: 0171 377 7367 / 0181 460 6295, Fax: 0171 377 7003 / 0181 460 6295.
- SPECIAL INTEREST: Hypertension; renal failure; urinary infections; nephritis.
- PRIVATE: London Independent Hospital, 1 Beaumont Square, Stepney Green, London E1 4NL. Tel: 0171 790 0990 Fax: 0171 265 9032

General Medicine. London

Dr Alfa Sa' adu BSc MSc PhD MBBS MRCP DTM & H
- NHS POST: Consultant Physician Watford General Hospital
- SPECIAL INTEREST:
- PRIVATE: Private Consulting Rooms, University College Hospital, 25 Grafton Way, London, WC1E 6DB. Tel: 0171 380 9311 Fax: 0171 380 9331

Professor Anthony W Segal MB ChB MD FRCP PhD DSc FRS
- NHS POST: Consultant Physician UCH / Middlesex Hospitals
- SPECIAL INTEREST: General medicine; immunology; post viral fatigue.
- PRIVATE: University College Hospital, 5 University Street, London WC1E 6JJ.
  Tel: 0171 209 6175 Fax: 0171 209 6211

Professor Stephen J G Semple MD FRCP
- SPECIAL INTEREST: General medicine; respiratory (thoracic) medicine.
- PRIVATE: Cromwell Hospital, Cromwell Road, London SW5 OTU.
  Tel: 0171 460 5700 Fax: 0171 460 5555
  The Middlesex Hospital Woolavington Wing, Mortimer Street, London W1N 8AA.
  Tel: 0171 504 9443 Fax: 0171 380 9117

Dr Edmund Peter Shephard BA MA(Oxon) MB BS MRCP MD
- YEAR QUALIFIED: 1970
- SPECIAL INTEREST: Diabetes thyroid; hypertension; diagnostic problems.
- PRIVATE: 80 Harley Street, London W1N 1AE.
  Tel: 0171 637 4962 Fax: 0171 637 4963

Dr Vera E Sutton MB ChB
- YEAR QUALIFIED: 1957
- NHS POST: Honorary Consultant Friern Hospital
- SPECIAL INTEREST: Psychiatry
- PRIVATE: 40 Holne Chase, Hampstead Garden Suburb, London N2 0QQ.
  Tel: 0181 455 0825 Fax: 0181 458 7188

Professor John Vallance-Owen MA MD FRCP FRCPI FRCPath FHKCP
- SPECIAL INTEREST: General (internal) medicine; diabetes; endocrinology.
- PRIVATE: London Independent Hospital, 1 Beaumont Square, Stepney Green, London E1 4NL.
  Tel: 0171 790 0990 Fax: 0171 265 9032

Dr Richard W E Watts MD DSc PhD FRCP
- NHS POST: Honorary Consultant Physician Hammersmith Hospital
- SPECIAL INTEREST: Endocrinology; metabolism; diabetes; renal medicine; general medicine.
- PRIVATE: Harley Street Clinic, 35 Weymouth Street, London, W1N 4BJ.
  Tel: 0171 935 7700, Appointments: 0171 586 5959 ext 2572
  Wellington Hospital,, Wellington Place, St John's Wood, London NW8 9LE.
  Tel: 0171 586 5959 xt 2572 Fax: 0171 483 0297 Aircall- 01459 126538.
  Highgate Private Clinic, 17-19 View Road, Highgate, London, N6.
  Tel: Appts.-0171 586 5959 xt 2572. 0181 341 4182 Fax: 0181 342 8347 Aircall- 01459 126538
  Sainsbury Wing, Hammersmith Hospital, Du Cane Road, London, W12 OHS.
  Tel: 0171 586 5959 ext.2572. Fax: 0171 483 0297
  E-mail: info@wellingtonchc.demon.co.uk

Middlesex

Dr Michael R Clements MD FRCP
- YEAR QUALIFIED: 1976
- NHS POST: Consultant Physician & Endocrinologist, Watford General Hospital.
- SPECIAL INTEREST: Endocrinology and metabolism including diabetes; thyroid; pituitary and adrenal disease; lipids; reproductive endocrinology and metabolic bone disease; osteoporosis and HRT.
- PRIVATE: Bishops Wood Hospital, Rickmansworth Road, Northwood, Middlesex HA6 2JW.
Tel: 01923 835 814 Fax: 01923 217455

North Wales

Dr Neville Hodges MD FRCP(London)
- YEAR QUALIFIED: 1964
- NHS POST: Consultant Physician, Northwest Wales NHS Trust; Ysbyty Gwynedd, Wales.
- SPECIAL INTEREST: All general internal medicine including respiratory and cardiovascular problems; somatization disorders and health screening. Particular interests also in asthma, obstructive sleep disorders and occupational lung disease.
- PRIVATE: The White House, Treborth Road, Bangor, North Wales LL57 2RJ.
Tel: 01248 355394, 384327 Fax: 01248 355394, 385093
E-mail: Sharon.Robinson@gwynh-tr.wales.nhs.uk

South Yorkshire

Dr John Leyshon Maddocks MD(Lond) FRCP(Lond)
- YEAR QUALIFIED: 1964
- SPECIAL INTEREST: Immunological disease; asthma; therapeutics; adverse drug reactions; drug errors; exposure to toxic substances.
- PRIVATE: Somersby, 3 Endcliffe Grove Avenue, Sheffield, South Yorkshire S10 3EJ.
Tel: 0114 266 7201 Fax: 0114 267 1210

Surrey

Dr Catherine Gleeson MBBS MRCGP
- YEAR QUALIFIED: 1985
- NHS POST: Honorary Consultant in Palliative Medicine, Surrey & Sussex NHS Trust, Mid Sussex Trust; St. Catherine's Hospice, West Sussex.
- SPECIAL INTEREST: Palliative medicine.
- PRIVATE: Gatwick Park Hospital, Povey Cross Road, Horley, Surrey RH6 0BB.
Tel: 01293 547333

General Medicine. Surrey

Dr Ronald K Knight MA MB BChir FRCP
YEAR QUALIFIED: 1970
NHS POST: Consultant in General and Respiratory Medicine, Frimley Park Hospital.
SPECIAL INTEREST: Adolescent asthma; cystic fibrosis - running one of the largest clinic in the country. I provide a desensitisation service for bee/wasp venom anaphylaxis and hay fever.
PRIVATE: Frimley Park Hospital, Portsmouth Road, Frimley, Camberley, Surrey GU16 5UJ.
Tel: 01276 604 122 Fax: 01276 604 148

Dr Geoffrey K Knowles MD FRCP
YEAR QUALIFIED: 1970
NHS POST: Consultant Physician, Kingston Hospital.
SPECIAL INTEREST: All aspects of respiratory medicine including asthma, allergy, infections and cancer.
PRIVATE: Coombe Wing, Kingston Hospital, Galsworthy Road, Kingston Upon Thames, Surrey, KT2 7QB. Tel: 0181 546 6677 Fax: 0181 541 5613
New Victoria Hospital, 184 Coombe Lane West, Kingston Upon Thames, Surrey, KT2 7EG. Tel: 0181 949 9000 Fax: 0181 949 9099

West Midlands

Dr Thomas Charles Dann MA MD MB BChir
YEAR QUALIFIED: 1957
SPECIAL INTEREST: ME (Chronic Fatigue Syndrome), aviation medicine.
PRIVATE: 37 Balsall Street East, Balsall Common, West Midlands CV7 7FQ.
Tel: 01676 532784

West Sussex

Dr Catherine Gleeson MBBS MRCGP
YEAR QUALIFIED: 1985
NHS POST: Honorary Consultant in Palliative Medicine, Surrey & Sussex NHS Trust, Mid Sussex Trust; St. Catherine's Hospice, West Sussex.
SPECIAL INTEREST: Palliative medicine.
PRIVATE: Ashdown Hospital, Burrell Road, Haywards Heath, West Sussex RH16 1UD.
Tel: 01293 547333

Dr Keith R Hine BSc MD FRCP
YEAR QUALIFIED: 1973
NHS POST: Consultant Physician, Princess Royal Hospital.
SPECIAL INTEREST: Gastroenterology
PRIVATE: Ashdown Nuffield Hospital, Burrell Road, Haywards Heath, West Sussex RH16 1UD.
Tel: 01444 456999 Fax: 01444 454 111; Secretary: 01273 843370

Genito-urinary Medicine

Berkshire

Dr Alan Tang MB BS(London) FRCP DipGUM DFFP
YEAR QUALIFIED: 1983
NHS POST: Consultant Physician in Genitourinary Medicine Royal Berkshire Hospital. Tel: 0118 987 7205.
SPECIAL INTEREST: Genital infections; penile dermatoses; hyfrecation; cryosurgery. HIV testing and treatment; erectile dysfunction; acupuncture.
PRIVATE: Berkshire Independent Hospital, Wensley Road, Coley Park, Reading, Berkshire RG1 6UZ. Tel: 0118 956 0056 (Mrs. Chris Toms) Fax: 0118 956 6333

Buckinghamshire

Dr Graz Luzzi BM BCh MA DM FRCP
NHS POST: Consultant in Genito-urinary Medicine, Wycombe General Hospital.
SPECIAL INTEREST: Genito-urinary infections; genital skin conditions; prostatitis; genital pain syndromes; HIV infection and testing.
PRIVATE: The Chiltern Hospital, London Road, Great Missenden, Buckinghamshire HP16 0EN. Tel: 01494 890 890 Fax: 01494 890 250
Wycombe General Hospital, High Wycombe, Buckinghamshire HP11 2TT. Tel: 01494 425 079 Fax: 01494 425 661

Derbyshire

Dr Dermot Murray T D MB ChB MRCP DipVen DFFP
YEAR QUALIFIED: 1962
SPECIAL INTEREST: Relapsing non specific urethritis; gulf war syndrome.
PRIVATE: Quarndon Medical Services, 10 Old Vicarage Lane, Quarndon, Derbyshire DE22 5B. Tel: 01332 553238
Military Medicine, Quarndon Medical Services, 10 Old Vicarage Lane, Quarndon, Derbyshire DE22 5B. Tel: 01332 553238

London

Dr Simon Barton BSc MBBS MD MRCOG
YEAR QUALIFIED: 1982
NHS POST: Consultant Physician and Clinical Director in Genitourinary Medicine, Chelsea & Westminster Hospital.
SPECIAL INTEREST: Genital infections in men and women; vulval conditions in women; HIV/AIDS testing and treatment.
PRIVATE: Lister Hospital, Chelsea Bridge Road, London, SW1W 8RH. Tel: 0171 730 8298 or 0181 846 6184 (sec) Fax: 0181 746 5611

Genito-urinary Medicine. London

Dr David A Hawkins BSc FRCP
- NHS POST: Consultant Physician in Genitourinary Medicine, Chelsea & Westminster Hospital.
- SPECIAL INTEREST: HIV testing and management; general genito-urinary medicine.
- PRIVATE: Cromwell Hospital, Cromwell Road, London SW5 OTU.
  Tel: Appointments: 0171 460 5700 Fax: 0181 846 6198; Enq/Secretary: 0181 846 6158

Dr Frederick Lim MBBS MRCP
- YEAR QUALIFIED: 1971
- SPECIAL INTEREST: Urinary tract infections; medical gynaecological infections including ureaplasma vaginitis; infections due to herpes and wart viruses; psycho-sexual counselling; male infertility.
- PRIVATE: Flat 6, 26 Devonshire Place, London, W1.
  Tel: 0171 487 3529 Fax: 0171 224 1784

Geriatrics

Enfield Middlesex

Dr Rodwin Jackson FCP(SA) MD FRCP
- NHS POST: Consultant Physician, Chase Farm Hospital.
- SPECIAL INTEREST: Diabetes and endocrinology.
- PRIVATE: Kings Oak Hospital, Chase Farm (North side), The Ridgeway, Enfield, Middlesex EN2 8SD. Tel: 0181 364 5520
North London Nuffield Hospital, Cavell Drive, Uplands Park Road, Enfield, EN2 7PR. Tel: 0181 366 2122

Hertfordshire

Dr Alfa Sa' adu BSc MSc PhD MBBS MRCP DTM & H
- NHS POST: Consultant Physician Watford General Hospital
- PRIVATE: BUPA Hospital Bushey, Heathbourne Rd, Bushey, Watford, Hertfordshire WD2 1RD. Tel: 0181 950 8550/01923 217 741 Fax: 0181 444 0919

London

Dr John Croker MA BM BCh FRCP
- YEAR QUALIFIED: 1970
- NHS POST: Consultant, Middlesex Hospital.
- SPECIAL INTEREST: Geriatrics; general medicine; gastroenterology.
- PRIVATE: 152 Harley Street, London W1N 1HH. Tel: 0171 935 8868 Fax: 0171 224 2574

Dr Rodwin Jackson FCP(SA) MD FRCP
- NHS POST: Consultant Physician, Chase Farm Hospital.
- SPECIAL INTEREST: Diabetes and endocrinology.
- PRIVATE: Hospital of St. John & St. Elizabeth, 60 Grove End Road, St Johns Wood, London, NW8 9NH. Tel: 0171 286 5126
The Garden Hospital, 46-50 Sunny Gardens Road, Hendon, London, NW4 1RX. Tel: 0181 203 6832

Dr John P D Keet MBBS MRCP
- YEAR QUALIFIED: 1968
- NHS POST: Consultant Physician since 1977, Mayday University Hospital, Croydon, CR7 7YE. Tel: 0181 401 3618. Fax: 0181 401 3620.
- SPECIAL INTEREST: Cognitive disorders; memory clinics; neurology; cardiology; nutrition medicine, primary prevention and rehabilitation in older people. General geriatrics and general medicine in older people. Medico-legal work. Telemedicine.
- PRIVATE: Private Consulting Rooms, 9 Upper Wimpole Street, London W1M 7TD. Tel: 0171 486 2729. 0171 486 9259 Fax: 0171 486 9259. Mobile: 0956 855 157. 0410 306 065 (GSM). Web site:www.medicalnet.co.uk/Dr_John_Keet

Geriatrics. London

Professor James Malone-Lee MD, FRCP
- YEAR QUALIFIED: 1974
- NHS POST: Consultant Physician, St. Pancras Hospital.
- SPECIAL INTEREST: Urodynamics and incontinence.
- PRIVATE: St. Pancras Hospital, 4 St. Pancras Way, London, NW1 0PE.
  Tel: 0171 530 3320 Fax: 0171 388 4364 E-mail: james.malone-lee@ucl.ac.uk

Surrey

Dr John P D Keet MBBS MRCP
- YEAR QUALIFIED: 1968
- NHS POST: Consultant Physician since 1977, Mayday University Hospital, Croydon, CR7 7YE.
  Tel: 0181 401 3618. Fax: 0181 401 3620.
- SPECIAL INTEREST: Cognitive disorders; memory clinics; neurology; cardiology; nutrition medicine, primary prevention and rehabilitation in older people. General geriatrics and general medicine in older people. Medico-legal work. Telemedicine.
- PRIVATE: Shirley Oaks Hospital, Poppy Lane, Shirley Oaks Village, Surrey, CR9 8AB.
  Tel: 0171 486 2729. 0171 486 9259 Fax: 0171 486 9259. Mobile: 0956 855 157. 0410 306 065(GSM). Web site:www.medicalnet.co.uk/Dr_John_Keet

Haematology

Berkshire

Dr Peter H Mackie MA BM FRCP FRCPath
NHS POST: Heatherwood & Wexham Park Hospitals Trust
SPECIAL INTEREST: Haematology
PRIVATE: HRH Princess Christian's Hospital, 12 Clarence Road, Windsor, Berkshire SL4 5AG.

Hampshire

Dr Alastair Gordon Smith BSc MBChB FRCP(Lond and Glas) FRCPath
YEAR QUALIFIED: 1974
NHS POST: Consultant Haematologist, Southampton University Hospitals NHS Trust.
SPECIAL INTEREST: Multiple myeloma; haematological oncology; iron deficiency anaemias and general haematology.
PRIVATE: BUPA Chalybeate Hospital, Chalybeate Close, Tremona Road, Southampton, Hampshire SO16 6UY.
Tel: 01703 825335 Fax: 01703 825338 E-mail: agsmith@tcp.co.uk

Hertfordshire

Dr Simon Ardeman MA BM PhD FRCPath
SPECIAL INTEREST: Coagulation; general haematology; haematological oncology.
PRIVATE: BUPA Hospital Bushey, Heathbourne Rd, Bushey, Watford, Hertfordshire WD2 1RD.
Tel: 0181 950 9090 Fax: 0181 950 7556

London

Dr Simon Ardeman MA BM PhD FRCPath
SPECIAL INTEREST: Coagulation; general haematology; haematological oncology.
PRIVATE: The Garden Hospital, 46-50 Sunny Gardens Road, Hendon, London, NW4 1RX.
Tel: 0181 203 0111

Dr Peter J Gravett MB BS MRCS FRCPath
SPECIAL INTEREST: Haematology, Oncology, Bone Marrow & Stem Cell Transplantation
PRIVATE: The London Clinic, 20 Devonshire Place, London, W1N 2DH.
Tel: 0171 935 4444 xt 3159 Fax: 0171 486 3782

Haematology. London

Dr Ian Hann MD FRCP FRCP(Glas) FRCPath
- NHS POST: Consultant Paediatric Haematologist, Great Ormond Street Childrens Hospital
- SPECIAL INTEREST: Paediatric haematology and oncology; childhood leukaemia and lymphoma; childhood blood and bleeding disorders; haemophilia.
- PRIVATE: Great Ormond Street Hospital for Children NHS Trust, Great Ormond Street, London WC1N 3JH.
  Tel: 0171 829 8831 Fax: 0171 813 8410 E-mail: Ian.Hann@gosh-tr.nthames.nhs.uk

Professor A Victor Hoffbrand MA DM FRCP FRCPath DSc
- YEAR QUALIFIED: 1959
- NHS POST: Honorary Consultant Haematologist, Royal Free Hospital.
- SPECIAL INTEREST: Anaemia; leukemia; lymphoma; myeloma; platelet disorders; general haematology.
- PRIVATE: Royal Free Hospital, Pond Street, Hampstead, London, NW3 2QG.
  Tel: 0171 435 1547 Fax: 0171 431 4537 E-mail: hoffbran@rfhsm.ac.uk

Professor H Grant Prentice MBBS(Lond) FRCP FRCPath
- YEAR QUALIFIED: 1968
- NHS POST: Professor of Haematological Oncology, Head of Haematology Dept, Director of bone marrow transplant programme. Royal Free and University College Medical School. Royal Free campus.
- SPECIAL INTEREST: Treatment of acute and chronic leukemias and other haematological malignancies by chemotherapy. Bone marrow and peripheral blood stem cell autologous and allogeneic transplantation for haematological malignancies, selected solid tumours and autoimmune diseases. General haematology.
- PRIVATE: Lyndhurst Rooms, Royal Free Hospital, Pond Street, Hampstead, London, NW3 2QG.
  Tel: 0171 830 2300 - appointments Fax: 0171 794 0645 - appointments

Merseyside

Dr Terence John Deeble MB ChB FRCPath
- YEAR QUALIFIED: 1964
- NHS POST: Consultant Haematologist, Arrowe Park Hospital.
- SPECIAL INTEREST: Haemato-oncology i.e. the treatment of the leukaemias and lymphomas and related disorders.
- PRIVATE: BUPA Murrayfield Hospital, Holmwood Drive, Thingwall, Wirral, Merseyside L61 1AU.
  Tel: 0151 929 5229 Fax: 0151 648 7000
  Park Suite, Arrowe Park Hospital, Upton, Wirral, Merseyside L49 5PE.
  Tel: 0151 678 5111 ext 2149

Oxfordshire

Dr T J Littlewood MBBCh FRCP FRCPath MD
- YEAR QUALIFIED: 1978
- NHS POST: Consultant Haematologist, John Radcliffe Hospital, Oxford.
- SPECIAL INTEREST: Haematological malignancy including lymphoma, leukaemia and myeloma; bone marrow transplantation; investigation of anaemia.
- PRIVATE: Department of Haematology, John Radcliffe Hospital, Oxford, Oxfordshire OX3 9DU.
  Tel: 01865 220364/220331 Fax: 01865 221778
  E-mail: tim.littlewood@mailgate.jr2.ox.ac.uk

Surrey

Dr Lydia Jones BSc MBBS FRCP FRCPath
 YEAR QUALIFIED: 1980
 NHS POST: Consultant Haematologist, Epsom General Hospital.
 SPECIAL INTEREST: Haematological malignancies.
 PRIVATE: Ashtead Hospital, The Warren, Ashtead, Surrey KT21 2SB.
 Tel: 01372 276 161/275 161-secretary Fax: 01372 277 494
 Epsom General Hospital (Trust), Dorking Road, Epsom, Surrey, KT18 7EG.
 Tel: 01372 735 144/735 735 xt 6096 Fax: 01372 748 802

Dr Jennifer Treleaven MD FRCP FRCPath
 NHS POST: Consultant Haematologist Royal Marsden Hospital
 SPECIAL INTEREST: Leukaemia treatment bone marrow transplantation; blood transfusion.
 PRIVATE: Royal Marsden Hospital, Downs Road, Sutton, Surrey, SM2 5PT.
 Tel: 0181 642 6011 Fax: 0181 643 7958

West Sussex

Dr Antoine Roques FRCP FRCPath
 NHS POST: Consultant Clinical Haematologist Worthing Hospital
 SPECIAL INTEREST: Lymphoproliferative disorders.
 PRIVATE: Goring Hall Hospital, Bodiam Avenue, Goring-By-Sea, West Sussex BN12 4UX.

Hypertension

East Sussex

Dr John C Kingswood FRCP
- NHS POST: Consultant Physician, Royal Sussex County Hospital.
- SPECIAL INTEREST: Nephrology & Hypertension
- PRIVATE: Sussex Diagnostic Centre, 13 New Church Road, Hove, East Sussex BN3 4AA.
  Tel: 01273 770044 Fax: 01273 726931

Infectious & Tropical Diseases

Leicestershire

Dr Martin Wiselka BM BCh MA MD PhD MRCP
- YEAR QUALIFIED: 1982
- NHS POST: Consultant in Infectious Diseases and General Medicine, Leicester Royal Infirmary.
- SPECIAL INTEREST: General medicine and all aspects of infectious diseases and tropical medicine including travel medicine and HIV / Hepatitis B and C.
- PRIVATE: BUPA Hospital, Gartree Road, Oadby, Leicester, Leicestershire LE2 2FF.
Tel: 0116 272 0888 Fax: 0116 272 0666 E-mail: mwiselka@lri.org.uk

London

Dr Robert N Davidson MD FRCP DTMH
- YEAR QUALIFIED: 1979
- NHS POST: Consultant in Infectious/Tropical Diseases, Northwick Park Hospital.
- SPECIAL INTEREST: Travel associated and parasitic infections; HIV related diseases; bacterial and viral infections; tuberculosis.
- PRIVATE: Charles Kingsley Suite, Northwick Park Hospital, Watford Road, Harrow, Middlesex, HA1 3UJ. Tel: 0181 869 2833, 869 2830 Fax: 0181 869 2836
E-mail: r.n.davidson@ic.ac.uk

Dr Stewart Goodwin MB BChir MD FRCPath FRCPA
- YEAR QUALIFIED: 1958
- SPECIAL INTEREST: Chronic fatigue syndrome (myalgic encephalo-myelitis); diet treatment that relieves 60% of symptoms in 60% of patients within 8 weeks, while recognising other aetiological factors.
- PRIVATE: P O Box 13683, Wimbledon, London SW19 7ZL.
Tel: 0410 416430 Fax: 0181 879 1611

Dr Felix I D Konotey-Ahulu MD(Lond) FRCP(Lond) DTMH(L'Pool)
- YEAR QUALIFIED: 1959
- SPECIAL INTEREST: Tropical medicine and haemoglobinopathy.
- PRIVATE: Cromwell Hospital, Cromwell Road, London SW5 OTU.
Tel: 0171 460 2000 Fax: 0171 460 5601
Consulting Rooms, 10 Harley Street, London W1N 1AA.
Tel: 0171 467 8300 Fax: 0171 460 5601

Infectious & Tropical Diseases. London

Dr Vas Novelli MBBS FRCP FRACP FRCPCH
- YEAR QUALIFIED: 1974
- NHS POST: Consultant in Paediatric Infectious Diseases Great Ormond Street Hospital for Children NHS Trust
- SPECIAL INTEREST: Infectious Diseases and HIV
- PRIVATE: Great Ormond Street Hospital for Children NHS Trust, Great Ormond Street, London WC1N 3JH. Tel: 0171 405 9200 ext 5946 Fax: 0171 813 8266
  E-mail: vnovelli@compuserve.com

Dr Stephen G Wright MB BS FRCP DCMT
- NHS POST: Consultant Physician Hospital for Tropical Diseases
- SPECIAL INTEREST: Infection: Parasitic diseases; Brucellosis: Gut diseases.
- PRIVATE: Private Patients Wing, University College Hospital, 25 Grafton Way, London, WC1E 6DB. Tel: 0171 387 8323 Fax: 0171 380 9816

Lipidology

Hertfordshire

Dr Michael R Clements MD FRCP
- YEAR QUALIFIED: 1976
- NHS POST: Consultant Physician & Endocrinologist, Watford General Hospital.
- SPECIAL INTEREST: Endocrinology and metabolism including diabetes; thyroid; pituitary and adrenal disease; lipids; reproductive endocrinology and metabolic bone disease; osteoporosis and HRT.
- PRIVATE: BUPA Hospital Bushey, Heathbourne Rd, Bushey, Watford, Hertfordshire WD2 1RD. Tel: 0181 901 5555 Fax: 01923 217455

London

Dr Ralph Abraham MA PhD BM BCh MRCP
- YEAR QUALIFIED: 1971
- SPECIAL INTEREST: Diabetes; endocrinology; lipid disorders; obesity; hypertension; impotence.
- PRIVATE: The London Diabetes & Lipid Centre, 14 Wimpole Street, London W1M 7AB. Tel: 0171 636 9901 Fax: 0171 636 9902

Dr Mary Seed BM BCh MA DM FRCPath
- NHS POST: Honorary Consultant / Senior Lecturer, Charing Cross Hospital, London W6 8RF
- SPECIAL INTEREST: Hyperlipidaemia - management; genetic hyperlipidaemia -(familial hypercholesterolaemia); use of HRT in reduction of cardiovascular risk and for patients with cardiovascular disease.
- PRIVATE: Charing Cross Hospital, Fulham Palace Road, London, W6 8RF. Tel: 0181 846 7901/7187 Fax: 0181 846 7999

Professor Gilbert Thompson MD FRCP
- YEAR QUALIFIED: 1956
- NHS POST: Honorary Consulting Physician Hammersmith Hospital.
- SPECIAL INTEREST: (1) Investigation and management of severe hyperlipidaemia, especially familial hypercholesterolaemia; (2) Prevention and treatment of atherosclerosis and vascular disease by lipid-lowering.
- PRIVATE: The Sainsbury Wing, Consulting Rooms, Hammersmith Hospital, Du Cane Road, London, W12 OHS. Tel /Fax: 0181 383 2322; Secretary 0181 383 3145

Dr Anthony Wierzbicki BA MA BMBCh DPhil
- NHS POST: Senior Lecturer / Consultant In Chemical Pathology St. Thomas' Hospital
- SPECIAL INTEREST: Lipids and cardiovascular disease prevention.
- PRIVATE: St. Thomas' Hospital, Lambeth Palace Road, London, SE1 7EH. Tel: 0171 928 9292 ext 1911 Fax: 0171 928 4226 E-mail: a.wierzbicki@umds.ac.uk

Middlesex

Dr Michael R Clements MD FRCP
- YEAR QUALIFIED: 1976
- NHS POST: Consultant Physician & Endocrinologist, Watford General Hospital.
- SPECIAL INTEREST: Endocrinology and metabolism including diabetes; thyroid; pituitary and adrenal disease; lipids; reproductive endocrinology and metabolic bone disease; osteoporosis and HRT.
- PRIVATE: Bishops Wood Hospital, Rickmansworth Road, Northwood, Middlesex HA6 2JW.
Tel: 01923 835 814 Fax: 01923 217455

West Sussex

Dr Mary Seed BM BCh MA DM FRCPath
- NHS POST: Honorary Consultant / Senior Lecturer, Charing Cross Hospital, London W6 8RF
- SPECIAL INTEREST: Hyperlipidaemia - management; genetic hyperlipidaemia -(familial hypercholesterolaemia); use of HRT in reduction of cardiovascular risk and for patients with cardiovascular disease.
- PRIVATE: Lipid Clinic, King Edward VII Hospital, Midhurst, West Sussex, GU29 0BL.
Tel: 01730 812 341

Medical Genetics

London

Professor Michael Patton MB MA MSc DCH FRCP FRCPCH
- YEAR QUALIFIED: 1974
- NHS POST: Consultant Clinical Geneticist, St. George's Hospital.
- SPECIAL INTEREST: Genetic diseases; counselling; congenital abnormalities.
- PRIVATE: Parkside Hospital, 53 Parkside, Wimbledon, London, SW19 5NX.
  Tel: 0181 946 4202 Fax: 0181 971 8002 E-mail: mpatton@sghms.ac.uk
  Portland Neurocare Ltd. (Child Neurology &, Neurodisability Services), 234 Great Portland Street, London W1N 5PH. Tel: 0171 390 8286 Fax: 0171 390 8287 E-mail: mpatton@sghms.ac.uk
  St. George's Hospital, Cranmer Terrace, London SW17 0RE.
  Tel: 0181 725 5335 (direct). 0181 725 2674 (appts.) Fax: 0181 725 3444
  E-mail: mpatton@sghms.ac.uk

Medico-Legal

Essex

Miss Janet Porter MB BChir FRCS FFAEM
YEAR QUALIFIED: 1971
NHS POST: Accident & Emergency Consultant, Southend Hospital.
SPECIAL INTEREST: Soft tissue injuries; shoulder and hand problems.
PRIVATE: 114 Woodside, Leigh-on-sea, Essex SS9 4RB.
Tel: 01702 421661 Fax: 01702 421661

London

Dr George Ikkos BSc LMSSA MRCPsych MInstGA
YEAR QUALIFIED: 1981
NHS POST: Consultant Psychiatrist, Barnet Healthcare Trust and Royal National Orthopaedic Hospital.
SPECIAL INTEREST: General psychiatry; stress secondary to injury and illness; psychiatric aspects of spinal injury; body image disorder; mental health of parents of abused children; interpersonal psychotherapy; Greek.
PRIVATE: Grovelands Priory Hospital, The Bourne, Southgate, London, N14 6RA.
Tel: 01426 917 231 Fax: 0181 444 1203
London Child & Family Consultation Service, 234 Great Portland Street, London W1N 5PH. Tel: 01426 917 231 Fax: 0181 444 1203

Assoc. Professor B Povlsen MD PhD
YEAR QUALIFIED: 1984
NHS POST: Consultant, Guy's and St Thomas' Hospital: St. Thomas' Hospital, Lambeth Palace Road, London SE1 7EH. Tel: 0171 928 9292. Guy's Hospital, St. Thomas Street, London SE1 9RT. Tel: 0171 955 5000.
SPECIAL INTEREST: Hand and upper limb.
PRIVATE: Churchill Clinic, 80 Lambeth Road, London, SE1 7PW.
Tel: 0171 620 1590 Fax: 0171 928 1702 E-mail: bo@povlsen.u-net.com

Mr Iynga Vanniasegaram MSc DLO FRCS(ENT)
NHS POST: Consultant Audiological Physician St. George's & Great Ormond Street Hospitals
SPECIAL INTEREST: Paediatric Audiology; Balance Disorders; Tinnitus Central Auditory Disorders; Noise Induced Hearing Loss (medico-legal). Glue Ear. Vertigo - Dizziness
PRIVATE: Depart. of Audiological Medicine, BMI Portland Hospital for Women & Children, 209 Great Portland Street, London, W1N 6AH.
Tel: 0171 390 8060 Fax: 0171 390 8053 E-mail: jx79@dial.pipex.com

Middlesex

Dr Stuart Blackie MB ChB BSc FRCPath
YEAR QUALIFIED: 1976
SPECIAL INTEREST: Mediation
PRIVATE: 28 Claremont Road, Teddington, Middlesex TW11 8DG.
Tel: 0181 977 1291 E-mail: RASBlackie@aol.com

Nottinghamshire

Mr S Ali FRCS DLO
YEAR QUALIFIED: 1972
NHS POST: Consultant ENT Surgeon, The King's Mill Centre.
SPECIAL INTEREST: Rhinology; paediatric ENT surgery and noise induced hearing loss.
PRIVATE: The Nottingham Nuffield Hospital, 748 Mansfield Road, Woodthorpe, Nottingham NG3 3FZ. Tel: 0115 920 9209 Fax: 0115 967 3005

South Yorkshire

Dr Christine I Harrington MB ChB(Hons) MD(Cam) FRCP(UK)
YEAR QUALIFIED: 1971
NHS POST: Consultant Dermatologist, Royal Hallmshire Hospital, Sheffield.
SPECIAL INTEREST: Vulval disease, skin and systemic disease, skin malignancy, eczema, psoriasis, acne, psycho-dermatology.
PRIVATE: Somersby, 3 Endcliffe Grove Avenue, Sheffield, South Yorkshire S10 3EJ.
Tel: 0114 266 7201 Fax: 0114 267 1210

Dr John Leyshon Maddocks MD(Lond) FRCP(Lond)
YEAR QUALIFIED: 1964
SPECIAL INTEREST: Immunological disease; asthma; therapeutics; adverse drug reactions; drug errors; exposure to toxic substances.
PRIVATE: Somersby, 3 Endcliffe Grove Avenue, Sheffield, South Yorkshire S10 3EJ.
Tel: 0114 266 7201 Fax: 0114 267 1210

West Yorkshire

Mr Keith Jepson MB FRCSE
YEAR QUALIFIED: 1965
NHS POST: Consultant Orthopaedic Surgeon, Royal Infirmary, Yorkshire.
SPECIAL INTEREST: Road traffic accidents.
PRIVATE: 1 Mornington Villas, Bradford, West Yorkshire BD9 7HB.
Tel: 01274 546861 Fax: 01274 487705

Metabolic Medicine

Cumbria

Dr Alan Taylor MA(Oxon) MB ChB FRCPath
YEAR QUALIFIED: 1977
NHS POST: Consultant Chemical Pathologist, Furness General Hospital.
SPECIAL INTEREST: Metabolic medicine; lipidology diabetes mellitus including impotence treatment; endocrinology investigations; health screening pre-employment.
PRIVATE: Pathology Directorate, Furness General Hospital, Dalton Lane, Barrow-in-Furness, Cumbria LA14 4LF.
Tel: 01229 491257, 01229 870870 ext 1257/4283 Fax: 01229 821098

Hertfordshire

Dr Michael R Clements MD FRCP
YEAR QUALIFIED: 1976
NHS POST: Consultant Physician & Endocrinologist, Watford General Hospital.
SPECIAL INTEREST: Endocrinology and metabolism including diabetes; thyroid; pituitary and adrenal disease; lipids; reproductive endocrinology and metabolic bone disease; osteoporosis and HRT.
PRIVATE: BUPA Hospital Bushey, Heathbourne Rd, Bushey, Watford, Hertfordshire WD2 1RD.
Tel: 0181 901 5555 Fax: 01923 217455

Kent

Dr Yvette I Lolin MD PhD FRCPath
YEAR QUALIFIED: 1978
NHS POST: Consultant in Chemical Pathology and Metabolic Medicine, Kent and Sussex Hospital.
SPECIAL INTEREST: Hyperlipidaemia, hyperhomocysteinaemia and other risk factors for coronary heart disease; lead poisoning; metabolic bone disease and/or hypercalcaemia; renal stones; endocrine disorders: particularly thyroid, pituitary and adrenal; fluid and electrolyte imbalance.
PRIVATE: Kent and Sussex Hospital, Mount Ephraim, Tunbridge Wells, Kent TN4 8AT.
Tel: 01892 526111 ext 2366 Fax: 01892 516698

Liverpool

Dr Eileen Manning MB BCh BAO MRCP MRCPath
YEAR QUALIFIED: 1982
NHS POST: Consultant Chemical Pathologist, Royal Liverpool and Broadgreen University Hospitals Trust.
SPECIAL INTEREST: Osteoporosis; Paget's disease; menopausal problems; disorders of calcium metabolism; hyperlipidaemia.
PRIVATE: Lourdes Hospital, 57 Greenbank Road, Liverpool, L18 1HQ.
Tel: 0151 706 4304 Fax: 0151 706 5813

London

Professor Carol Seymour MSc PhD FRCPath FRCP
- YEAR QUALIFIED: 1969
- NHS POST: Honorary Consultant Physician St. George's Hospital. Professor of Clinical Biochemistry & Metabolic Medicine, Division of Cardiological Sciences (Metabolic Medicine), St George's Hospital Medical School, Cranmer Terrace, Tooting London SW17 0RE.
- SPECIAL INTEREST: Metabolic Medicine: Lipid Disorders (acquired and genetic): Liver disease (Wilson's disease, haemochromatosis and other inborn errors).
- PRIVATE: Knightsbridge Wing, St. George's Hospital, Blackshaw Road, London, SW17 0QT. Tel: 0181 725 1407appts. 0181 725 1416consult

  Division of Cardiological Sciences (Metabolic Medicine), St. George's Hospital Medical School, Cranmer Terrace, Tooting, London, SW17 0RE.
  Tel: 0181 725 5926 Fax: 0181 725 2582 E-mail: cseymour@sghms.ac.uk
  Lansborough Wing, St. George's Hospital, Blackshaw Road, London, SW17 0QT.
  Tel: 0181 725 1407appts. 0181 725 1416cons.

Middlesex

Dr Michael R Clements MD FRCP
- YEAR QUALIFIED: 1976
- NHS POST: Consultant Physician & Endocrinologist, Watford General Hospital.
- SPECIAL INTEREST: Endocrinology and metabolism including diabetes; thyroid; pituitary and adrenal disease; lipids; reproductive endocrinology and metabolic bone disease; osteoporosis and HRT.
- PRIVATE: Bishops Wood Hospital, Rickmansworth Road, Northwood, Middlesex HA6 2JW.
  Tel: 01923 835 814 Fax: 01923 217455

Nephrology

East Sussex

Dr John C Kingswood FRCP
NHS POST: Consultant Physician, Royal Sussex County Hospital.
SPECIAL INTEREST: Nephrology & Hypertension
PRIVATE: Sussex Diagnostic Centre, 13 New Church Road, Hove, East Sussex BN3 4AA.
Tel: 01273 770044 / 724174 Fax: 01273 726931
Esperance House, Esperance Private Hospital, Esperance House, Hartington Place, Eastbourne BN21 3BG. Tel: 01323 410 717 Fax: 01323 730 313

Hertfordshire

Dr Andrew B D Palmer MBBS FRCP
NHS POST: Consultant Nephrologist St. Mary's Hospital
SPECIAL INTEREST: Nephrology; hypertension; renal failure.
PRIVATE: BUPA Hospital Bushey, Heathbourne Rd, Bushey, Watford, Hertfordshire WD2 1RD.
Tel: 0181 950 8550 Fax: 0181 421 8514

London

Dr Laurence R I Baker MA MD FRCP FRCPE
YEAR QUALIFIED: 1963
NHS POST: Consultant Physician and Nephrologist, St. Bartholomew's Hospital / Royal London Hospital, London.
SPECIAL INTEREST: Nephrology
PRIVATE: The London Clinic, 20 Devonshire Place, London, W1N 2DH.
Tel: 0171 224 5234 Fax: 0171 486 8706

Dr Edwina A Brown MA (Oxon) DM FRCP
YEAR QUALIFIED: 1973
NHS POST: Consultant Physician and Nephrologist, Charing Cross Hospital, London.
SPECIAL INTEREST: Hypertension; renal failure; all types of renal disease.
PRIVATE: Charing Cross Hospital, Fulham Palace Road, London, W6 8RF.
Tel: 0181 846 1754 Fax: 0181 846 7589

Dr Frank Marsh MA FRCP MB B Chir
YEAR QUALIFIED: 1960
NHS POST: Consultant Physician & Nephrologist, Royal London Hospital, Whitechapel, London E1 1BB. Tel: 0171 377 7367 / 0181 460 6295, Fax: 0171 377 7003 / 0181 460 6295.
SPECIAL INTEREST: Hypertension; renal failure; urinary infections; nephritis.
PRIVATE: London Independent Hospital, 1 Beaumont Square, Stepney Green, London E1 4NL.
Tel: 0171 790 0990 Fax: 0171 265 9032

Dr Andrew B D Palmer MBBS FRCP
NHS POST: Consultant Nephrologist St. Mary's Hospital
SPECIAL INTEREST: Nephrology; hypertension; renal failure.
PRIVATE: St. Mary's Hospital, Praed Street, Paddington, London, W2 1NY.
Tel: 0171 402 7784 Fax: 0171 402 7784

Middlesex

Dr Andrew B D Palmer MBBS FRCP
NHS POST: Consultant Nephrologist St. Mary's Hospital
SPECIAL INTEREST: Nephrology; hypertension; renal failure.
PRIVATE: The Clementine Churchill Hospital, Sudbury Hill, Harrow, Middlesex, HA1 3RX.
Tel: 0181 872 3939 Fax: 0181 872 3871

Neurology

Berkshire

Dr Ralph Peter Gregory FRCP
YEAR QUALIFIED: 1982
NHS POST: Consultant Neurologist, Royal Berkshire Hospital Reading/Radcliffe Infirmary Oxford.
SPECIAL INTEREST: General neurologist with particular interest in Parkinson's disease and other movement disorders; experience in various neurosurgical procedures for PD and botulinum toxin therapy.
PRIVATE: Berkshire Independent Hospital, Wensley Road, Coley Park, Reading, Berkshire RG1 6UZ. Tel: 0118 956 0056 Fax: 0118 956 6333

Dr Russell J M Lane BSc MD FRCP
YEAR QUALIFIED: 1973
NHS POST: Consultant Neurologist, Charing Cross & Ashford & St. Peter's Hospital.
SPECIAL INTEREST: Neuromuscular disorders; headache; epilepsy.
PRIVATE: The Princess Margaret Hospital, Osborne Road, Windsor, Berkshire SL4 3SJ. Tel: 01784 884617 Fax: 01784 884273 E-mail: r.lane@ic.ac.uk

Essex

Dr Margaret Barrie MB BS FRCP
NHS POST: Honorary Consultant Neurologist, The Royal London Hospitals.
SPECIAL INTEREST: Migraine; epilepsy; Parkinson's disease; Alzheimer's; multiple sclerosis; medicolegal cases.
PRIVATE: The London Independent Hospital, 21 Bourne Court, Southend Road, Woodford, Essex IG8 8HD. Tel: 0800 328 8057 Fax: 0181 551 5446 Private secretary (Mrs M J Austin) Tel/Fax: 01992 574167

Holly House Hospital, High Road, Buckhurst Hill, Essex, IG9 5HX. Tel: 0181 505 3311 Fax: 0181 506 1013 Private secretary (Mrs M J Austin) Tel/Fax: 01992 574167

Dr Giles Elrington MBBS(Hons) MD FRCP
YEAR QUALIFIED: 1980
NHS POST: Consultant Neurologist, Royal London Hospital, Colchester General Hospital.
SPECIAL INTEREST: Headache and migraine, rehabilitation, especially of multiple sclerosis, epilepsy, neurology/psychiatry interface.
PRIVATE: Oaks Hospital, Oaks Place, Colchester, Essex CO4 5XR. Tel: 01206 753206 Fax: 01206 753240

21 Bourne Court, Southend Road, Woodford Green, Essex IG8 8HD. Tel: 0800 328 8057

Professor Leslie Findley TD MD FRCP FACP DCH
YEAR QUALIFIED: 1968
NHS POST: Consultant Neurologist, Essex Neurosciences Unit, Oldchurch Hospital, Essex and Professor, South Bank University, London.
SPECIAL INTEREST: Movement disorders; botulinum toxin; fatigue syndromes; headache.
PRIVATE: Essex Nuffield Hospital, Shenfield Road, Brentwood, Essex CM15 8EH.
Tel: 01277 263 263/01708 722 826 -appts. Fax: 01708 736 323
E-mail:ljfindley@uk-consultants.co.uk
BUPA Hartswood Hospital, Eagle Way, Brentwood, Essex, CM13 3LE.
Tel: 01277 232 525/01708 722 826 -appts. Fax: 01708 736 323
BUPA Roding Hospital, Roding Lane South, Redbridge, Ilford, Essex IG4 5PZ.
Tel: 081 551 1100/01708 722 826 -appointments Fax: 01708 736 323

Hampshire

Dr William Gibb MD FRCP
YEAR QUALIFIED: 1979
NHS POST: Consultant Neurologist, Southampton and Portsmouth NHS Hospitals.
SPECIAL INTEREST: Parkinson's disease; movement disorders and neurodegenerations.
PRIVATE: BUPA Hospital, Bartons Road, Havant, Hampshire PO9 5NP.
Tel: 01705 456004 Fax: 01705 456100
BUPA Chalybeate Hospital, Chalybeate Close, Southampton, Hampshire SO9 4AX.
Tel: 01703 775544 Fax: 01703 701160

Hertfordshire

Dr Margaret Barrie MB BS FRCP
NHS POST: Honorary Consultant Neurologist, The Royal London Hospitals.
SPECIAL INTEREST: Migraine; epilepsy; Parkinson's disease; Alzheimer's; multiple sclerosis; medicolegal cases.
PRIVATE: The Rivers Hospital, High Wych Road, Sawbridgeworth, Hertfordshire CM21 6HH.
Tel: 01279 600 282. appointments - 01992 574 167 Fax: 01279 600 212 Private secretary (Mrs M J Austin) Tel/Fax: 01992 574167

London

Dr Margaret Barrie MB BS FRCP
NHS POST: Honorary Consultant Neurologist, The Royal London Hospitals.
SPECIAL INTEREST: Migraine; epilepsy; Parkinson's disease; Alzheimer's; multiple sclerosis; medicolegal cases.
PRIVATE: The Royal London Hospital, Whitechapel, London, E1 1BB.
St. Bartholomew's Hospital, West Smithfield, London, EC1A 7BE.

Neurology. London

Dr Marion Crouchman FRCP DCH FRCPCH
- YEAR QUALIFIED: 1967
- NHS POST: Consultant Neuro-Developmental Paediatrician, King's College Hospital.
- SPECIAL INTEREST: Acquired brain injury: Causation, assessment, management, rehabilitation. Botulinum toxin treatment in cerebral palsy. Fluent in French.
- PRIVATE: BMI Portland Hospital for Women & Children, 205-209 Great Portland Street, London, W1N 6AH. Tel: 0171 580 4400 Fax: 0171 610 5553
E-mail: marioncrouchman@rowanroad.demon.co.uk
Variety Club Children's Hospital, King's College Hospital, Denmark Hill, London, SE5 9RS. Tel: 0171 346 3690 Fax: 0171 610 5553

Dr Giles Elrington MBBS(Hons) MD FRCP
- YEAR QUALIFIED: 1980
- NHS POST: Consultant Neurologist, Royal London Hospital, Colchester General Hospital.
- SPECIAL INTEREST: Headache and migraine, rehabilitation, especially of multiple sclerosis, epilepsy, neurology/psychiatry interface.
- PRIVATE: London Independent Hospital, 1 Beaumont Square, Stepney Green, London E1 4NL. Tel: 0170 790 0990

Dr Michael Espir MA MB FRCP
- SPECIAL INTEREST: Epilepsy.
- PRIVATE: Wellington Hospital South, Wellington Place, London NW8 9LE.
Hospital of St. John & St. Elizabeth, 60 Grove End Road, St Johns Wood, London, NW8 9NH.
The Lister Hospital, Chelsea Bridge Road, London, SW1W 8RH.
Cromwell Hospital, Cromwell Road, London SW5 0TU.

Dr Simon Francis Farmer MB ChB BSc PhD MRCP
- YEAR QUALIFIED: 1986
- NHS POST: Consultant Neurologist, St Mary's Hospital NHS Trust and National Hospital for Neurology and Neurosurgery.
- SPECIAL INTEREST: General neurology; movement disorders; neuro-ophthalmology.
- PRIVATE: The Lindo Wing, St. Mary's Hospital, Praed Street, Paddington, London, W2 1NY. Tel: 0171 886 1389 Fax: 0171 886 1422

Dr Jeffrey Gawler MBBS(Hons) FRCP
- YEAR QUALIFIED: 1968
- NHS POST: Consultant Royal London Hospital And St. Bartholomew's Hospital
- SPECIAL INTEREST:
- PRIVATE: 149 Harley Street, London W1N 2DE.
Tel: 0171 224 0640 Fax: 0171 935 7245

Dr Roberto J Guiloff MD FRCP
- NHS POST: Consultant Neurologist, Charing Cross and Chelsea & Westminster Hospitals.
- SPECIAL INTEREST: Neuromuscular diseases; neurology of HIV disease; motor neurone diseases.
- PRIVATE: Cromwell Hospital, Cromwell Road, London SW5 0TU.
Tel: 0181 746 8319 Fax: 0181 746 8420

Neurology. London

Dr Gwilym Hosking MBBS FRCP FRCPCH FFPM
YEAR QUALIFIED: 1969
NHS POST: Honorary Consultant Paediatric Neurologist, Hospital For Sick Children, Great Ormond Street, Charing Cross Hospital & Southend NHS Trust.
SPECIAL INTEREST: Child neurology; epilepsy; cerebral palsy; head injury; neuro metabolic disorders; attention deficit disorder. Medico-legal practice.
PRIVATE: Portland Neurocare Ltd. (Child Neurology &, Neurodisability Services), 234 Great Portland Street, London W1N 5PH.
Tel: 0171 390 8286 Fax: 0171 390 8287
E-mail: admin@portlandneurocare.com Web: www.portlandneurocare.com

Dr Robin Howard MA MB BChir FRCP PhD
YEAR QUALIFIED: 1980
NHS POST: Consultant Neurologist, St. Thomas' Hospital And National Hospital For Neurology And Neurosurgery.
SPECIAL INTEREST: General neurology; neuromuscular diseases (particularly neuropathy, myasthenia gravis and motor neurone disease); sleep medicine; cerebrovascular disease and respiratory complications of neurological disorders.
PRIVATE: York House Consulting Rooms, 199 Westminster Bridge Road, London SE1 7UT.
Tel: 0171 928 5485 Fax: 0171 922 8263
The Consulting Rooms, 23 Queen Square, London WC1N 3BY.
Tel: 0171 829 9732 Fax: 0171 833 8658

Dr Peter Kaufmann MBBS FRCP
YEAR QUALIFIED: 1969
NHS POST: Honorary Consultant Neurologist, Chalfont Centre For Epilepsy (NSE).
SPECIAL INTEREST: Epilepsy and other causes of blackouts; multiple sclerosis; disorders of vision.
PRIVATE: 99 Harley Street, London W1N 1DF.
Tel: 0171 935 5944 Fax: 01494 483424
The Garden Hospital, 46-50 Sunny Gardens Road, Hendon, London, NW4 1RX.
Tel: 0181 203 0111

Dr Russell J M Lane BSc MD FRCP
YEAR QUALIFIED: 1973
NHS POST: Consultant Neurologist, Charing Cross & Ashford & St. Peter's Hospital.
SPECIAL INTEREST: Neuromuscular disorders; headache; epilepsy.
PRIVATE: Cromwell Hospital, Cromwell Road, London SW5 0TU.
Tel: 0171 370 4233 ext 5224/5/6 Fax: 0171 370 4063 E-mail: r.lane@ic.ac.uk

Dr Nigel John Legg MB BS FRCP
YEAR QUALIFIED: 1959
NHS POST: Consultant Neurologist, Hammersmith Hospital, London W12 0HS. 0181 383 1000.
SPECIAL INTEREST: Migraine and other headaches; epilepsy; peripheral nerve disorders.
PRIVATE: 152 Harley Street, London W1N 1HH.
Tel: 0171 935 8868
Hospital of St. John & St. Elizabeth, 60 Grove End Road, St Johns Wood, London, NW8 9NH. Tel: 0171 286 3370 Fax: 0171 286 6202

Dr John Michael Oxbury MB BChir MA PhD FRCP
- YEAR QUALIFIED: 1963
- NHS POST: Consultant Neurologist, Radcliffe Infirmary, Oxford.
- SPECIAL INTEREST: Epilepsy, including chronic epilepsy possibly amenable to surgical treatment; higher cerebral function disorders - e.g. amnesia, apraxia, aphasia.
- PRIVATE: Cromwell Hospital, Cromwell Road, London SW5 0TU.
Tel: 0171 460 5700 Fax: 0171 460 5731

Dr Richard Peatfield MD FRCP
- YEAR QUALIFIED: 1973
- NHS POST: Consultant Neurologist Charing Cross Hospital & Mount Vernon Hospital
- SPECIAL INTEREST: Headache
- PRIVATE: Charing Cross Hospital, Fulham Palace Road, London, W6 8RF.
Tel: 0181 846 1194

Dr G D Perkin BA FRCP
- YEAR QUALIFIED: 1966
- NHS POST: Consultant Neurologist Charing Cross & Hillingdon Hospitals
- SPECIAL INTEREST: Multiple sclerosis; cerebro-vascular disease.
- PRIVATE: Charing Cross Hospital, Fulham Palace Road, London, W6 8RF.
Tel: 0181 846 1153 Fax: 0181 846 7487
Cromwell Hospital, Cromwell Road, London SW5 0TU.
Tel: 0171 460 2000

Dr Gordon Plant MA(Cantab) MD(Cantab) FRCP
- YEAR QUALIFIED: 1977
- NHS POST: Consultant Neurologist National Hospital for Neurology & Neurosurgery, Moorfields Eye Hospital, St. Thomas' Hospital
- SPECIAL INTEREST: Visual disorders; neuro-ophthalmology.
- PRIVATE: Private Consulting Rooms, National Hospital for Neurology and Neurosurgery, Queen Square, London, WC1N 3BG. Tel: 0171 829 8741 Fax: 0171 833 8658

Professor Anthony Schapira BSc MB BS MD FRCP DSc
- NHS POST: Consultant Neurologist Royal Free Hospital and National Hospital, Queen Square
- SPECIAL INTEREST: Parkinson's disease; muscle disease; migraine.
- PRIVATE: Royal Free Hospital, Pond Street, Hampstead, London, NW3 2QG.
Tel: 0171 830 2012 Fax: 0171 431 1577

Professor P K Thomas CBE MD DSc FRCP FRCPath
- NHS POST: Honorary Consultant Neurologist Royal Free Hospital and National Hospital for Neurology and Neurosurgery.
- SPECIAL INTEREST: Neuromuscular disease.
- PRIVATE: Royal Free Hospital, Pond Street, Hampstead, London, NW3 2QG.
Tel: 0171 794 0500 ext 4966 Fax: 0171 431 1577

Middlesex

Dr Russell J M Lane BSc MD FRCP
- YEAR QUALIFIED: 1973
- NHS POST: Consultant Neurologist, Charing Cross & Ashford & St. Peter's Hospital.
- SPECIAL INTEREST: Neuromuscular disorders; headache; epilepsy.
- PRIVATE: Ashford Hospital, London Road, Ashford, TW15 3AA.
Tel: 01784 884617 Fax: 01708 884273 E-mail: r.lane@ic.ac.uk

Dr Richard Peatfield MD FRCP
- YEAR QUALIFIED: 1973
- NHS POST: Consultant Neurologist Charing Cross Hospital & Mount Vernon Hospital
- SPECIAL INTEREST: Headache
- PRIVATE: Bishops Wood Private Hospital, Rickmansworth Road, Northwood, Middlesex HA6 2JW. Tel: 01923 835 814

Oxfordshire

Dr Ralph Peter Gregory FRCP
- YEAR QUALIFIED: 1982
- NHS POST: Consultant Neurologist, Royal Berkshire Hospital Reading/Radcliffe Infirmary Oxford.
- SPECIAL INTEREST: General neurologist with particular interest in Parkinson's disease and other movement disorders; experience in various neurosurgical procedures for PD and botulinum toxin therapy.
- PRIVATE: Radcliffe Infirmary, Woodstock Road, Oxford, Oxfordshire OX2 6HE.
Tel: 01865 224537 Fax: 01865 224303

Dr John Michael Oxbury MB BChir MA PhD FRCP
- YEAR QUALIFIED: 1963
- NHS POST: Consultant Neurologist, Radciffe Infirmary, Oxford.
- SPECIAL INTEREST: Epilepsy, including chronic epilepsy possibly amenable to surgical treatment; higher cerebral function disorders - e.g. amnesia, apraxia, aphasia.
- PRIVATE: Felstead House, 23 Banbury Road, Oxford, Oxon OX2 6NX.
Tel: 01865 558532 Fax: 01865 558532

Surrey

Dr Patrick Trend MA PhD FRCP
- YEAR QUALIFIED: 1979
- NHS POST: Consultant Neurologist, Royal Surrey County Hospital, Guildford, GU2 5XX.
Tel: 01483 406762 . Mobile: 0370 820177
- SPECIAL INTEREST: Parkinson's disease and other movement disorders, the dementias, motor system disorders, neuro-ophthalmology and neuro-oncology.
- PRIVATE: Guildford Nuffield Hospital, Stirling Road, Guildford, Surrey GU2 6RF.
Tel: 01483 555800 Fax: 01483 555832 Secretary: Mrs. J. Worthington 01483 555830.
Mobile: 0370 820177

  Ashtead Hospital, The Warren, Ashtead, Surrey KT21 2SB.
Tel: 01372 276161 ext 376 Fax: 01372 278704 Mobile: 0370 820177

  BUPA Gatwick Park Hospital, Povey Cross Road, Horley, Surrey RH6 0BB.
Tel: 01293 785511 Fax: 01293 774883 Mobile: 0370 820177

Neurophysiology (Clinical)

London

Dr Noel Rudolf MA BM BCh
SPECIAL INTEREST: Consultant Clinical Neurophysiologist; electroencephalography (EEG), electromyography (EMG) and nerve conduction studies (NCS).
PRIVATE: 22 Devonshire Place, London W1N 1PD.
Tel: 0171 935 1825 Fax: 0171 224 7220

Staffordshire

Dr Peter Desmond Heath FRCP DM(Oxon)
YEAR QUALIFIED: 1978
NHS POST: Consultant in Clinical Neurophysiology, North Staffordshire Hospital (NHS Trust), Stoke-on-Trent.
SPECIAL INTEREST: Diagnosis of peripheral nerve entrapments.
PRIVATE: Department of Clinical Neurophysiology, North Staffs Hospital (NHS Trust), Stoke-on-Trent, Staffs ST4 7LN. Tel: 01782 554554 Fax: 01782 555315

Nuclear Medicine

London

Dr Durval Costa MD MSc PhD FRCR
NHS POST: Consultant Physician, University College London Hospitals NHS Trust, The Middlesex Hospital
SPECIAL INTEREST: Nuclear Medicine, particularly applications in neurology; psychiatry; oncology; neuro endocrinology; nuclear cardiology and nephro urology. Nuclear medicine applied to sports medicine.
PRIVATE: Institute of Nuclear Medicine, UCL, Royal Free & UCL Medical School The Middlesex Hospital, Mortimer Street, London, W1N 8AA.
Tel: 0171 380 9425 Fax: 0171 436 0603/E-mail:d.costa@nucmed.ucl.ac.uk
Harley Street Clinic, 35 Weymouth Street, London, W1N 4BJ.
Tel: 0171 323 0365 Fax: 0171 323 0340/E-mail:d.costa@nucmed.ucl.ac.uk

Norfolk

Dr John Bannerman Latham MB ChB FRCR
YEAR QUALIFIED: 1966
NHS POST: Consultant Radiologist, Norfolk and Norwich.
SPECIAL INTEREST: General radiology including CT, MRI, ultrasound and mammography.
PRIVATE: Norfolk & Norwich Hospital, Brunswick Road, Norwich, Norfolk NR1 3SR.
Tel: 01603 286807 Fax: 01603 286806

Obstetrics & Gynaecology

Berkshire

Mr Rajat K Goswamy MBBS FRCOG
YEAR QUALIFIED: 1976
NHS POST: Consultant Gynaecologist, Royal Berkshire Hospital, Reading.
SPECIAL INTEREST: Infertility Investigations, Treatment Including IVF, IUI, Egg/Sperm Donation, Ultrasound Research Into Failed IVF Patients
PRIVATE: Royal Berkshire Hospital, London Road, Reading, Berkshire RG1 5AN.
Tel: 01734 875111
BUPA Dunedin Hospital, 16 Bath Road, Reading, Berkshire RG1 6NB.
Tel: 01734 587 676 Fax: 01734 393 063

Birmingham

Mr J Michael Emens MD FRCOG
YEAR QUALIFIED: 1964
NHS POST: Consultant Gynaecologist, Womens Hospital Birmingham NHS Trust.
SPECIAL INTEREST: Consultant gynaecologist, special interests gynae urology and management of female incontinence, colposcopy and vaginal infections especially Candida.
PRIVATE: 14 Church Road, Edgbaston, Birmingham B15 3SR.
Tel: 0121 454 7576 Fax: 0121 454 7576

Bristol

Professor Michael G R Hull MD FRCOG
YEAR QUALIFIED: 1962
NHS POST: Consultant Obstetrician and Gynaecologist (Hon), St Michael's Hospital.
SPECIAL INTEREST: Reproductive medicine within consultant team with full specialist support in dedicated, accredited tertiary referral centre covering: complete male and female infertility; assisted conception; reproductive endocrinology; postmenopausal endocrinology; recurrent miscarriage; sexual medicine.
PRIVATE: University of Bristol Centre for Reproductive Medicine, 4 Priory Road, Bristol BS8 1TY.
Tel: 0117 902 1100 Fax: 0117 902 1101 E-mail: m.g.r.hull@bristol.ac.uk

Mr Fraser Neil McLeod FRCOG
YEAR QUALIFIED: 1974
NHS POST: Consultant Obstetrician and Gynaecologist, Frenchay and Southmead Hospitals, Bristol.
SPECIAL INTEREST: Vaginal and minimal access surgery (Hysteroscopic and Laparoscopic); the menopause; incontinence surgery.
PRIVATE: Cavendish Lodge, 7 Percival Road, Clifton, Bristol BS8 3LE.
Tel: 0117 974 1396 Fax: 0117 973 3809

Obstetrics & Gynaecology. Bristol

Mr Peter Ashley R Niven MA MB BChir FRCS FRCOG
YEAR QUALIFIED: 1962
NHS POST: Consultant Obstetrician and Gynaecologist, United Bristol Healthcare Trust, St Michael's Hospital, Bristol.
SPECIAL INTEREST: General obstetrics and gynaecology; vaginal surgery; endoscopic surgery.
PRIVATE: 2 Clifton Park, Clifton, Bristol, BS8 3BS. Tel: 0117 923 8206

Buckinghamshire

Mr Martin Usherwood MBBS MRCS LRCP FRCOG MFFP
YEAR QUALIFIED: 1977
NHS POST: Consultant Obstetrician & Gynaecologist Stoke Mandeville Hospital
SPECIAL INTEREST: Gynaecological oncology; colposcopy; endometrial ablation and laparoscopic laser surgery.
PRIVATE: The Chiltern Hospital, London Road, Great Missenden, Buckinghamshire HP16 0EN. Tel: 01494 890 890 Fax: 01296 330 477

Cambridgeshire

Mr John G Williamson MB FRCS FRCOG
YEAR QUALIFIED: 1963
NHS POST: Consultant in Obstetrics and Gynaecology, Addenbrooke's Hospital, Cambridge.
SPECIAL INTEREST: Urogynaecology (prolapse and urinary incontinence); oncology (including colposcopy); endoscopic surgery: hysterectomy, colposuspension, adhesiolysis and hysteroscopic procedures.
PRIVATE: Evelyn Hospital, 4 Trumpington Road, Cambridge, Cambridgeshire CB2 2AF. Tel: Appointments-01223 360380 Fax: 01223 510021

Cleveland

Mr Philip Taylor MRCOG
YEAR QUALIFIED: 1970
NHS POST: Consultant gynaecologist, South Cleveland Hospital.
SPECIAL INTEREST: Reproductive medicine (male and female); assisted conception (including IVF, donor sperm, donor eggs, ICSI); tubal microsurgery; minimally invasive surgery; HRT.
PRIVATE: Spring House, Great Broughton, Middlesbrough, Cleveland TS9 7HX. Tel: 01642 778239 Fax: 01642 854891

Derbyshire

Mr Howard Jenkins DM FRCOG
YEAR QUALIFIED: 1971
NHS POST: Consultant Obstetrician and Gynaecologist, Derby City General Hospital.
SPECIAL INTEREST: Menstrual disorders; minimal access surgery;ovarian carcinoma.
PRIVATE: 14 Vernon Street, Derby DE1 1FT. Tel: 01332 347314 Fax: 01332 206461

Devon

Mr John M Morsman FRCS FRCS(Ed) FRCOG
- YEAR QUALIFIED: 1970
- NHS POST: Consultant Obstetrician and Gynaecologist, Derriford Hospital, Devon.
- SPECIAL INTEREST: Gynaecological; oncology (especially ovarian carcinoma); colposcopy; menopause and HRT; perimenopausal bleeding/symptoms; medico-legal opinions given.
- PRIVATE: Nuffield Hospital, Derriford Road, Plymouth, Devon PL6 8BG.
Tel: 01752 790482 Fax: 01752 778421

Dorset

Mr Richard Henry MB FRCS FRACOG FRCOG
- YEAR QUALIFIED: 1976
- NHS POST: Consultant Obstetrician and Gynaecologist, Poole Hospital NHS Trust and Royal Bournemouth NHS Trust.
- SPECIAL INTEREST: General gynaecology; gynaecological oncology; endometriosis; colposcopy; minimally invasive gynaecological surgery; surgery for pelvic prolapse and urinary incontinence.
- PRIVATE: 1 Chaucer Road, Canford Cliffs, Poole, Dorset BH13 7HB.
Tel: 01202 701122 Fax: 01202 701909

Down

Dr Paul Fogarty MD FRCOG
- YEAR QUALIFIED: 1981
- NHS POST: Consultant Obstetrician and Gynaecologist, Ulster Hospital.
- SPECIAL INTEREST: Antenatal care; holistic gynaecology with special expertise in HRT, minimal access surgery and treatment of incontinence.
- PRIVATE: Glen House, Crawfordsburn, Down BT19 1HY.
Tel: 01232 561401 Fax: 01232 561402

Essex

Mr Henry Annan MA(Cantab) MBBChir FRCOG MFFP
- NHS POST: Consultant Obstetrician and Gynaecologist, Whipps Cross Hospital.
- SPECIAL INTEREST: Premalignant lesions of cervix and vulva. Conservative surgery for fibroids and endometriosis. Management of menorrhagia, including laser endometrial ablation surgery for urinary incontinence and prolapse. Obstetric care and clinical risk management.
- PRIVATE: Holly House Hospital, High Road, Buckhurst Hill, Essex, IG9 5HX.
Tel: 0181 505 3311 Fax: 0181 508 9349
BUPA Roding Hospital, Roding Lane South, Redbridge, Ilford, Essex IG4 5PZ.
Tel: 0181 551 1100 Fax: 0181 508 9349

Obstetrics & Gynaecology. Essex

Mr Geoffrey W Cochrane MBBS FRCOG
- NHS POST: Consultant, King George Hospital.
- SPECIAL INTEREST: Gynaecology; minimal access surgery; gynae urology.
- PRIVATE: Holly House Hospital, High Road, Buckhurst Hill, Essex, IG9 5HX.
  Tel: 0181 505 3311
  BUPA Roding Hospital, Roding Lane South, Redbridge, Ilford, Essex IG4 5PZ.
  Tel: 0181 551 1100

Mr Antony Hollingworth MBChB PhD MBA FRCS(Ed) MRCOG
- NHS POST: Consultant in Obstetrics and Gynaecology Whipps Cross Hospital
- SPECIAL INTEREST: Colposcopy
- PRIVATE: Holly House Hospital, High Road, Buckhurst Hill, Essex, IG9 5HX.
  Tel: 0181 505 3311 Fax: 0181 506 1013

Mr Cheng-Lian Lee MB ChB MD FRCS FRCOG
- YEAR QUALIFIED: 1981
- NHS POST: Consultant, Southend Hospital.
- SPECIAL INTEREST: Vaginal hysterectomy and bilateral salpingo-oophorectomy with early discharge and quick recovery.
- PRIVATE: BUPA Wellesley Hospital, Eastern Avenue, Southend on Sea SS2 4XH.
  Tel: 01702 462 944 Fax: 01702 600 160

Mr Michael Martin FRCOG MB BS
- NHS POST: Consultant Obstetrician and Gynaecologist Basildon Hospital
- SPECIAL INTEREST: General gynaecology; no private obstetrics.
- PRIVATE: Essex Nuffield Hospital, Shenfield Road, Brentwood, Essex, CM15 8EH.
  Tel: 01277 263263 Fax: 01277 261 924

Mr Satha-M Sathanandan MPhil FRCS FRCOG MFFP
- NHS POST: Consultant Obstetrician & Gynaecologist Haroldwood Hospital and Senior Lecturer at University College London and St. Bartholomew's Hospital and Royal London School of Medicine & Dentistry
- SPECIAL INTEREST: Infertility and assisted conception inc. IVF and donor insemination. Gynaecological endocrinology inc. menopause and family planning. All forms of menstrual disorders.
- PRIVATE: Essex Nuffield Hospital, Shenfield Road, Brentwood, Essex, CM15 8EH.
  Tel: 01277 263363 / 260824 Fax: 01277 260824

Miss Isabel Helen Tebbutt FRCOG
- YEAR QUALIFIED: 1977
- NHS POST: Consultant Obstetrician and Gynaecologist, Harold Wood Hospital.
- SPECIAL INTEREST: Oncology; laparoscopic surgery.
- PRIVATE: BUPA Hartswood Hospital, Eagle Way, Brentwood, Essex, CM13 3LE.
  Tel: 01268 542580 Fax: 01268 542580

Hampshire

Miss Claire Iffland MBBS MRCOG
YEAR QUALIFIED: 1982
NHS POST: Consultant Obstetrician & Gynaecologist, The North Hampshire Hospital.
SPECIAL INTEREST: General gynaecologist.
PRIVATE: The Hampshire Clinic, Basing Road, Basingstoke, Hampshire RG24 7AL.
Tel: 01256 357111 Fax: 01256 329986

Hertfordshire

Dr Brenda E Bean MBBS DCH MFFP RCOG
YEAR QUALIFIED: 1964
NHS POST: Consultant in Family Planning and Reproductive Healthcare, East Hertfordshire NHS Trust.
SPECIAL INTEREST: Menopause; contraception; infertility.
PRIVATE: Queen Victoria Memorial Hospital, School Lane, Welwyn, Hertfordshire AL6 9PW.
Tel: 01707 365 291

Mr Nicholas C Drew FRCOG
YEAR QUALIFIED: 1968
NHS POST: Consultant in Obstetrics & Gynaecology, Queen Elizabeth II Hospital.
SPECIAL INTEREST: Urogynaecology; general gynaecological abdominal surgery; vaginal surgery.
PRIVATE: BUPA Hospital Harpenden, Ambrose Lane, Harpenden, Herts, AL5 4BP.
Tel: 01582 769067 or Freephone 0800 585112 Fax: 01582 712 312 Secretary:01707 365050-appointments. 01438 798099-(Tel/Fax).
Elizabeth House, Queen Elizabeth II Hospital, Howlands, Welwyn Garden City, Hertfordshire, AL7 4HQ.
Tel: 01707 365 111 Secretary:01707 365050-appointments. 01438 798099-(Tel/Fax).

Mr Owen Owens MD MRCOG MRCPI
YEAR QUALIFIED: 1980
NHS POST: Consultant Obstetrician/Gynaecologist Luton & Dunstable NHS Trust
SPECIAL INTEREST: Colposcopy; laparoscopic surgery; vaginal surgery; diseases of the vulva; general gynaecology.
PRIVATE: BUPA Hospital Harpenden, Ambrose Lane, Harpenden, Herts, AL5 4BP.
Tel: 01582 763 191 Fax: 01582 712 312
BUPA Hospital Bushey, Heathbourne Rd, Bushey, Watford, Hertfordshire WD2 1RD.
Tel: 0181 950 9090 Fax: 0181 950 7556

Kent

Mr Rajat K Goswamy MBBS FRCOG
- YEAR QUALIFIED: 1976
- NHS POST: Consultant Gynaecologist, Royal Berkshire Hospital, Reading.
- SPECIAL INTEREST: Infertility Investigations, Treatment Including IVF, IUI, Egg/Sperm Donation, Ultrasound Research Into Failed IVF Patients
- PRIVATE: Nuffield Hospital Tunbridge Wells, Kingswood Road, Tunbridge Wells, Kent TN2 4UL. Tel: 01892 531 111 Fax: 01892 515 689

Mr Laurence M A Shaw MBBS MRCS LRCP FHSM FRCOG
- YEAR QUALIFIED: 1978
- NHS POST: East Kent Hospitals NHS Trust.
- SPECIAL INTEREST: Obstetrics & Gynaecology (Endoscopic Surgery, Reproductive Medicine).
- PRIVATE: The Chaucer Hospital, Nackington Road, Canterbury, Kent CT4 7AR. Tel: 01227 455466 Fax: 01227 762733
  The Spencer Wing, Queen Elizabeth the Queen Mother Hospital, St. Peters Road, Margate, Kent CT9 4AN. Tel: 01843 234555 Fax: 01843 296333

Lancashire

Mr Ian William Mahady MB ChB FRCOG
- YEAR QUALIFIED: 1966
- NHS POST: Consultant Obstetrician and Gynaecologist, Burnley General.
- SPECIAL INTEREST: Urogynaecology/female incontinence; diabetes in pregnancy.
- PRIVATE: 56 Bank Parade, Burnley, Lancashire BB11 1TS. Tel: 01282 429432

Leeds

Mr Adam H Balen MB BS MRCOG MFFP MD
- YEAR QUALIFIED: 1983
- NHS POST: Consultant Obstetrician/Gynaecologist and Subspecialist Reproductive Medicine, Leeds General Infirmary.
- SPECIAL INTEREST: Reproductive medicine, infertility, polycystic ovary syndrome, ovulation induction, IVF, adolescent gynaecology (intersex problems etc) and menopause.
- PRIVATE: Clarendon Wing, Leeds General Infirmary, Leeds LS2 9NS. Tel: 0113 392 2728 Fax: 0113 392 2446

Lincolnshire

Mr Martin Piers Lamb MBBS FRCOG
 YEAR QUALIFIED: 1969
 NHS POST: Consultant Gynaecologist and Obstetrician, Lincoln and Louth NHS (T), Greetwell Road, Lincoln LN2 5QY.
 SPECIAL INTEREST: Minimal access surgery; gynaecological oncology and colposcopy.
 PRIVATE: Dunston House, Front Street, Dunston, Lincoln, Lincolnshire LN4 2ES.
 Tel: 01526 320175 Fax: 01526 323239 E-mail: mplamb@uk-consultants.co.uk

Mr Arabinda Saha MRCOG
 YEAR QUALIFIED: 1980
 NHS POST: Consultant Obstetrician and Gynaecologist, Grimsby Hospital.
 SPECIAL INTEREST: Colposcopy; gynaecological cancers; menstrual disorders; genital prolapse; hysteroscopic and laparoscopic surgery.
 PRIVATE: St Hugh's Hospital, Peaks Lane, Grimsby, NE Lincs DN32 9RP.
 Tel: 01472 251100 Fax: 01472 251130

London

Mr Hossam Abdalla MRCOG
 NHS POST: Consultant Gynaecologist, Chelsea & Westminster Hospital.
 SPECIAL INTEREST: IVF; infertility; endoscopic surgery.
 PRIVATE: IVF Unit, Lister Hospital, Chelsea Bridge Road, London, SW1W 8RH.
 Tel: 0171 730 5932 Fax: 0171 259 9039

Mrs Roxana Chapman MD LMSSA FRCOG FRACOG
 YEAR QUALIFIED: 1963
 SPECIAL INTEREST: Laser surgery; infertility including IVF, and endocrinology.
 PRIVATE: Suite 10, 103-105 Harley Street, London W1N 1HD.
 Tel: 0171 224 3011 Fax: 0171 487 3680 E-mail: yi28@dial.pipex.com
 Cromwell Hospital, Cromwell Road, London SW5 0TU.
 Tel: 0171 460 2000

Mr Dickinson B Cowan FRCS FRCOG
 YEAR QUALIFIED: 1970
 SPECIAL INTEREST: IVF & ICSI; donor insemination; egg and embryo donation; embryo freezing; reproductive failure; obstetrics; benign and check up gynaecology.
 PRIVATE: Portland Hospital for Women & Children, First Floor Consulting Rooms, 212-214 Great Portland Street, London W1N 5HG.
 Tel: Consultations 0171 390 8081/2/3. Fax: 0171 383 4162

Ms Friedericke Eben MRCOG
 NHS POST: Consultant Obstetrician and Gynaecologist, Whittington Hospital.
 SPECIAL INTEREST: General and high risk obstetrics and general gynaecology.
 PRIVATE: Portland Hospital for Women & Children, 205-209 Gt. Portland Street, London W1N 6AH. Tel: 0171 390 8089 Fax: 0171 390 8478

Obstetrics & Gynaecology. London

Mr Alan Farthing MBBS MD MRCOG
- YEAR QUALIFIED: 1986
- NHS POST: Consultant in Obstetrics & Gynaecology, St. Mary's Hospital, Paddington, London.
- SPECIAL INTEREST: Laparoscopic gynaecology and gynaecological oncology.
- PRIVATE: Lindo Wing, St. Mary's Hospital, South Wharf Road, Paddington, London W2 1NY.
Tel: 0171 886 1673. Emergencies-0171 886 1624. Fax: 0171 886 6770

Professor Nicholas Fisk MBBS PhD FRACOG FRCOG DDU
- YEAR QUALIFIED: 1980
- NHS POST: Honorary Consultant Obstetrician & Gynaecologist, Queen Charlotte's & Chelsea Hospital.
- SPECIAL INTEREST: Fetal medicine; ultrasound; invasive procedures; multiple pregnancy; high risk obstetrics.
- PRIVATE: Centre for Fetal Care, Queen Charlotte's & Chelsea Hospital, Goldhawk Road, London, W6 0XG. Tel: 0181 383 3190 Fax: 0181 748 6311   E-mail: nfisk@rpms.ac.uk

Mr Malcolm G Gillard MB (Hons)FRCS FRCOG
- YEAR QUALIFIED: 1972
- NHS POST: Previously - Consultant at St. Bartholomew's & Homerton Hospitals.
- SPECIAL INTEREST: Obstetrics and benign gynaecology.
- PRIVATE: First Floor Suite, 1 Devonshire Place, London W1N 1PA.
Tel: 0171 486 2856 Fax: 0171 486 2858

Mr Yehudi Gordon MB BCh FRCOG FCOG SA MD
- SPECIAL INTEREST: Obstetrics with an accent on active birth. Infertility using assisted conception techniques and nutritional support. Menstrual and menopausal disorders, support and treatment.
- PRIVATE: 27A Queens Terrace, London NW8 6EA.
Tel: 0171 483 0099 Fax: 0171 483 3899   E-mail: whc@btconnect.com
Hospital of St. John & St. Elizabeth, 60 Grove End Road, St Johns Wood, London, NW8 9NH. Tel: 0171 286 5126 E-mail: whc@btconnect.com

Mr Rajat K Goswamy MBBS FRCOG
- YEAR QUALIFIED: 1976
- NHS POST: Consultant Gynaecologist, Royal Berkshire Hospital, Reading.
- SPECIAL INTEREST: Infertility Investigations, Treatment Including IVF, IUI, Egg/Sperm Donation, Ultrasound Research Into Failed IVF Patients
- PRIVATE: Churchill Clinic, 80 Lambeth Road, London, SE1 7PW.
Tel: 0171 928 5633 ext 294 Fax: 0171 401 9942

Miss Marion Hatton BSc FRCS(Ed) MRCOG LLM
- YEAR QUALIFIED: 1978
- NHS POST: Consultant Obstetrician & Gynaecologist, West Midlands.
- SPECIAL INTEREST: Obstetrics, medical and surgical gynaecology (including the menopause).
- PRIVATE: The Consulting Suite, 214 Great Portland Street, London W1N 5HG.
Tel: 0171 383 2626 Fax: 0171 390 8428

Obstetrics & Gynaecology. London

Dr Maurice Katz FCP(SA) FRCP
- YEAR QUALIFIED: 1963
- NHS POST: Consultant Endocrinologist, University College London Hospitals.
- SPECIAL INTEREST: Reproductive endocrinology; menstrual disorders; androgenised females; PCO.; premenstrual syndrome; menopause; osteoporosis; male and female infertility; psychosexual problems and endocrinology of ageing; pituitary; thyroid; adrenal.
- PRIVATE: 148 Harley Street, London W1N 1AH.
Tel: 0171 383 7911 Fax: 0171 380 9816

Mr Adrian Lower BMedSc BM BS MRCOG
- YEAR QUALIFIED: 1983
- NHS POST: Consultant Gynaecologist, St. Bartholomew's Hospital, London.
- SPECIAL INTEREST: Endoscopic surgery; fertility and reproductive medicine.
- PRIVATE: 136 Harley Street, London W1N 1AA.
Tel: 0171 486 2440 Fax: 0171 487 4488

Mr Roger P Marwood MSc FRCOG
- YEAR QUALIFIED: 1969
- NHS POST: Consultant Obstetrician & Gynaecologist, Chelsea & Westminster Hospital.
- SPECIAL INTEREST: High risk pregnancy; prolapse; colposcopy; vulval disease.
- PRIVATE: 96 Harley Street, London W1N 1AF.
Tel: 0171 637 7977 Fax: 0171 486 2022

Miss Angela M Mills MA BM BCh FRCOG MFFP MFPHM
- YEAR QUALIFIED: 1972
- SPECIAL INTEREST: Gynaecology and colposcopy.
- PRIVATE: 80 Harley Street, London W1N 1AE.
Tel: 0171 637 0584

Mr Karl Murphy MD MRCOG MRCPI DCH
- YEAR QUALIFIED: 1981
- NHS POST: Consultant, St Mary's Hospital NHS Trust.
- SPECIAL INTEREST: High risk obstetrics; prenatal diagnosis; fetal medicine; general gynaecology.
- PRIVATE: Lindo Wing, St. Mary's Hospital, South Wharf Road, Paddington, London W2 1NY.
Tel: 0171 886 1692 Fax: 0171 886 6141

Mr Owen Owens MD MRCOG MRCPI
- YEAR QUALIFIED: 1980
- NHS POST: Consultant Obstetrician/Gynaecologist Luton & Dunstable NHS Trust
- SPECIAL INTEREST: Colposcopy; laparoscopic surgery; vaginal surgery; diseases of the vulva; general gynaecology.
- PRIVATE: Hospital of St. John & St. Elizabeth, 60 Grove End Road, St Johns Wood, London, NW8 9NH. Tel: 0171 286 5126 Fax: 0171 266 4813

Obstetrics & Gynaecology. London

Mr Nigel Perks MBBS MRCOG
- NHS POST: Consultant Obstetrician And Gynaecologist Greenwich Hospital And The Royal Hospitals Trust
- SPECIAL INTEREST: General gynaecology with special expertise in infertility, assisted conception (including IVF And ICSI) and minimal access surgery.
- PRIVATE: The Bridge Centre, 1 St. Thomas Street, London SE1
  Tel: 0171 403 3363 Fax: 0171 403 8552
  The Blackheath Hospital, 40-42 Lee Terrace, Blackheath, London, SE3 9UD.
  Tel: 0181 318 7722 Fax: 0181 318 2542

Mr Alvan Priddy MBChB MRCOG MD
- YEAR QUALIFIED: 1983
- NHS POST: Consultant obstetrician and gynaecologist Northwick Park Hospital
- SPECIAL INTEREST: Infertility; minimal access surgery including endometrial ablation.
- PRIVATE: Consulting Rooms (Obst & Gynae), The Clementine Churchill Hospital, Sudbury Hill, Harrow, Middlesex, HA1 3RX.
  Tel: 0181 872 3939 Fax: 0181 872 3871

Mr Talha Shawaf MB ChB FRCS(Ed) FRCOG
- NHS POST: St. Bartholomews Hospital, 2nd floor KGV Block, West Smithfield, London EC1A 7BE.
  Tel: 0171 601 7176.
- SPECIAL INTEREST: Reproductive medicine from nutritional support to assisted conception. Obstetrics with an accent on active birth. Menstrual and menopausal disorders, support and treatment.
- PRIVATE: 27A Queens Terrace, London NW8 6EA.
  Tel: 0171 483 0099 Fax: 0171 483 3988
  Hospital of St. John & St. Elizabeth, 60 Grove End Road, St Johns Wood, London, NW8 9NH. Tel: 0171 286 5126

Mr John Shepherd FRCS FRCOG FACOG
- YEAR QUALIFIED: 1971
- NHS POST: Consultant Gynaecological Surgeon & Oncologist St. Bartholomew's and The Royal Marsden Hospitals
- SPECIAL INTEREST: Gynaecological oncology; gynaecological surgery; colposcopy.
- PRIVATE: The London Clinic, 149 Harley Street, London, W1N 2DE.
  Tel: 0171 935 4444 Fax: 0171 935 6224

Professor Albert Singer PhD DPhil FRCOG
- NHS POST: Consultant Gynaecologist, Whittington Hospital Trust, London N19 5NF.
- SPECIAL INTEREST: Colposcopy and gynaecological oncology; medical and surgical gynaecology including menopause; menorrhagia; vulval diseases.
- PRIVATE: Portland Hospital for Women & Children, First Floor Consulting Rooms, 212-214 Great Portland Street, London W1N 5HG.
  Tel: Appointments-0171 3908442. Secretary-0181 4585925. Fax: 0181 458 0168

Mr J Richard Smith MB ChB MD MRCOG
- YEAR QUALIFIED: 1917
- NHS POST: Senior Consultant/Lecturer, Gynaecology, Chelsea & Westminster Hospital.
- SPECIAL INTEREST: Oncology, infection and immunity.
- PRIVATE: Lister Hospital, Chelsea Bridge Road, London, SW1W 8RH.
  Tel: 0171 730 0431 Fax: 0171 730 6861

Obstetrics & Gynaecology. London

Mr William P Soutter MD FRCOG
- NHS POST: Reader in Gynaecology Hammersmith Hospitals Trust
- SPECIAL INTEREST: Gynaecological oncology; colposcopy; gynaecology.
- PRIVATE: Robert & Lisa Sainsbury Wing, Hammersmith Hospital, Du Cane Road, London, W12 0HS. Tel: 0181 740 3267 Fax: 0181 259 8056

Mr Clive Spence-Jones FRCS MRCOG
- YEAR QUALIFIED: 1981
- NHS POST: Consultant in Obstetrics & Gynaecology The Whittington Hospital
- SPECIAL INTEREST: Incontinence prolapse and endoscopic surgery.
- PRIVATE: The London Clinic, 149 Harley Street, London, W1N 2DE. Tel: 0171 935 4444 Fax: 0171 486 2580

Mr Stuart Steele MA FRCS FRCOG MFFP
- NHS POST: Honorary Consultant UCL Hospitals
- SPECIAL INTEREST: Paediatric and adolescent gynaecology; infertility.
- PRIVATE: The London Women's Clinic, 113-115 Harley Street, London W1N 1DG. Tel: 0171 487 5050 Fax: 0171 487 5850

Mr John W W Studd DSc MD FRCOG
- NHS POST: Consultant Gynaecologist, Chelsea and Westminster Hospital, London.
- SPECIAL INTEREST: Gynaecology; hormone replacement therapy; menopause; PMS; postnatal depression; osteoporosis.
- PRIVATE: Lister Hospital, Chelsea Bridge Road, London, SW1W 8RH. Tel: 0171 730 5433 Fax: 0171 823 6108
  120 Harley Street, London W1N 1AN. Tel: 0171 486 0497 Fax: 0171 224 4190

Mr T G Teoh MD MSc MRCOG MRCPI
- YEAR QUALIFIED: 1987
- NHS POST: Consultant Obstetrician and Gynaecologist, Specialist in Maternal and Fetal Medicine, St Mary's Hospital NHS Trust.
- SPECIAL INTEREST: Medical complications of pregnancy, fetal medicine (ultrasound and prenatal diagnosis), labour and delivery.
- PRIVATE: Lindo Wing, St. Mary's Hospital, South Wharf Road, Paddington, London W2 1NY. Tel: 0171 886 1484 Fax: 0171 706 7302

Mr Geoffrey Trew MBBS MRCOG
- NHS POST: Consultant In Reproductive Medicine And Surgery, Hammersmith Hospital.
- SPECIAL INTEREST: Infertility, covering the full range of treatment options from open tubal microsurgery, laparoscopic surgery, hysteroscopic surgery through to all forms of assisted conception; IVF, ICSI, MESA and preimplantation diagnosis.
- PRIVATE: Sainsbury Wing, Hammersmith Hospital, Du Cane Road, London, W12 0HS. Tel: 0181 383 2372 Fax: 0181 383 2371

Obstetrics & Gynaecology. London

Mr Patrick Walker MD FRCOG
YEAR QUALIFIED: 1973
NHS POST: Consultant Gynaecologist Royal Free Hospital
SPECIAL INTEREST: Colposcopy and gynaecological cancer. Laser surgery
PRIVATE: 78 Harley Street, London W1N 1AE.
Tel: 0171 637 4312

Mr Charles Wright MA MB BChir FRCOG
YEAR QUALIFIED: 1968
NHS POST: Consultant, Hillingdon Hospital.
SPECIAL INTEREST: General and high risk obstetrics; general gynaecology.
PRIVATE: 152 Harley Street, London W1N 1HH.
Tel: 0171 935 2477 Fax: 0181 810 5098

Middlesex

Mr E A Dermot Manning MBBS FRCOG
YEAR QUALIFIED: 1974
NHS POST: Consultant Obstetrician & Gynaecologist, Central Middlesex Hospital NHS Trust.
SPECIAL INTEREST: Colposcopy; minimal access gynaecological surgery; gynaecological oncology.
PRIVATE: Clementine Churchill Hospital, Sudbury Hill, Harrow, Middlesex, HA1 3RX.
Tel: 0181 872 3838/3872 Fax: 0181 872 3871

Shropshire

Mr Andrew John S Tapp MBBS MRCOG
YEAR QUALIFIED: 1982
NHS POST: Consultant Obstetrician and Gynaecologist, Royal Shrewsbury Hospital.
SPECIAL INTEREST: Minimal access surgery; pelvic floor reconstruction; urogynaecology and high risk obstetrics.
PRIVATE: Shropshire Nuffield Hospital, Longden Road, Shrewsbury, Shropshire SY3 9DP.
Tel: 01743 353441 Fax: 01743 247575

Surrey

Mr Michael Booker MB ChB MRCOG
YEAR QUALIFIED: 1978
NHS POST: Consultant Obstetrician & Gynaecologist, Mayday University Hospital.
SPECIAL INTEREST: Infertility; assisted conception including IVF; reproductive medicine; endometriosis; fibroids; laparoscopic surgery; menopause & HRT; transvaginal scanning.
PRIVATE: Shirley Oaks Hospital, Poppy Lane, Shirley Oaks Village, Surrey, CR9 8AB.
Tel: 0181 657 6155 Fax: 0181 657 0755

Obstetrics & Gynaecology. Surrey

Mr Philip Toplis MB ChB FRCS FRCOG
- YEAR QUALIFIED: 1973
- NHS POST: Consultant Obstetrician and Gynaecologist, Frimley Park Hospital
- SPECIAL INTEREST: Urogynaecology; colposcopy; minimal access surgery; general gynaecology..
- PRIVATE: Parkside Suite, Frimley Park Hospital, Portsmouth Road, Frimley, Camberley, Surrey GU16 5UJ.
 BUPA Hospital Clare Park, Crondall Lane, Crondall, Farnham, Surrey GU10 5XX. Tel: Appointments - 01252 615886 Fax: 01252 629426
 Windmill House, Hagley Road, Fleet, Hampshire GU13 8LH. Tel: 01252 615886 Fax: 01252 629426

Tyne & Wear

Miss Maureen Dalton MRCS LRCP MBBS FRCOG
- YEAR QUALIFIED: 1976
- NHS POST: Consultant in Obstetrics and Gynaecology, Sunderland Royal Hospital.
- SPECIAL INTEREST: Gynaecology - infertility and gynaecological endocrinology.
- PRIVATE: Hillside Lodge, Tunstall Road, Sunderland, Tyne & Wear SR3 1AA. Tel: 0191 528 9259 Fax: 0191 528 5789

West Sussex

Mr Zaky H Z Ibrahim MRCOG ChM
- YEAR QUALIFIED: 1979
- SPECIAL INTEREST: Obstetrics & gynaecology with special interest in infertility.
- PRIVATE: The Sherburne Hospital, 78 Broyle Road, Chichester, West Sussex PO19 4BE. Tel: 01243 530 600

Mr Richard J D Pyper FRCS(Ed) MRCOG
- YEAR QUALIFIED: 1978
- NHS POST: Consultant Obstetrician & Gynaecologist, Worthing & Southlands Hospitals NHS Trust.
- SPECIAL INTEREST: Female incontinence and prolapse; hysteroscopy and hysteroscopic surgery.
- PRIVATE: Goring Hall Hospital, Bodiam Avenue, Goring-By-Sea, West Sussex BN12 4UX. Tel: 01903 700 775 Fax: 01903 700 782
 Hareswith House, West Chiltington Road, Storrington, West Sussex RH20 4BP. Tel: 01903 740 670 Fax: 01903 745 788

Oncology

East Sussex

Dr George P Deutsch FRCP FRCR
YEAR QUALIFIED: 1967
NHS POST: Consultant Clinical Oncologist, Royal Sussex County Hospital.
SPECIAL INTEREST: Breast; head and neck; urological and gastro-intestinal malignancy.
PRIVATE: Hove Nuffield Hospital, 55 New Church Road, Hove, East Sussex BN3 4BG.
Tel: 01273 720217 Fax: 01273 220919

Kent

Dr David Pickering MBBS MRCP FRCR
NHS POST: Consultant Clinical Oncologist Mid Kent Oncology Centre
SPECIAL INTEREST: Breast Cancer; Gastro-intestinal Cancer; Gynaecological Cancer.
PRIVATE: Nuffield Hospital Tunbridge Wells, Kingswood Road, Tunbridge Wells, Kent TN2 4UL.
Tel: /Fax 01892 618977
Somerfield Hospital, 63-77 London Road, Maidstone, Kent, ME16 0DU.
Tel: /Fax 01892 618977 (Secretary)

London

Dr Ronald Beaney BSc MB ChB FRCP FRCR MD
YEAR QUALIFIED: 1974
NHS POST: St Thomas' Hospital, London. 0171 928 9292.
SPECIAL INTEREST: Neuro-oncology; genitourinary and gynaecological tumours.
PRIVATE: Radiotherapy Department, Cromwell Hospital, Cromwell Road, London SW5 0TU.
Tel: 0171 460 5626 Fax: 0171 460 5622

Dr Peter Blake MBBS BSc MD FRCR
YEAR QUALIFIED: 1976
NHS POST: Consultant Clinical Oncologist, Royal Marsden Hospital, London.
SPECIAL INTEREST: Gynaecological cancer especially radiotherapy and brachytherapy.
PRIVATE: Royal Marsden Hospital, Fulham Road, London, SW3 6JJ.
Tel: 0171 808 2581 Fax: 0171 349 0786

Dr Christopher H Collis MD FRCP FRCR
NHS POST: Consultant & Honorary Senior Lecturer, Royal Free Hospital.
SPECIAL INTEREST: Radiotherapy and general oncology including breast, gastro intestinal, gynaecological, endocrine, head & neck and lymphomas.
PRIVATE: Royal Free Hospital, Pond Street, Hampstead, London, NW3 2QG.
Tel: 0171 794 0500 ext 3157/4476. Direct line: 0171 830 2396 Fax: 0171 830 2968

Oncology. London

Dr Iain W F Hanham FRCP FRCR
NHS POST: Consultant Radiotherapy & Oncology, Charing Cross Hospital
SPECIAL INTEREST: Breast cancer; head and neck cancer; urological cancer - gastrointestinal cancer.
PRIVATE: Dept. Radiotherapy & Clinical Oncology, Cromwell Hospital, Cromwell Road, London SW5 OTU. Tel: 0171 460 5626/7 Fax: 0171 460 5555

Dr Ian Hann MD FRCP FRCP(Glas) FRCPath
NHS POST: Consultant Paediatric Haematologist, Great Ormond Street Childrens Hospital
SPECIAL INTEREST: Paediatric haematology and oncology; childhood leukaemia and lymphoma; childhood blood and bleeding disorders; haemophilia.
PRIVATE: Great Ormond Street Hospital for Children NHS Trust, Great Ormond Street, London WC1N 3JH. Tel: 0171 829 8831 Fax: 0171 813 8410
E-mail: Ian.Hann@gosh-tr.nthames.nhs.uk

Dr Len Price MD(Lond) MRCP(UK)
SPECIAL INTEREST: Breast Cancer, Stem cell transplant therapy. UK representative, International Advisory Council, New York Chemotherapy Foundation.
PRIVATE: 147 Harley Street, London, W1N IDL. Tel: 0171 486 2545 Fax: 0171 935 6324

Dr Pat Price MB BChir MA MD FRCP FRCR
NHS POST: Consultant Oncologist & Reader in Clinical Oncology Hammersmith Hospital
SPECIAL INTEREST: Gastrointestinal cancer.
PRIVATE: Sainsbury Wing, Hammersmith Hospital, Du Cane Road, London W12 0NN. Tel: 0181 383 3357 Fax: 0181 383 1532

Dr Maurice L Slevin MBChB MD FRCP
YEAR QUALIFIED: 1973
NHS POST: Consultant Medical Oncologist, St. Bartholomew's Hospital, London.
SPECIAL INTEREST: GI oncology; gynae oncology; breast cancer.
PRIVATE: 149 Harley Street, London W1N 1HG. Tel: 0171 224 0685 Fax: 0171 224 1722

Dr Margaret F Spittle MSc FRCP FRCR
YEAR QUALIFIED: 1963
NHS POST: Consultant Clinical Oncologist Middlesex Hospital
SPECIAL INTEREST: Head & neck, breast, skin, and AIDS related cancers; general oncology.
PRIVATE: The Harley Street Clinic, 35 Weymouth Street, London W1N 4BJ. Tel: 0171 880 9090
The Cromwell Hospital, RT Dept, Cromwell Road, London, SW5. Tel: 0171 380 9090 Fax: 0171 436 0160

Middlesex

Dr Robert Glynne-Jones BA MB BS FRCP FRCR
- YEAR QUALIFIED: 1978
- NHS POST: Consultant, Mount Vernon Hospital.
- SPECIAL INTEREST: Gastrointestinal and colorectal cancer; the use of synchronous chemotherapy and radiation.
- PRIVATE: The Cancer Centre, Mount Vernon Hospital, Northwood, Middlesex, HA6 2RN. Tel: 01923 844012

Ophthalmology

Avon

Mr Jonathan Luck FRCS FRCOphth
YEAR QUALIFIED: 1985
NHS POST: Consultant Ophthalmologist and Clinical Director, The Royal United Hospital.
SPECIAL INTEREST: Small incision 'Phako'; cataract surgery under topical anaesthesia.
PRIVATE: The Bath Clinic, Claverton Down Road, Combe Down, Bath BA2 7BR.
Tel: 01225 835555 Fax: 01225 840708

Mr Michael Potts PhD FRCS FRCOphth
YEAR QUALIFIED: 1981
NHS POST: Consultant Ophthalmic Surgeon, Bristol Eye Hospital.
SPECIAL INTEREST: Cataracts; oculoplastics.
PRIVATE: 2 Clifton Park, Clifton, Bristol, BS8 3BS.
Tel: 0117 973 5904 Fax: 0117 973 0887

Bedfordshire

Mr ffolliott Francis Fisher FRCS FRCOphth
NHS POST: Consultant Ophthalmologist, Bedford.
SPECIAL INTEREST: Cataract surgery (phacoemulsification).
PRIVATE: The Manor Hospital, Biddenham, Bedford, Bedfordshire MK40 4AW.
Tel: 01234 364252 Fax: 01234 772423 E-mail: ffollalulu@compuserve.com

Birmingham

Mr Peter McDonnell FRCP FRCS FRCOphth DO
YEAR QUALIFIED: 1978
NHS POST: Consultant Ophthalmic Surgeon, Birmingham and Midland Eye Centre, Birmingham.
SPECIAL INTEREST: Small incision cataract surgery; corneal surgery including transplant surgery and refractive surgery; external eye disease including ocular surface problems and general ophthalmology.
PRIVATE: 38 Harborne Road, Edgbaston, Birmingham B15 3HE.
Tel: 0121 455 8066 Fax: 0121 454 7960

Buckinghamshire

Mr Nicholas Lee BsC MB BS FRCS FRCOphth
YEAR QUALIFIED: 1983
NHS POST: Consultant Ophthalmologist, Hillingdon and Western Eye Hospitals.
SPECIAL INTEREST: Diabetic, age related macular degeneration and other medical retinal diseases of the eye. Small incision cataract surgery.
PRIVATE: Harrold's Medical Eye Centre, 4 Station Approach, Gerrards Cross, Buckinghamshire SL9 8PP. Tel: Appointments - 01895 835 144 or 0800 0266344
E-mail: nicklee@leemedical.co.uk

Cheshire

Mr Nicholas P Jones BSc MB ChB FRCS FRCOphth
YEAR QUALIFIED: 1981
NHS POST: Consultant Ophthalmic Surgeon, Manchester Royal Eye Hospital.
SPECIAL INTEREST: Cataract and anterior segment microsurgery; uveitis and intraocular inflammatory disease; trauma.
PRIVATE: 3 Ridgeway, Wilmslow, Cheshire SK9 2BP.
Tel: 0161 276 5582 Fax: 0161 272 6618

Mr Brian Leatherbarrow BSc MB ChB DO FRCS FRCOphth
YEAR QUALIFIED: 1982
NHS POST: Consultant Ophthalmic Surgeon, Manchester Royal Eye Hospital, Manchester.
SPECIAL INTEREST: Oculoplastic, orbital and lacrimal surgery - ptosis, eyelid tumour and reconstruction hydroxyapatite implants, brow lifts, blepharoplasty, thyroid eye disease, entropion, ectropion, watering eye, phacoemulsification (cataracts).
PRIVATE: The Cheshire Eye Clinic, 75 Alderley Road, Wilmslow, Cheshire SK9 1PA.
Tel: 01625 531000 Fax: 01625 535533

Mr Anthony Peter Moriarty MA MB BChir FRCS FRCOphth
YEAR QUALIFIED: 1983
NHS POST: Consultant Ophthalmologist/Cataract Surgeon, Stepping Hill Hospital, Stockport.
SPECIAL INTEREST: Micro-incision cataract and laser surgery; glaucoma and squint surgery; surgical and laser treatment of cataract and refractive errors (astigmatism, short and long sightedness); eyelid surgery.
PRIVATE: Highfield House, 442 Buxton Road, Stockport, Cheshire SK2 7JB.
Tel: 0161 483 9512 Fax: 0161 487 3492
Alexandra Hospital, Mill Lane, Cheadle, Cheshire SK8 2PX.
Tel: 0161 428 3656
Regency Hospital, West Street, Macclesfield, Cheshire SK11 8DW.
Tel: 01625 501150
Knutsford Cataract Clinic Woodvale Clinic, The Lodge, Toft Road, Knutsford, Cheshire WA16 9SS. Tel: 01565 632889 Fax: 01565 632889

Devon

Mr Peter Reginald Simcock MB ChB DO FRCSEng MRCP(UK) FRCOphth
YEAR QUALIFIED: 1983
NHS POST: Consultant, Royal Devon and Exeter Hospital.
SPECIAL INTEREST: Cataract surgery; vitreoretinal surgery; oculoplastic surgery.
PRIVATE: 4 Manston Terrace, Exeter, Devon EX2 4NP.
Tel: 01392 434141 Fax: 01392 435301

Dorset

Mr David Dorrell FRCS FRCOphth MBBS
YEAR QUALIFIED: 1965
NHS POST: Consultant Ophthalmologist, Royal Bournemouth Hospital.
SPECIAL INTEREST: Neuro-ophthalmology.
PRIVATE: Bournemouth Nuffield Consulting Rooms, 65 Lansdowne Road, Bournemouth, Dorset BH1 1RN. Tel: 01202 316555

Enfield Middlesex

Mr Rhodri D Daniel BSc FRCS DO
YEAR QUALIFIED: 1979
NHS POST: Consultant Ophthalmologist, Moorfields Eye Hospital NHS Trust.
SPECIAL INTEREST: General and medical ophthalmology. Excimer laser refractive surgery.
PRIVATE: Kings Oak Hospital, Chase Farm (North side), The Ridgeway, Enfield, Middlesex EN2 8SD. Tel: 0181 366 0036 Fax: 0181 366 0075

Essex

Mr Charles Claoué MA MD DO FRCS FRCOphth
NHS POST: Consultant Ophthalmic Surgeon, Whipps Cross Hospital and Havering Hospital.
SPECIAL INTEREST: Viral eye disease; corneal and refractive surgery; small incision cataract surgery (phakoemulsification). Consultations en Francais.
PRIVATE: BUPA Hartswood Hospital, Eagle Way, Brentwood, Essex, CM13 3LE.
Tel: 01277 232 525 Fax: 01277 200 128   Secretary Tel/Fax: 0181 852 8522. E-mail: eyes@dbcg.co.uk
Essex Nuffield Hospital, Shenfield Road, Brentwood, Essex, CM15 8EH.
Tel: 01277 263 363 Fax: 01277 201 158
The Roding Hospital, Roding Lane South, Redbridge, Ilford, Essex IG4 5PZ.
Tel: 0181 551 1100 Fax: 0181 551 6515

Ophthalmology. Essex.

Mr Reginald Daniel MBBS FRCS DO FRCOphth
- YEAR QUALIFIED: 1964
- NHS POST: Consultant St. Thomas' Hospital & Guy's Hospital
- SPECIAL INTEREST: Cataract; glaucoma; squint; corneal and lacrimal diseases.
- PRIVATE: Holly House Hospital, High Road, Buckhurst Hill, Essex, IG9 5HX.
  Tel: 0181 505 3311 Fax: 0181 506 1013

Mr Ivan Fawcett FRCS FRCOphth
- YEAR QUALIFIED: 1980
- NHS POST: Consultant Ophthalmic Surgeon, Princess Alexandra Hospital.
- SPECIAL INTEREST: Retina surgery; cataract surgery.
- PRIVATE: Holly House Hospital, High Road, Buckhurst Hill, Essex, IG9 5HX.
  Tel: 0181 505 3311

Mr Russell Pearson BSc MB BS MRCP FRCS FRCOphth
- YEAR QUALIFIED: 1980
- NHS POST: Consultant Ophthalmic Surgeon Southend, Basildon and Orsett Hospitals
- SPECIAL INTEREST: Small incision cataract; medical and surgical retina; glaucoma.
- PRIVATE: BUPA Hartswood Hospital, Eagle Way, Brentwood, Essex, CM13 3LE.
  Tel: 01277 232525 Fax: 01277 200128
  Essex Nuffield Hospital, Shenfield Road, Brentwood, Essex, CM15 8EH.
  Tel: 01277 263363 Fax: 01277 201158

Mr Hamish Towler MBChB MRCP FRCS(Ed) FRCOphth
- YEAR QUALIFIED: 1979
- NHS POST: Consultant Ophthalmology Whipps Cross Hospital, Whipps Cross Road, London E11 1NR
- SPECIAL INTEREST: Ocular inflammatory diseases; medical retina; vitreoretinal surgery; small incision cataract surgery.
- PRIVATE: BUPA Roding Hospital, Roding Lane South, Redbridge, Ilford, Essex IG4 5PZ.
  Tel: 0181 551 1100 Fax: 0181 551 6415
  Holly House Hospital, High Road, Buckhurst Hill, Essex, IG9 5HX.
  Tel: 0181 505 3311 Fax: 0181 506 1013

Glamorgan

Mr Manzoor S Hashmi MBBS DO FRCS FRCOphth
- YEAR QUALIFIED: 1964
- NHS POST: Consultant Ophthalmologist, Princess of Wales Hospital, Costy Road, Bridgend, CF31 1RQ.
- SPECIAL INTEREST: Cataract surgery, glaucoma and glaucoma surgery, squint surgery, corneal transplantation.
- PRIVATE: 69 Priory Oak, Brackla, Bridgend, Glamorgan CF31 2HZ.
  Tel: 01656 658574, 752100 (Bridgend Clinic) Fax: 01656 658574
  E-mail: m_h@talk21.com

Gloucestershire

Mr James Nairne MA MB BChir FRCOphth FRACS FRACO
YEAR QUALIFIED: 1976
NHS POST: Consultant Ophthalmic Surgeon, Gloucestershire Royal Hospital and Cheltenham General Hospital.
SPECIAL INTEREST: Minimally invasive small incision cataract surgery (phacoemulsification and intraocular lens); glaucoma - all forms of modern management including laser techniques and surgery.
PRIVATE: Winfield Hospital, Tewkesbury Road, Longford, Gloucester, Gloucestershire GL2 9EE.
Tel: 01452 331111 Fax: 01452 331200

Hertfordshire

Mr Ivan Fawcett FRCS FRCOphth
YEAR QUALIFIED: 1980
NHS POST: Consultant Ophthalmic Surgeon, Princess Alexandra Hospital.
SPECIAL INTEREST: Retina surgery; cataract surgery.
PRIVATE: The Rivers Hospital, High Wych Road, Sawbridgeworth, Hertfordshire CM21 6HH.
Tel: 01279 600 282 Fax: 01279 600 212

Kent

Mr Charles G.F. Munton FRCS FRCOphth MB ChB DO
YEAR QUALIFIED: 1960
SPECIAL INTEREST: Micro surgical cataract surgery; glaucoma; diabetic retinopathy; neuro-ophthalmology.
PRIVATE: 36 Marsham Street, Maidstone, Kent ME14 1HG.
Tel: 01622 756 038 Fax: 01622 756 038

Mr David Trew FRCS FRCOphth
YEAR QUALIFIED: 1983
NHS POST: Consultant Ophthalmic Surgeon, Farnborough Hospital, Orpington, Kent BR6 8ND.
Tel:01689 814407.
SPECIAL INTEREST: Small incision cataract surgery; Glaucoma.
PRIVATE: Sloane Hospital, 125 Albermarle Road, Beckenham, Kent BR3 5HS.
Tel: 0181 466 6911 Fax: 0181 464 1443
Chelsfield Park Hospital, Bucks Cross Road, Chelsfield, Kent, BR6 7RG.
Tel: 01689 877 855 Fax: 01689 837 439
Beadle House Clinic, London Road, Sevenoaks, Kent TN13 2JD.
Tel: 01732 741 641 Fax: 01734 455 919

Lancashire

Mr Annaswami Vijaykumar MBBS FRCS(E) FRCOphth DO
- YEAR QUALIFIED: 1972
- NHS POST: Consultant Ophthalmologist, Blackburn Royal Infirmary and Burnley General Hospital.
- SPECIAL INTEREST: Small incision phacoemulsification cataract surgery; glaucoma diagnosis and management including surgery, diabetic retinopathy and all general ophthalmology.
- PRIVATE: The Beardwood Hospital, Preston New Road, Blackburn, Lancashire BB2 7AE. Tel: 01254 56421 Fax: 01254 695032
Abbey Gisburn Park Hospital, Gisburn, Lancashire BB7 4HX. Tel: 01200 445693 Fax: 01200 445688

Leicestershire

Mr Gerald T Fahy MB MD FRCS(Ed) FRCOphth
- YEAR QUALIFIED: 1979
- NHS POST: Consultant Ophthalmologist, Leicester Royal Infirmary.
- SPECIAL INTEREST: Cataract surgery, corneal surgery, lid lacrimal and orbit surgery.
- PRIVATE: BUPA Hospital Leicester, Gartree Road, Oadby, Leicester, Leicestershire LE2 2FF.

London

Mr David Abrams MA(Oxon) DM FRCS FRCOphth
- SPECIAL INTEREST: Cataract & Lid Surgery
- PRIVATE: Hospital of St. John & St. Elizabeth, 60 Grove End Road, St Johns Wood, London, NW8 9NH. Tel: 0171 286 5126, Direct line-0171 266 1797 Fax: 0171 603 8807

Mr James Acheson BM MRCP(UK) DO(RCS) FRCS(Glas) FRCOphth
- YEAR QUALIFIED: 1980
- NHS POST: Consultant Ophthalmologist, National Hospital For Neurology And Neurosurgery and Moorfields Eye Hospital
- SPECIAL INTEREST: Neuro-ophthalmology and strabismus; general ophthalmology.
- PRIVATE: 149 Harley Street, London W1N 2DE. Tel: 0171 486 1592 Fax: 0171 486 1592

Mr G William Aylward MB BChir FRCS FRCOphth MD
- NHS POST: Consultant Ophthalmic Surgeon, Moorfields Eye Hospital, London.
- SPECIAL INTEREST: Medical and surgical retina (vitreoretinal surgery).
- PRIVATE: 114 Harley Street, London, W1N 1AG. Tel: 0171 935 1565 Fax: 0171 224 1752 E-mail: bill@promed.compulink.co.uk
Lower Corridor Suite, Moorfields Eye Hospital, City Road, London, EC1V 2PD. Tel: 0171 566 2604 Fax: 0171 566 2603 E-mail: bill@promed.compulink.co.uk

Ophthalmology. London

Mr John D L Beare MRCP FRCS FRCOphth
- YEAR QUALIFIED: 1976
- NHS POST: Consultant Ophthalmologist, Kingston Hospital NHS Trust (The Royal Eye Unit).
- SPECIAL INTEREST: Cataract surgery; glaucoma; eyelid surgery including blepharoplasty; lacrimal drainage surgery; general ophthalmology problems.
- PRIVATE: Parkside Hospital, 53 Parkside, Wimbledon, London, SW19 5NX.
  Tel: 0181 971 8000 Fax: 0181 971 8002
  148 Harley Street, London W1N 1AH.
  Tel: 0171 935 1900

Mr James Chesterton MA FRCS FRCOphth DO
- YEAR QUALIFIED: 1961
- NHS POST: Consultant Ophthalmic Surgeon, Greenwhich District Hospital.
- SPECIAL INTEREST: Cataracts; glaucoma; neuro-ophthalmology and squints.
- PRIVATE: Consulting Rooms, BMI Blackheath Hospital, 40-42 Lee Terrace, London, SE3 9UD.
  Tel: 0181 318 7722 Fax: 0181 318 2542
  148 Harley Street, London W1N 1AH.
  Tel: 0171 935 1900 Fax: 0171 226 0726

Mr Charles Claoué MA MD DO FRCS FRCOphth
- NHS POST: Consultant Ophthalmic Surgeon, Whipps Cross Hospital and Havering Hospital.
- SPECIAL INTEREST: Viral eye disease; corneal and refractive surgery; small incision cataract surgery (phakoemulsification). Consultations en Francais.
- PRIVATE: The Blackheath Hospital, 40-42 Lee Terrace, Blackheath, London, SE3 9UD.
  Tel: 0181 318 7722 Fax: 0181 318 2542
  Cromwell Hospital, Cromwell Road, London SW5 OTU.
  Tel: 0171 460 2000 Fax: 0171 460 5555

Mr Roger Coakes FRCS FRCOphth
- YEAR QUALIFIED: 1967
- NHS POST: Consultant Ophthalmic Surgeon, King's College Hospital.
- SPECIAL INTEREST: Glaucoma and cataract surgery.
- PRIVATE: 148 Harley Street, London W1N 1AH.
  Tel: 0171 935 1207 Fax: 0181 761 7229
  Guthrie Clinic, King's College Hospital, Denmark Hill, London, SE5 9RS.
  Tel: 0171 346 3572 Fax: 0171 738 6089

Mr Reginald Daniel MBBS FRCS DO FRCOphth
- YEAR QUALIFIED: 1964
- NHS POST: Consultant St. Thomas' Hospital & Guy's Hospital
- SPECIAL INTEREST: Cataract; glaucoma; squint; corneal and lacrimal diseases.
- PRIVATE: 152 Harley Street, London W1N 1HH.
  Tel: 0171 935 3834 Fax: 0171 224 2574
  Suite 101, Emblem House London Bridge Hospital, 27 Tooley Street, London, SE1 2PR.
  Tel: 0171 403 4884 xt 2106 Fax: 0171 407 3162

Ophthalmology. London

Mr Rhodri D Daniel BSc FRCS DO
- YEAR QUALIFIED: 1979
- NHS POST: Consultant Ophthalmologist, Moorfields Eye Hospital NHS Trust.
- SPECIAL INTEREST: General and medical ophthalmology. Excimer laser refractive surgery.
- PRIVATE: John Saunders Suite, Moorfields Eye Hospital, City Road, London, EC1V 2PD.
Tel: 0171 566 2829 Fax: 0171 566 2608
Highgate Private Hospital, 17 View Road, Highgate, London N6 4DJ.
Tel: 0181 341 5163 Fax: 0181 342 8347

Dr David Darby MB BS MRCS LRCP DO MRCOphth
- YEAR QUALIFIED: 1960
- NHS POST: Consultant Ophthalmologist, Moorfields Eye Hospital.
- SPECIAL INTEREST: General and medical ophthalmology; contact lenses.
- PRIVATE: 73 Harley Street, London W1N 1DE.
Tel: 0171 487 4025 Fax: 0171 224 6381

Mr John K G Dart MA DM FRCS FRCOphth
- YEAR QUALIFIED: 1976
- NHS POST: Consultant Ophthalmic Surgeon, Moorfields Eye Hospital, London.
- SPECIAL INTEREST: Corneal & external disease; inflammatory and infectious disease; corneal graft surgery; small incision cataract surgery; anterior segment reconstruction.
- PRIVATE: 8 Upper Wimpole Street, London W1M 7TD.
Tel: 0171 486 2257 Fax: 0171 487 3764 E-mail: jdart@dial.pipex.com

Miss Clare Davey MB BS BSc FRCS FCOphth
- YEAR QUALIFIED: 1978
- NHS POST: Consultant, Royal Free Hospital and Whittington Hospital, London.
- SPECIAL INTEREST: Cataract; medical retina.
- PRIVATE: Hospital of St. John & St. Elizabeth, 60 Grove End Road, St Johns Wood, London, NW8 9NH. Tel: 0171 286 5126/266 2316

Mr Sheraz M Daya MD FACP FACS FRCS(Ed.)
- YEAR QUALIFIED: 1984
- NHS POST: Director & Consultant Ophthalmic Surgeon, Corneo Plastic Unit, Queen Victoria Hospital.
- SPECIAL INTEREST: Cornea; corneal transplantation; small incision cataract; Keratorefractive surgery & laser surgery (LASIK)
- PRIVATE: 57 Harley Street, London W1N 1DD.
Tel: 0171 580 7660 Fax: 0171 580 7547

Mr Michael Falcon MA MB BChir MRCP FRCS FRCOphth
- NHS POST: Consultant Ophthalmologist, St. Thomas Hospital.
- SPECIAL INTEREST: Cornea; cataract; glaucoma.
- PRIVATE: Private Consulting Rooms, 25 Wimpole Street, London W1M 7AD.
Tel: 0171 580 7199 Fax: 0171 580 6855

Ophthalmology. London

Mr Timothy Fallon MD FRCS FRCOphth
- NHS POST: Consultant Ophthalmologist Central Middlesex Hospital
- SPECIAL INTEREST: Diabetes. Cataract. Retinal Detachment.
- PRIVATE: Hospital of St. John & St. Elizabeth, 60 Grove End Road, St Johns Wood, London, NW8 9NH. Tel: 0171 286 5126
  The Garden Hospital, 46-50 Sunny Gardens Road, Hendon, London, NW4 1RX.
  Tel: 0181 203 0111 Fax: 0181 203 4343

Mrs Veronica M G Ferguson MB BS FRCS FRCOphth
- YEAR QUALIFIED: 1983
- NHS POST: Consultant Ophthalmic Surgeon, Charing Cross Hospital, London.
- SPECIAL INTEREST: Ophthalmic surgeon with a special interest in cataract and strabismus surgery.
- PRIVATE: 115a Harley Street, London, W1N 1DG.
  Tel: 0171 487 5581 Fax: 0171 486 0211
  King Edward VII Hospital, Beaumont Street, London, W1N 2AA.
  Tel: 0171 486 4411

Miss Linda Anne Ficker BSc FRCS FRCOphth
- YEAR QUALIFIED: 1977
- NHS POST: Consultant, Moorfields Eye Hospital.
- SPECIAL INTEREST: Cataract and small incision phacoemulsification; corneal and ocular surface disease and trauma; corneal transplantation and excimer laser surgery including LASIK for myopia and hypermetropia.
- PRIVATE: John Saunders Suite, Moorfields Eye Hospital, City Road, London, EC1V 2PD.
  Tel: 0171 566 2599 Fax: 0171 566 2608

Mr Zdenek J Gregor FRCS FCOphth
- YEAR QUALIFIED: 1971
- NHS POST: Consultant Surgeon, Moorfields Eye Hospital.
- SPECIAL INTEREST: Vitreo-retinal surgery; macular disorders; diabetic retinopathy.
- PRIVATE: 94 Harley Street, London, W1N 1AF.
  Tel: 0171 935 0777 Fax: 0171 935 6860 E-mail: zjgregor@aol.com

Mr Philip G Hykin BSc FRCS FRCOphth
- YEAR QUALIFIED: 1984
- NHS POST: Consultant Ophthalmologist, Moorfields Eye Hospital, London.
- SPECIAL INTEREST: Retinal disease, including diabetic retinopathy and macular degeneration; small incision cataract surgery, especially if complicated by diabetic retinopathy, retinal disorders and uveitis.
- PRIVATE: 149 Harley Street, London W1N 2DE.
  Tel: 0171 935 4444 Fax: 0171 486 3782

Mr Jonathan Jagger FRCS DO FRCOphth
- NHS POST: Consultant Ophthalmic Surgeon, Royal Free Hospital.
- SPECIAL INTEREST: Cataract surgery; diabetic retinopathy; lasers; general ophthalmology.
- PRIVATE: 149 Harley Street, London W1N 2DE.
  Tel: 0171 935 4444 Fax: 0171 935 3934

Ophthalmology. London

Mr Paul Kinnear MBBS FRCS FRCOphth
- YEAR QUALIFIED: 1975
- NHS POST: Consultant Ophthalmologist, Hammersmith Hospital NHS Trust.
- SPECIAL INTEREST: Cataract surgery; diabetic eye disease; paediatric ophthalmology.
- PRIVATE: 62 Wimpole Street, London W1M 7DE.
Tel: 0171 935 5416 Fax: 0171 460 5934
Cromwell Hospital, Cromwell Road, London SW5 OTU.
Tel: 0171 460 5700 Fax: 0171 460 5943

Mr Nicholas Lee BsC MB BS FRCS FRCOphth
- YEAR QUALIFIED: 1983
- NHS POST: Consultant Ophthalmologist, Hillingdon and Western Eye Hospitals.
- SPECIAL INTEREST: Diabetic, age related macular degeneration and other medical retinal diseases of the eye. Small incision cataract surgery.
- PRIVATE: The Western Eye Hospital Private Consulting Rooms, Marylebone Road, London NW1 5YE. Tel: 0800 0266344 Fax: 01895 835404 E-mail: nicklee@leemedical.co.uk

Mr Timothy J K Leonard MRCP FRCS FRCOphth
- NHS POST: Consultant Ophthalmic Surgeon Charing Cross Hospital
- SPECIAL INTEREST: Cataract by phacoemulsification; glaucoma; strabismus; neuro-retina.
- PRIVATE: The London Clinic, 149 Harley Street, London, W1N 2DE.
Tel: 0171 935 4444 Fax: 0171 486 3782

Mr Dominic McHugh MBBS DO FRCS FRCOphth MD
- NHS POST: Consultant Ophthalmologist, King's College Hospital.
- SPECIAL INTEREST: Cataract; retinal laser therapy; retinal surgery.
- PRIVATE: 73 Harley Street, London W1N 1DE.
Tel: 0171 935 5874 or 07000 DMcHUGH(362484). Fax: 0171 224 5210

Mr Clive Migdal MD FRCS FRCOphth
- NHS POST: Consultant Ophthalmologist, The Western Eye Hospital (St. Mary's NHS Trust).
- SPECIAL INTEREST: Glaucoma and cataracts.
- PRIVATE: The London Clinic, 149 Harley Street, London, W1N 2DE.
Tel: 0171 935 4444 Fax: 0171 486 3782

Dr Gordon Plant MA(Cantab) MD(Cantab) FRCP
- YEAR QUALIFIED: 1977
- NHS POST: Consultant Neurologist National Hospital for Neurology & Neurosurgery, Moorfields Eye Hospital, St. Thomas' Hospital
- SPECIAL INTEREST: Visual disorders; neuro-ophthalmology.
- PRIVATE: Private Consulting Rooms, National Hospital for Neurology and Neurosurgery, Queen Square, London, WC1N 3BG. Tel: 0171 829 8741 Fax: 0171 833 8658

Mr Paul Rosen BSc(Hons) MB ChB FRCS FRCOphth
- YEAR QUALIFIED: 1980
- NHS POST: Consultant Ophthalmic Surgeon, Oxford Eye Hospital and Radcliffe Infirmary, Oxford.
- SPECIAL INTEREST: Cataract and refractive surgery; trauma; vitreoretinal surgery.
- PRIVATE: Highgate Ophthalmologists, Highgate Private Clinic, 17-19 View Road, Highgate, London, N6. Tel: 0181 341 5163 Fax: 0181 341 3771

Ophthalmology. London

Mr Chad K Rostron MBBS DO FRCS FRCOphth
YEAR QUALIFIED: 1975
NHS POST: Consultant Ophthalmologist St George's Hospital
SPECIAL INTEREST: Corneal transplantation including penetrating, lamellar, and epikeratoplasty, for keratoconus etc. Keratorefractive surgery for myopia or hypermetropia, excimer laser in situ keratomileusis (LASIK), and intraocular contact lens (ICL). Cataract surgery by phakoemulsification.
PRIVATE: 10 Harley Street, London W1N 1AA.
Tel: 0171 483 4921 Fax: 0171 467 8312 E-mail: rostron@sghms.ac.uk
Parkside Hospital, 53 Parkside, Wimbledon, London, SW19 5NX.
Tel: 0181 971 8026 Fax: 0181 971 8002 E-mail: rostron@sghms.ac.uk

Mr Edmund Schulenburg FRCS FRCOphth
YEAR QUALIFIED: 1980
NHS POST: Consultant Ophthalmic Surgeon St. Mary's Hospital and Hammersmith Hospital
SPECIAL INTEREST: Vitreo-retinal, diabetic eye disease. Small incision cataract surgery.
PRIVATE: 8 Upper Wimpole Street, London, W1M 7TD.
Tel: 0171 486 2257 Fax: 0171 487 3764

Mr David S I Taylor FRCOphth FRCPCH
NHS POST: Consultant Ophthalmologist, Great Ormond Street Hospital for Children.
SPECIAL INTEREST: Paediatric ophthalmology and strabismus.
PRIVATE: 234 Great Portland Street, London W1N 5PH.
Tel: 0171 935 7916 Fax: 0171 323 5430 E-mail: d.taylor@vissci.ion.ucl.ac.uk

Mr Hamish Towler MBChB MRCP FRCS(Ed) FRCOphth
YEAR QUALIFIED: 1979
NHS POST: Consultant Ophthalmology Whipps Cross Hospital, Whipps Cross Road, London E11 1NR
SPECIAL INTEREST: Ocular inflammatory diseases; medical retina; vitreoretinal surgery; small incision cataract surgery.
PRIVATE: 149 Harley Street, London W1N 2DE.
Tel: 0171 935 4444 Fax: 0171 486 3782

Mr Calver Townsend MB BS FRCS FRCOphth DO
YEAR QUALIFIED: 1967
NHS POST: Honorary Consultant Ophthalmic Surgeon The Western Eye Hospital & St. Mary's Hospital
SPECIAL INTEREST: Cataract surgery; laser treatment of diabetic retinopathy and vascular diseases of the retina.
PRIVATE: 114 Harley Street, London W1N 1AG.
Tel: 0171 935 1565 Fax: 0171 224 1752

Mr David M Watson FRCS FRCOphth
SPECIAL INTEREST: Cataract anterior segment surgery and glaucoma.
PRIVATE: 115A Harley Street, London W1N 1DG.
Tel: 0171 935 8922 Fax: 0171 486 0211

Ophthalmology. London

Mr Rodger Whitelocke MB BS PhD FRCS FRCOphth
- YEAR QUALIFIED: 1968
- NHS POST: Consultant Ophthalmic Surgeon, St. Bartholomew's Hospital and Royal Marsden Hospital.
- SPECIAL INTEREST: Cataract surgery; laser treatment of diabetic retinopathy; general ophthalmic surgery.
- PRIVATE: 152 Harley Street, London W1N 1HH.
  Tel: 0171 935 3834 Fax: 0171 224 2574

Mr Hugh Williams FRCS FRCOphth
- YEAR QUALIFIED: 1961
- NHS POST: Consultant Surgeon, Moorfields Eye Hospital, London.
- SPECIAL INTEREST: Cataract surgery and external eye disease.
- PRIVATE: 5 Harmont House, 20 Harley Street, London W1N 1AL.
  Tel: 0171 636 4406 Fax: 0171 636 5150

Mr Keith Williams FRCSC FACS FRCOphth MB BS MRCS LRCP
- SPECIAL INTEREST: Excimer laser treatments and small incision phaco. cataract surgery; LASIK
- PRIVATE: Laser Vision, 22 Harley Street, London W1N 2AP.
  Tel: 0171 580 1200 Fax: 0171 580 1201

Lothian

Dr Alistair Adams MBCB BSc DO FRISEI
- YEAR QUALIFIED: 1967
- NHS POST: Consultant Ophthalmic Surgeon, Princess Alexandra Eye Pavilion, Edinburgh.
- SPECIAL INTEREST: Cataract and lens implant surgery.
- PRIVATE: Moray Consulting Rooms, 14 Moray Place, Edinburgh, Lothian FH3 6DT.
  Tel: 0131 225 8059 Fax: 0131 225 6749

Manchester

Mr Christopher Dodd FRCS FRCOphth
- NHS POST: Consultant Ophthalmologist, Manchester Royal Eye Hospital.
- SPECIAL INTEREST: Cataract, glaucoma, vitreo-retinal problems.
- PRIVATE: Russell House, Russell Road, Whalley Range, Manchester M16 8AR.
  Tel: 0161 862 9564 Fax: 0161 232 2588
  8 Old Hall Road, Whitefield, Manchester M45 7QW.
  Tel: 0161 862 9564 Fax: 0161 232 2588

Mr Brian Leatherbarrow BSc MB ChB DO FRCS FRCOphth
- YEAR QUALIFIED: 1982
- NHS POST: Consultant Ophthalmic Surgeon, Manchester Royal Eye Hospital, Manchester.
- SPECIAL INTEREST: Oculoplastic, orbital and lacrimal surgery - ptosis, eyelid tumour and reconstruction hydroxyapatite implants, brow lifts, blepharoplasty, thyroid eye disease, entropion, ectropion, watering eye, phacoemulsification (cataracts).
- PRIVATE: BMI Victoria Park Hospital, Daisy Bank Road, Victoria Park, Manchester M14 5QH.
  Tel: 0161 257 2233 Fax: 0161 256 3128

Ophthalmology. Manchester

Mrs Joan L Noble MB ChB DO FRCSE FRCOphth
YEAR QUALIFIED: 1971
NHS POST: Consultant Ophthalmic and Orbital Surgeon, Manchester Royal Eye Hospital.
SPECIAL INTEREST: Orbital including thyroid eye disease; lacrimal and orbital disease; paediatric ophthalmology.
PRIVATE: BUPA Hospital, Russell Road, Whalley Range, Manchester M16 8AJ.
Tel: 0161 276 5524 Fax: 01565 722871

Merseyside

Mr Louis Clearkin ChM FRCS FRCOphth DO
YEAR QUALIFIED: 1978
NHS POST: Consultant Ophthalmic Surgeon, Arrowe Park Hospital, Wirral.
SPECIAL INTEREST: Cataract surgery; management of the complications of cataract surgery; macular degeneration; diabetic eye disease; medical retina; uveitis and inflammatory eye disease.
PRIVATE: BUPA Murrayfield Hospital, Holmwood Drive, Thingwall, Wirral, Merseyside L61 1AU.
Tel: 0151 604 7047 Fax: 0151 604 7152 E-mail: l.clearkin@liverpool.ac.uk

Middlesex

Mr Nicholas Lee BsC MB BS FRCS FRCOphth
YEAR QUALIFIED: 1983
NHS POST: Consultant Ophthalmologist, Hillingdon and Western Eye Hospitals.
SPECIAL INTEREST: Diabetic, age related macular degeneration and other medical retinal diseases of the eye. Small incision cataract surgery.
PRIVATE: The Hillingdon Consulting Rooms, Pield Heath Road, Hillingdon, Middlesex UB8 3NN.
Tel: 01895 835144 or 0800 0266344 E-mail: nicklee@leemedical.co.uk
The Clementine Churchill Hospital, Sudbury Hill, Harrow, Middlesex, HA1 3RX.
Tel: 0800 0266344 E-mail: nicklee@leemedical.co.uk
Bishops Wood Private Hospital, Rickmansworth Road, Northwood, Middlesex HA6 2JW. Tel: 0800 0266344 Fax: 01895 835404 E-mail: nicklee@leemedical.co.uk

Mr Calver Townsend MB BS FRCS FRCOphth DO
YEAR QUALIFIED: 1967
NHS POST: Honorary Consultant Ophthalmic Surgeon The Western Eye Hospital & St. Mary's Hospital
SPECIAL INTEREST: Cataract surgery; laser treatment of diabetic retinopathy and vascular diseases of the retina.
PRIVATE: Northwood Consulting Rooms, 25B Green Lane, Northwood, Middlesex, HA6 2UZ.
Tel: 01923 826 948 Fax: 01923 835 794

North Yorkshire

Mr David Ivor Bowen MB BChir FRCS(Eng) FRCS(Edin) FRCophth
YEAR QUALIFIED: 1961
NHS POST: Consultant Ophthalmic Surgeon, Harrogate District Hospital.
SPECIAL INTEREST: Cataract and glaucoma.
PRIVATE: Duchy Nuffield Hospital, Queens Road, Harrogate, North Yorkshire HG2 0HF.
Tel: 01423 567136

Mr Robert Taylor MBBS FRCS FRCOphth
YEAR QUALIFIED: 1985
NHS POST: Consultant Ophthalmologist, York District Hospital.
SPECIAL INTEREST: Cataract; adult ocular motility; strabismus; paediatric ophthalmology.
PRIVATE: Purey Cust Nuffield Hospital, Precentors Court, York, North Yorkshire YO1 2EL.
Tel: 01904 641571 Fax: 01904 453397

Oxfordshire

Professor Gordon J Johnson MD BChir FRCS(C) FRCOphth
YEAR QUALIFIED: 1960
NHS POST: Honorary Consultant, Moorfields Eye Hospital.
SPECIAL INTEREST: Glaucoma; external eye disease; general ophthalmology.
PRIVATE: Felstead House, 23 Banbury Road, Oxford, Oxon OX2 6NX.
Tel: 01869 35082; 01865 515036

Mr Paul Rosen BSc(Hons) MB ChB FRCS FRCOphth
YEAR QUALIFIED: 1980
NHS POST: Consultant Ophthalmic Surgeon, Oxford Eye Hospital and Radcliffe Infirmary, Oxford.
SPECIAL INTEREST: Cataract and refractive surgery; trauma; vitreoretinal surgery.
PRIVATE: Felstead House, 23 Banbury Road, Oxford, Oxon OX2 6NX.
Tel: 01865 513483 Fax: 01865 510238

Somerset

Mr Kim Neal Hakin MB BS FRCS FRCOphth
YEAR QUALIFIED: 1983
NHS POST: Consultant Ophthalmic Surgeon, Musgrove Park Hospital, Taunton.
SPECIAL INTEREST: Cataract surgery; oculoplastic and lacrimal disorders; skin laser resurfacing and cosmetic eyelid surgery.
PRIVATE: Somerset Nuffield Hospital, Staplegrove Elm, Taunton, Somerset TA2 6AN.
Tel: 01823 286991 Fax: 01823 338951

Surrey

Mr John D L Beare MRCP FRCS FRCOphth
- YEAR QUALIFIED: 1976
- NHS POST: Consultant Ophthalmologist, Kingston Hospital NHS Trust (The Royal Eye Unit).
- SPECIAL INTEREST: Cataract surgery; glaucoma; eyelid surgery including blepharoplasty; lacrimal drainage surgery; general ophthalmology problems.
- PRIVATE: Ashtead Hospital, The Warren, Ashtead, Surrey KT21 2SB.
  Tel: 01372 276 161 Fax: 01372 278 704
  St. Anthony's Hospital, London Road, North Cheam, Surrey, SM3 9DW.
  Tel: 0181 337 6691 Fax: 0181 337 0816

Mr Roger Coakes FRCS FRCOphth
- YEAR QUALIFIED: 1967
- NHS POST: Consultant Ophthalmic Surgeon, King's College Hospital.
- SPECIAL INTEREST: Glaucoma and cataract surgery.
- PRIVATE: Ashtead Hospital, The Warren, Ashtead, Surrey KT21 2SB.
  Tel: 01372 276161 Fax: 0181 761 7229

Mr Richard W Condon FRCS(Ed) FRCOphth
- YEAR QUALIFIED: 1973
- NHS POST: Consultant, St. Peter's Hospital, Chertsey. Royal Surrey Hospital, Guildford.
- SPECIAL INTEREST: Small incision cataract surgery; anterior segment surgery; glaucoma; cornea and general ophthalmology.
- PRIVATE: Guildford Nuffield Hospital, Stirling Road, Guildford, Surrey GU2 6RF.
  Tel: 01483 555800 Fax: 01483 555888
  Runnymede Hospital, Guildford Road, Ottershaw, Surrey, KT16 0RQ.
  Tel: 01932 872007 Fax: 01932 875433
  Woking Nuffield Hospital, Shores Road, Woking, Surrey, GU21 4BY.
  Tel: 01483 763511

Mr Charles Cory FRCS FRCOphth
- SPECIAL INTEREST: Cataract surgery (Gatwick Park Hospital) and excimer refractive surgery. General ophthalmology including glaucoma and contact lenses (Private Practice).
- PRIVATE: The Cory Eye Clinic, 43 Alma Road, Reigate, Surrey RH2 0DN.
  Tel: 01737 247855 Fax: 01737 247855 E-mail: coryeye@mcmail.com

Mr Chad K Rostron MBBS DO FRCS FRCOphth
- YEAR QUALIFIED: 1975
- NHS POST: Consultant Ophthalmologist St George's Hospital
- SPECIAL INTEREST: Corneal transplantation including penetrating, lamellar, and epikeratoplasty, for keratoconus etc. Keratorefractive surgery for myopia or hypermetropia, excimer laser in situ keratomileusis (LASIK), and intraocular contact lens (ICL). Cataract surgery by phakoemulsification.
- PRIVATE: St. Anthony's Hospital, London Road, North Cheam, Surrey, SM3 9DW.
  Tel: 0181 337 6691 Fax: 0181 330 1037 E-mail: rostron@sghms.ac.uk

West Glamorgan

Mr Michael William Austin MB Bch FRCS FRCOphth
YEAR QUALIFIED: 1983
NHS POST: Consultant Ophthalmologist, Singleton Hospital, Swansea.
SPECIAL INTEREST: Small incision cataract surgery (phacoemulsification), glaucoma.
PRIVATE: Sancta Maria Hospital, Ffynone Road, Uplands, Swansea, West Glamorgan SA1 6DF. Tel: 01792 479040 Fax: 01792 641452

West Sussex

Mr Sheraz M Daya MD FACP FACS FRCS(Ed.)
YEAR QUALIFIED: 1984
NHS POST: Director & Consultant Ophthalmic Surgeon, Corneo Plastic Unit, Queen Victoria Hospital.
SPECIAL INTEREST: Cornea; corneal transplantation; small incision cataract; Keratorefractive surgery & laser surgery (LASIK)
PRIVATE: Corneo Plastic Unit & Eye Bank, Queen Victoria Hospital, Holtye Road, East Grinstead, West Sussex RH19 2PU. Tel: 01342 410 210 xt 217/216 Fax: 01342 317 907

Mr Robert Williams FRCS FRCOphth MRCP DO MBBS
SPECIAL INTEREST: Small incision cataract surgery.
PRIVATE: Southdowns House, 48 West Street, Storrington, West Sussex RH20 4EE.
Tel: 01903 742 266 Fax: 01903 746 395
Goring Hall Hospital, Bodiam Avenue, Goring-By-Sea, West Sussex BN12 5AT.
Tel: 01903 742 266 Fax: 01903 746 395
King Edward VII Hospital, Midhurst, West Sussex, GU29 0BL.
Tel: 01903 742 266 Fax: 01903 746 395
Sherburne Hospital, 78 Broyle Road, Chichester, West Sussex PO19 4BE.
Tel: 01903 742 266 Fax: 01903 746 395

West Yorkshire

Mr Annaswami Vijaykumar MBBS FRCS(E) FRCOphth DO
YEAR QUALIFIED: 1972
NHS POST: Consultant Ophthalmologist, Blackburn Royal Infirmary and Burnley General Hospital.
SPECIAL INTEREST: Small incision phacoemulsification cataract surgery; glaucoma diagnosis and management including surgery, diabetic retinopathy and all general ophthalmology.
PRIVATE: 'Logan House', Main Road, Eastburn, NR Keighley, W. Yorks BD20 7SJ.
Tel: 01535 633356 Fax: 01535 633356

Orthopaedics

Avon

Mr Christopher E Ackroyd MA MB BChir FRCS
YEAR QUALIFIED: 1967
NHS POST: Consultant Orthopaedic Surgeon, Avon Orthopaedic Centre, Southmead Hospital.
SPECIAL INTEREST: General orthopaedic surgery especially lower limb arthroplasty and special interest in knee surgery.
PRIVATE: 2 Clifton Park, Clifton, Bristol, BS8 3BS.
Tel: 0117 973 0958 Fax: 0117 923 7672

Mr John Howard Newman MB BChir FRCS
YEAR QUALIFIED: 1968
NHS POST: Consultant Orthopaedic Surgeon, Bristol Royal Infirmary and Southmead.
SPECIAL INTEREST: Knee and hip surgery; sports injuries.
PRIVATE: 2 Clifton Park, Clifton, Bristol, BS8 3BS.
Tel: 0117 973 4262 Fax: 0117 973 0887

Berkshire

Mr Jonathan R Jones BSc FRCS
YEAR QUALIFIED: 1977
NHS POST: Consultant Orthopaedic Surgeon, Heatherwood & Wexham Park Trust.
SPECIAL INTEREST: Lower limb joint replacement; revision surgery; arthroscopic surgery; surgery for lumbar disc prolapse; spinal stenosis.
PRIVATE: Consulting Rooms, 9 Beaumont Road, Windsor, Berks SL4 1HY.
Tel: 01753 854659 Fax: 01753 850128

Bristol

Mr Ian Geoffrey Winson MB ChB FRCS
YEAR QUALIFIED: 1978
NHS POST: Consultant ortopaedic and Trauma Surgeon, Avon Orthopaedic Centre, Bristol.
SPECIAL INTEREST: Foot and ankle surgery.
PRIVATE: St. Mary's Hospital, Upper Byron Place, Clifton, Bristol BS8 1JU.
Tel: 0117 987 2727 Fax: 01454 228779

Buckinghamshire

Mr John Lourie MA BM BCh PhD FRCS
YEAR QUALIFIED: 1973
NHS POST: Consultant Orthopaedic Surgeon, Milton Keynes Hospital.
SPECIAL INTEREST: Shoulder; upper limb; foot and joint replacement surgery.
PRIVATE: Saxon Clinic, Saxon Street, Eaglestone, Milton Keynes, Buckinghamshire MK6 5LR.
Tel: 01908 665533 Fax: 01908 608112; Secretary (T/F): 01908 642411

Cambridgeshire

Mr Richard Villar MB BS BSc(Hons) MA MS FRCS
YEAR QUALIFIED: 1977
NHS POST: Consultant Hip And Knee Surgeon Addenbrooke's Hospital
SPECIAL INTEREST: Hip and knee surgery.
PRIVATE: Cambridge Hip & Knee Unit, Cambridge Lea Hospital, 30 New Road, Impington, CB4 9EL. Tel: 01223 235888 Fax: 01223 235884 E-mail: rvillar@uk-consultants.co.uk

Devonshire

Mr David Jameson Evans FRCS FRCS(C)
YEAR QUALIFIED: 1965
SPECIAL INTEREST: Joint replacement surgery; arthroscopic surgery; foot surgery; childrens orthopaedics.
PRIVATE: 45 Denmark Road, Exeter, Devonshire EX1 1SQ.
Tel: 01392 256444 Fax: 01392 427872

East Sussex

Mr Barry Fearn TD MA MB BChir FRCS FRCS(Ed)
NHS POST: Honorary Consultant Orthopaedic And Accident Surgeon, Royal Sussex County Hospital, Brighton And Princess Royal Hospital, Haywards Heath.
SPECIAL INTEREST: Hand and upper limb - open and arthroscopic rheumatoid surgery; knee surgery - open and arthroscopic; hip and knee replacements; osteoporosis - diagnosis and treatment (DEXA); sports injury and rehabilitation; dancers and musicians injuries; elbow and shoulder arthroplasties.
PRIVATE: The Sussex Osteoporosis Clinic, 40 Wilbury Road, Hove BN3 3JP.
Tel: 01273 206 206 Fax: 01273 721 411

Mr Charles Gallannaugh MS FRCS(Eng) FRCS(Ed)
NHS POST: Formerly, Consultant Orthopaedic Surgeon, Hastings.
SPECIAL INTEREST: Hip and knee replacement and surgery of rheumatoid arthritis hip; knee revision surgery using impaction grafting and reconstruction techniques.
PRIVATE: Surgical Director, The Horder Centre For Arthritis, St. John's Road, Crowborough, East Sussex TN6 1XP. Tel: 01892 665577 Fax: 01892 662142
BUPA Hospital Hastings, The Ridge, St. Leonards-on-sea, East Sussex TN37 7RE.
Tel: 01424 757400 Fax: 01424 757424

Essex

Mr Derek A Boston FRCS
- YEAR QUALIFIED: 1972
- NHS POST: Consultant Orthopaedic Surgeon, Southend Hospital.
- SPECIAL INTEREST: General orthopaedic surgery; knee surgery; joint replacement surgery.
- PRIVATE: BUPA Wellesley Hospital, Eastern Avenue, Southend on Sea SS2 4XH. Tel: 01702 462944 Fax: 01702 600160

Mr Jamie Flanagan FRCS FRCS(Ed)
- YEAR QUALIFIED: 1970
- NHS POST: Consultant Orthopaedic Surgeon
- SPECIAL INTEREST: Knee surgery, including arthroscopy, ligament reconstruction osteotomy and arthroplasty, hip surgery
- PRIVATE: Chelmsford Knee Clinic, Springfield Hospital, Lawn Lane, Springfield, Chelmsford, Essex CM1 7GU. Tel: 01245 462331 Fax: 01245 460169

Mr Richard King MBBS FRCS
- YEAR QUALIFIED: 1969
- NHS POST: Consultant Orthopaedic Surgeon, Oldchurch Hospital, Romford, Essex. (Havering Hospitals)
- SPECIAL INTEREST: General orthopaedics; shoulder surgery - arthroplasty, rotator cuff repair, frozen shoulder; cervical rib thoracic outlet; arthroscopic knee surgery and join replacements. Medico-legal work.
- PRIVATE: Private Patients Office, Oldchurch Hospital, Oldchurch Road, Romford, Essex, RM7 OBE. Tel: 01708 708492 Fax: 01708 752883

Mr Andrew Lang-Stevenson MB ChB BSc FRCS FRCSE
- YEAR QUALIFIED: 1974
- NHS POST: Consultant In Charge, Havering Trust Knee Unit Oldchurch Hospital and Harold Wood Hospital.
- SPECIAL INTEREST: Acute and chronic reconstructive knee surgery in the young and old.
- PRIVATE: BUPA Roding Hospital, Roding Lane South, Redbridge, Ilford, Essex IG4 5PZ. Tel: 0181 551 1100 Fax: 0181 551 6415/9452

  BUPA Hartswood Hospital, Eagle Way, Brentwood, Essex, CM13 3LE. Tel: 01277 232 525 Fax: 01277 200 128

  The Essex Nuffield Hospital, Shenfield Road, Brentwood, Essex, CM15. Tel: 01277 263363 Fax: 01277 201158

  Direct Contact Address,, P.O. Box 234, Brentwood, Essex CM15 8EP. Tel: 01277 234123 Fax: 01277 234123

Mr Tom McAuliffe MA FRCS
- NHS POST: Consultant Orthopaedic Surgeon, Whipps Cross Hospital.
- SPECIAL INTEREST: Knee; shoulder and revision hip surgery.
- PRIVATE: Holly House Hospital, High Road, Buckhurst Hill, Essex, IG9 5HX. Tel: 0181 498 9931

  BUPA Roding Hospital, Roding Lane South, Redbridge, Ilford, Essex IG4 5PZ. Tel: 0181 551 1100

Mr R Julien J Wenger MBBS LRCP DRCOG FRCS
YEAR QUALIFIED: 1968
NHS POST: Consultant Trauma & Orthopaedic Surgeon Havering Hospitals Trust
SPECIAL INTEREST: Hand surgery.
PRIVATE: Essex Nuffield Hospital, Shenfield Road, Brentwood, Essex, CM15 8EH.
Tel: 01277 263 263 Fax: 01277 375 299

Hertfordshire

Mr Stephen R Cannon MB MCh (Orth) FRCS
YEAR QUALIFIED: 1974
NHS POST: Consultant Orthopaedic Surgeon, Royal National Orthopaedic Hospital, Stanmore.
SPECIAL INTEREST: Bone tumours and knee surgery.
PRIVATE: BUPA Hospital Bushey, Heathbourne Rd, Bushey, Watford, Hertfordshire WD2 1RD.
Tel: 0181 950 9090

Kent

Mr Paul R Allen MB LRCP FRCS
YEAR QUALIFIED: 1970
NHS POST: Consultant Orthopaedic Surgeon, Bromley NHS Hospitals Trust.
SPECIAL INTEREST: Knee surgery (arthroscopic surgery).
PRIVATE: BMI Sloane Hospital, 125 Albermarle Road, Beckenham, Kent BR3 2HS.
Tel: 0181 460 6998/466 6911 Fax: 0181 464 1443
Chelsfield Park Hospital, Bucks Cross Road, Chelsfield, Kent, BR6 7RG.
Tel: 01689 877 855 Fax: 01689 837 439
Beadle House Clinic, London Road, Sevenoaks, Kent TN13 2JD.
Tel: 01732 741 641 Fax: 01732 455 919

Mr Michael Fordyce MBBS FRCS
YEAR QUALIFIED: 1980
NHS POST: Consultant Orthopaedic Surgeon, Kent & Sussex Hospital, Tunbridge Wells.
SPECIAL INTEREST: Primary and revision total hip replacement; arthroscopic knee surgery; foot surgery.
PRIVATE: BUPA Hospital Tunbridge Wells, Fordcombe Road, Fordcombe, Tunbridge Wells, Kent TN3 0RD. Tel: 01892 740 047 xt 450 Fax: 01892 740 046

Mr Bipin Gopalji MRCS LRCP FRCS(Ed)
NHS POST: Consultant Orthopaedic Surgeon, Medway Hospital.
SPECIAL INTEREST: Joint replacement and hand surgery.
PRIVATE: BUPA Alexandra Hospital, Impton Lane, Walderslade, Chatham, Kent ME5 9PG.
Tel: 01634 687 166 Fax: 01634 686 162

Mr Soli Lam FRCS FRCSE FICS FACS
 YEAR QUALIFIED: 1957
 NHS POST: Hon. Emeritus Consultant Orthopaedic Surgeon Bromley Hospital NHS Trust
 SPECIAL INTEREST: Anterior knee pain; ligament repairs/reconstruction; hand surgery; peripheral nerve compression syndrome; peripheral constrictive conditions e.g. deQuervains, Triggers etc. Surgery of rheumatoid disease; silastic & all joint replacement; cervical rib syndromes.
 PRIVATE: (Room 178), Beckenham Hospital, 379 Croydon Road, Beckenham, Kent BR3 3QL.

Mr John E Nixon MA(Oxon) ChM FRCS
 NHS POST: Consultant Orthopaedic Surgeon Charing Cross Hospital
 SPECIAL INTEREST: General orthopaedics; arthroscopy; joint replacement and lumbar spine surgery (minimally invasive).
 PRIVATE: BMI Sloane Hospital, 125 Albermarle Road, Beckenham, Kent BR3 2HS. Tel: 0181 466 6911

Mr Sudhir Rao MCh(Orth) FRCS FRCS(Ed) FRCS(Orth)
 YEAR QUALIFIED: 1985
 NHS POST: Consultant Orthopaedic Surgeon, University Hospital, Lewisham, London.
 SPECIAL INTEREST: Knee surgery; arthroscopy; sports surgery; joint replacement; revision joint replacement; shoulder surgery and trauma surgery.
 PRIVATE: Chelsfield Park Hospital, Bucks Cross Road, Chelsfield, Kent, BR6 7RG. Tel: 01689 877855 Fax: 01689 837439

Mr Paul W Skinner MBBS FRCS
 YEAR QUALIFIED: 1977
 NHS POST: Consultant Orthopaedic Surgeon Kent & Sussex Hospitals
 SPECIAL INTEREST: Arthroscopic Surgery Knee & Shoulder
 PRIVATE: BUPA Hospital Tunbridge Wells, Fordcombe Road, Fordcombe, Tunbridge Wells, Kent TN3 0RD. Tel: 01892 740 039 Fax: 01892 740 046

Mr Neil Slater MA FRCS(Ed) FRCS (Orth)
 YEAR QUALIFIED: 1983
 NHS POST: Consultant Orthopaedic Surgeon The Maidstone Hospital
 SPECIAL INTEREST: Joint replacement; trauma; back surgery; foot and ankle surgery.
 PRIVATE: Somerfield Hospital, 63-77 London Road, Maidstone, Kent ME16 0DU. Tel: 01622 208 000 Fax: 01622 674 706

Lancashire

Mr Peter Wood MB BS FRCS
 YEAR QUALIFIED: 1971
 NHS POST: Consultant Orthopaedic Surgeon, Wrightington Hospital, Wigan.
 SPECIAL INTEREST: Total ankle and knee replacement; surgery for arthritis of the lower limb and foot including arthroplasty.
 PRIVATE: Wrightington Hospital, Wigan, Lancashire WN6 9EP.

London

Mr Hassan B Al-Haddad MD(Germany) FRCS
- YEAR QUALIFIED: 1969
- SPECIAL INTEREST: Hip replacement; femur osteotomy; reconstruction of bone deformity after fracture; arthroscopic surgery; knee replacement.
- PRIVATE: Cromwell Hospital, Cromwell Road, London SW5 OTU.
Tel: 0171 460 2000 ext 5914-Secretary. ext 5700-Appts. Fax: 0171 460 5709
E-mail: feisal1@compuserve.com

Miss Swee Ang MBBS MSc FRCS(Eng)
- YEAR QUALIFIED: 1973
- NHS POST: Consultant Orthopaedic Surgeon, Royal London Hospital.
- SPECIAL INTEREST: Trauma and general orthopaedic replacements (more than 500 hips and 200 knee replacements). Sub-specialty: hand and upper limb surgery especially shoulders and arthritic hands.
- PRIVATE: London Independent Hospital, 1 Beaumont Square, Stepney Green, London E1 4NL.
Tel: 0171 790 0990. Private secretary:0171 790 0990 ext 2273 Fax: 0171 265 9032

Mr Peter Baird MB BChir FRCS
- YEAR QUALIFIED: 1968
- NHS POST: Consultant Orthopaedic Surgeon, Chelsea and Westminster Hospital.
- SPECIAL INTEREST: Knees - arthroscopic and ligament reconstruction; joint replacement, hip, knee. Shoulder reconstructive and arthroscopic surgery
- PRIVATE: 1A Pennant Mews, London W8 5JN.
Tel: 0171 460 5596 Fax: 0171 460 5598 E-mail: Bairdorth@aol.com

Mr Simon Bridle FRCS FRCS(Orth)
- NHS POST: Consultant Orthopaedic Surgeon, St. George's Hospital.
- SPECIAL INTEREST: Hip and knee replacement; revision surgery; sports injuries.
- PRIVATE: Parkside Hospital, 53 Parkside, Wimbledon, London, SW19 5NX.
Tel: 0181 971 8000. Private secretary-0181 947 9524. Fax: 0181 947 0490
Lister Hospital, Chelsea Bridge Road, London, SW1W 8RH.
Tel: 0171 730 3417. Private secretary-0181 947 9524. Fax: 0181 947 0490

Mr John Peter Browett FRCS
- NHS POST: Consultant Orthopaedic Surgeon, St. Bartholomew's Hospital.
- SPECIAL INTEREST: Surgery of the knee, especially knee instabilities.
- PRIVATE: 95 Harley Street, London, W1N 1DF.
Tel: 0171 486 9323 Fax: 01707 876218

Mr Stephen R Cannon MB MCh (Orth) FRCS
- YEAR QUALIFIED: 1974
- NHS POST: Consultant Orthopaedic Surgeon, Royal National Orthopaedic Hospital, Stanmore.
- SPECIAL INTEREST: Bone tumours and knee surgery.
- PRIVATE: 32 Wimpole Street, London W1M 7AE.
Tel: 0171 580 1650/01923 828 898-secretary
Royal National Orthopaedic Hospital, Brockley Hill, Stanmore, Middlesex, HA7 4LP.
Tel: 0181 954 2300

Orthopaedics. London

Mr Anthony Catte MChir FRCS
- YEAR QUALIFIED: 1960
- NHS POST: Consultant Orthopaedic Surgeon, Royal National Orthopaedic Hospital Trust.
- SPECIAL INTEREST: Particular interest in children's orthopaedics, leg length inequality and the young adult hip.
- PRIVATE: 149 Harley Street, London W1N 2DE.
  Tel: 0171 935 4444 Fax: 0171 486 4700

Mr Anthony Catterall MChir FRCS
- YEAR QUALIFIED: 1970
- NHS POST: Consultant Orthopaedic Surgeon Royal National Orthopaedic Hospital
- SPECIAL INTEREST: Paediatric orthopaedics; hip surgery.
- PRIVATE: 149 Harley Street, London W1N 2DE.
  Tel: 0171 935 4444 Fax: 0171 486 4700

Mr Justin Cobb MCh(Oxon) FRCS
- NHS POST: Consultant Orthopaedic Surgeon University College London Hospitals
- SPECIAL INTEREST: Lower Limb Surgery and Musculoskeletal Oncology
- PRIVATE: The London Clinic, 149 Harley Street, London, W1N 2DE.
  Tel: 0171 224 0326 Fax: 0171 487 5997

Mr Brian Cohen MD FRCS FRCS(Orth)
- YEAR QUALIFIED: 1982
- NHS POST: Consultant Orthopaedic Surgeon, The Middlesex Hospital and University College Hospital, London.
- SPECIAL INTEREST: Surgery of the shoulder, elbow wrist and hand.
- PRIVATE: The Princess Grace Hospital, 42-52 Nottingham Place, London W1M 3FD.
  Tel: 0171 486 2349 Fax: 0171 486 2349

Mr Richard R H Coombs MA DM MCh MRCP FRCS FRCS(Ed)ORTH
- YEAR QUALIFIED: 1969
- NHS POST: Consultant Orthopaedic Surgeon, Charing Cross Hospital, Fulham Palace Road, London W6 8RF.
- SPECIAL INTEREST: Knee, hip and spinal surgery with a particular interest in minimally invasive surgery and arthroscopic surgery.
- PRIVATE: 22 Harley Street, London W1N 2AP.
  Tel: 0181 546 1778 Fax: 0181 549 1254

Mr Roger J H Emery MS FRCS
- NHS POST: Consultant Orthopaedic Surgeon, St Mary's Hospital.
- SPECIAL INTEREST: Shoulder and elbow surgery.
- PRIVATE: Hospital of St. John & St. Elizabeth, 60 Grove End Road, St Johns Wood, London, NW8 9NH. Tel: 0171 286 5126 xt 500

Orthopaedics. London

Mr Michael John Evans MB ChB FRCS
- **NHS POST:** Consultant Orthopaedic, Surgeon Charing Cross Hospital.
- **SPECIAL INTEREST:** General orthopaedics: back, hips, knee, upper Limb surgery; trauma.
- **PRIVATE:** 144 Harley Street, London W1N 1AH.
  Tel: 0171 935 0023 Fax: 0181 967 5630 E-mail: mje@evanorth.demon.co.uk
  Charing Cross Hospital, Fulham Palace Road, London, W6 8RF.
  Tel: 0181 846 1479 Fax: 0181 846 1439 E-mail: mje@evanorth.demon.co.uk

Mr Adrian C Fairbank MA FRCS FRCS(Orth)
- **YEAR QUALIFIED:** 1986
- **NHS POST:** Consultant Orthopaedic Surgeon, St. George's Hospital, Blackshaw Road, London SW17 0QT.
- **SPECIAL INTEREST:** General orthopaedics with a special interest in hip and knee surgery.
- **PRIVATE:** The London Clinic, 149 Harley Street, London W1N 2DE.
  Tel: 0171 935 4444 Fax: 0181 971 5096
  Parkside Hospital, 53 Parkside, Wimbledon, London, SW19 5NX.
  Tel: 0181 971 5096 Fax: 0181 971 5096

Mr Anthony John Hall MB BS FRCS
- **YEAR QUALIFIED:** 1962
- **NHS POST:** Consultant Orthopaedic Surgeon, Chelsea and Westminster Hospital.
- **SPECIAL INTEREST:** Knee surgery - sports and arthritic disorders.
- **PRIVATE:** 126 Harley Street, London W1N 1AH.
  Tel: 0171 486 1096 Fax: 0171 224 2520

Mr Robert A Hill BSc MBBS FRCS
- **NHS POST:** Consultant Orthopaedic Surgeon, Great Ormond Street Hospital & Princess Alexandra Hospitals Trust.
- **SPECIAL INTEREST:** Paediatric and general orthopaedics; length discrepancy; correction of limb deformity.
- **PRIVATE:** Private Consulting Rooms, Great Ormond Street Hospital for Children NHS Trust, Great Ormond Street, London WC1N 3JH.
  Tel: 0171 829 8632/813 8240-secretary Fax: 0171 813 8243
  Hospital of St. John & St. Elizabeth, 60 Grove End Road, St Johns Wood, London, NW8 9NH. Tel: 0171 286 5126 Fax: 0171 266 2316
  Portland Hospital for Women & Children, 205-209 Gt. Portland Street, London W1N 6AH. Tel: 0171 390 8351 Fax: 0171 390 8362

Professor Sean Hughes MS FRCS(Ed)Orth FRCS FRCSI
- **YEAR QUALIFIED:** 1966
- **NHS POST:** Honorary Consultant Orthopaedic Surgeon, Hammersmith Hospitals.
- **SPECIAL INTEREST:** Spinal surgery and musculo-skeletal infections.
- **PRIVATE:** Hammersmith Hospital, Du Cane Road, London, W12 OHS.
  Tel: 0181 846 1477 Fax: 0181 383 0468

Orthopaedics. London

Mr Andrew Jackson MBBS FRCS
- NHS POST: Consultant Orthopaedic Surgeon St. George's Hospital, Tooting
- SPECIAL INTEREST: Knee Surgery And Arthroscopy. Children's Orthopaedics As Well As More Generalised Orthopaedic Problems.
- PRIVATE: 107 Harley Street, London W1. Tel: 0171 935 9521 Fax: 0171 486 0956
  Parkside Hospital, 53 Parkside, Wimbledon, London, SW19 5NX.
  Tel: 0181 971 8000

Mr Jonathan R Johnson MB BS FRCS (Eng)
- NHS POST: Consultant Orthopaedic & Spinal Surgeon St Mary's Hospital & Royal National Orthopaedic Hospital, Stanmore
- SPECIAL INTEREST: Spinal surgery
- PRIVATE: Consulting Rooms, Princess Grace Hospital, 42-52 Nottingham Place, London, W1M 3FD. Tel: 0171 935 6485 Fax: 0171 487 4476

Mr Richard King MBBS FRCS
- YEAR QUALIFIED: 1969
- NHS POST: Consultant Orthopaedic Surgeon, Oldchurch Hospital, Romford, Essex. (Havering Hospitals)
- SPECIAL INTEREST: General orthopaedics; shoulder surgery - arthroplasty, rotator cuff repair, frozen shoulder; cervical rib thoracic outlet; arthroscopic knee surgery and join replacements. Medico-legal work.
- PRIVATE: 126 Harley Street, London W1N 1AH. Tel: 0171 935 2030 Fax: 0171 224 2520

Mr Soli Lam FRCS FRCSE FICS FACS
- YEAR QUALIFIED: 1957
- NHS POST: Hon. Emeritus Consultant Orthopaedic Surgeon Bromley Hospital NHS Trust
- SPECIAL INTEREST: Anterior knee pain; ligament repairs/reconstruction; hand surgery; peripheral nerve compression syndrome; peripheral constrictive conditions e.g. deQuervains, Triggers etc. Surgery of rheumatoid disease; silastic & all joint replacement; cervical rib syndromes.
- PRIVATE: 10 Harley Street, London W1N 1AA. Tel: 0171 467 8300 Fax: 0171 637 5227

Mr Simon Moyes MB FRCS FRCS.Orth D.Sports Med
- YEAR QUALIFIED: 1982
- SPECIAL INTEREST: Minimally invasive surgery of the knee, shoulder, foot and ankle.
- PRIVATE: 86 Harley Street, London W1N 1AE.
  Tel: 0171 323 0040 Fax: 0171 323 0080 E-mail:simonmoyes@aol.com

Mr John E Nixon MA(Oxon) ChM FRCS
- NHS POST: Consultant Orthopaedic Surgeon Charing Cross Hospital
- SPECIAL INTEREST: General orthopaedics; arthroscopy; joint replacement and lumbar spine surgery (minimally invasive).
- PRIVATE: Charing Cross Hospital, Fulham Palace Road, London, W6 8RF.
  Tel: 0181 846 1148 Fax: 0181 846 1150
  148 Harley Street, London W1N 1AH.
  Tel: 0171 935 1207 Fax: 0171 224 1528
  Lister Hospital, Chelsea Bridge Road, London, SW1W 8RH.
  Tel: 0171 730 3417 xt 210
  Cromwell Hospital, Cromwell Road, London SW5 0TU.
  Tel: 0171 460 2000

Orthopaedics. London

Mr J Mark H Paterson MBBS FRCS
  YEAR QUALIFIED: 1977
  NHS POST: Consultant Royal London Hospital
  SPECIAL INTEREST: Paediatric orthopaedics.
  PRIVATE: London Independent Hospital, 1 Beaumont Square, Stepney Green, London E1 4NL.
  Tel: 0171 790 9989 Fax: 0171 790 9989 E-mail: 101343,541@compuserve.com
  The Portland Hospital, 205-209 Great Portland Street, London W1N 6AH.
  Tel: 0171 790 9989 Fax: 0171 790 9989 E-mail: 101343,541@compuserve.com

Mr Anthony J L Percy MBBS MRCS LRCP FRCS(Eng) FRCS(Ed)
  YEAR QUALIFIED: 1964
  NHS POST: Consultant Orthopaedic & Trauma Queen Mary's Hospital, Sidcup, Kent.
  SPECIAL INTEREST: Hand surgery; joint replacements; children's orthopaedics; surgery for rheumatoid arthritis. Medico-legal reporting - personal accident claims and medical negligence.
  PRIVATE: BMI Blackheath Hospital, 40-42 Lee Terrace, London, SE3 9UD.
  Tel: 0181 318 7722 Fax: 0181 460 6513

Dr John Price MBBS MRCS LRCP DRCOB DPhMed
  YEAR QUALIFIED: 1958
  SPECIAL INTEREST: Cervical and lumbo-sacral disc lesions and spondylosis; joint injuries and sports injuries; rehabilitation for degenerative joint disease.
  PRIVATE: 144 Harley Street, London, W1N 1AH.
  Tel: 0171 935 0023 Fax: 0171 935 5972

Mr Sudhir Rao MCh(Orth) FRCS FRCS(Ed) FRCS(Orth)
  YEAR QUALIFIED: 1985
  NHS POST: Consultant Orthopaedic Surgeon, University Hospital, Lewisham, London.
  SPECIAL INTEREST: Knee surgery; arthroscopy; sports surgery; joint replacement; revision joint replacement; shoulder surgery and trauma surgery.
  PRIVATE: The Blackheath Hospital, 40-42 Lee Terrace, Blackheath, London, SE3 9UD.
  Tel: 0181 318 7722 ext 2371 Fax: 0181 300 9294
  The London Bridge Hospital, 27 Tooley Street, London, SE1 2PR.
  Tel: 0171 815 3653 Fax: 0171 815 3654

Mr Gareth Scott MBBS FRCS(Ed) FRCS(Eng)
  NHS POST: Consultant Orthopaedic Surgeon Royal London Hospital
  SPECIAL INTEREST: Adult reconstructive surgery. i.e. joint replacement and revision surgery for arthritis at the hip and knee.
  PRIVATE: 149 Harley Street, London W1N 2DE.
  Tel: 0171 935 4444 Fax: 0171 486 3782

Mr John D Spencer MS MRCP FRCS
  NHS POST: Reader/Honorary Consultant Trauma & Orthopaedic Surgeon, Guy's Hospital.
  SPECIAL INTEREST: Hand Surgery
  PRIVATE: Guy's Nuffield House, Newcomen Street, London, SE1 1YR.
  Tel: 0171 955 4479

Orthopaedics. London

Mr Roger Vickers MA BM BCh FRCS
YEAR QUALIFIED: 1970
SPECIAL INTEREST: Orthopaedics and hand surgery.
PRIVATE: The London Clinic, 149 Harley Street, London, W1N 2DE.
Tel: 0171 935 4444 Fax: 0171 935 5742

Mr David A Ward FRCSOrth FRCS(Ed)
YEAR QUALIFIED: 1985
NHS POST: Consultant Orthopaedic & Trauma Surgeon, Queen Mary's University Hospital, Roehampton and Kingston Hospital. NHS sec.
Tel: 0181 546 7711 ext 3240.
SPECIAL INTEREST: Lower limb joint replacement and revision surgery; trauma and reconstructive surgery; foot surgery; amputation surgery.
PRIVATE: Parkside Hospital, 53 Parkside, Wimbledon, London, SW19 5NX.
Tel: 0181 971 8026 Fax: 0181 944 8461 Private Secretary, Tel. & Fax:01932 336 676.

Mr Johan Witt MBBS FRCS FRCSOrth
YEAR QUALIFIED: 1983
NHS POST: Consultant Orthopaedic Surgeon, The Middlesex Hospital.
SPECIAL INTEREST: Hip surgery: joint replacement, pelvic osteotomy for dysplasia; knee surgery: joint replacement, arthroscopic surgery, ligament reconstruction.
PRIVATE: Private Consulting Rooms, University College Hospital, 25 Grafton Way, London, WC1E 6DB.
Tel: 0171 383 7916 Fax: 0171 380 9816
Sports Injuries Clinic, The London Clinic, 149 Harley Street, London, W1N 2DE.
Tel: 0171 935 4444 Fax: 0171 486 3782

Manchester

Mr Jonathan Noble MB ChM FRCS FRCSE
YEAR QUALIFIED: 1966
NHS POST: Consultant Orthopaedic Surgeon, Hope Hospital, Manchester.
SPECIAL INTEREST: Knee surgery including arthroscopy, total knee replacement and ligament surgery; hand surgery and sports injuries.
PRIVATE: BUPA Hospital Manchester, Russell Road, Manchester M16 8AJ.
Tel: 0161 226 0112 Fax: 0161 226 1187

Merseyside

Mr Richard W Parkinson MB ChB FRCS(Ed) FRCS(Orth)
YEAR QUALIFIED: 1981
NHS POST: Consultant Orthopaedic Surgeon, Arrowe Park Hospital.
SPECIAL INTEREST: All aspects of knee surgery - primary and revision knee arthroplasty, arthroscopy, ligament reconstruction; hip replacement; all aspects of general trauma surgery.
PRIVATE: BUPA Murrayfield Hospital, Holmwood Drive, Thingwall, Wirral, Merseyside L61 1AU.
Tel: 0151 639 3546 Fax: 0151 639 3546

Middlesbrough

Mr Michael Peter M Stewart MBChB FRCS FRCS(Orth)
- YEAR QUALIFIED: 1979
- NHS POST: Consultant Orthopaedic Surgeon, The Duchess of Kent's Hospital, Catterick Garrison, North Yorkshire.
- SPECIAL INTEREST: Surgery of the shoulder/upper limb/hand, soft tissues injuries of the knee.
- PRIVATE: The Park View Medical Clinic, 276 Marton Road, Middlesbrough TS4 2NS.
Tel: 01642 242357

Middlesex

Mr Stephen R Cannon MB MCh (Orth) FRCS
- YEAR QUALIFIED: 1974
- NHS POST: Consultant Orthopaedic Surgeon, Royal National Orthopaedic Hospital, Stanmore.
- SPECIAL INTEREST: Bone tumours and knee surgery.
- PRIVATE: Clementine Churchill Hospital, Sudbury Hill, Harrow, Middlesex, HA1 3RX.
Tel: 0181 872 3872

Norfolk

Mr John Keith Tucker MB BS BRCPMRCS FRCS
- YEAR QUALIFIED: 1968
- NHS POST: Consultant Orthopaedic Surgeon, Norfolk Norwich NHS Trust.
- SPECIAL INTEREST: General orthopaedics; hip; children spine.
- PRIVATE: 77 Newmarket Road, Norwich, Norfolk NR2 2HW.
Tel: 01603 614016 Fax: 01603 766469

North Yorkshire

Mr Michael Peter M Stewart MBChB FRCS FRCS(Orth)
- YEAR QUALIFIED: 1979
- NHS POST: Consultant Orthopaedic Surgeon, The Duchess of Kent's Hospital, Catterick Garrison, North Yorkshire.
- SPECIAL INTEREST: Surgery of the shoulder/upper limb/hand, soft tissues injuries of the knee.
- PRIVATE: St John of Gods Hospital, Scorton, Richmond, North Yorkshire DL10 6EB.
Tel: 01748 811535

Oxfordshire

Mr Hamish Simpson BA(Hons) BM BCh MA FRCS DM
NHS POST: Honorary Consultant Orthopaedic Surgeon, Nuffield Orthopaedic Centre and Oxford University.
SPECIAL INTEREST: Limb reconstruction including the treatment of fractures that are healing badly (non union/malunion); correction of deformity; limb lengthening; bone and joint infection; joint replacement; Ilizarov for adults and children (also olliers, pseudoarthrosis, neurofibromatosis, hemimelia).
PRIVATE: N.D.O.S., Nuffield Orthopaedic Centre, Windmill Road, Headington, Oxford, Oxfordshire OX3 7LD. Tel: 01865 227374 Fax: 01865 227354

South Wales

Mr Witer Mintowt-Czyz MB BS FRCS(Ed) FRCS(Eng)
YEAR QUALIFIED: 1971
NHS POST: Consultant Orthopaedic Surgeon, Royal Gwent Hospital.
SPECIAL INTEREST: Surgery of the lower limb, in particular the knee, both sporting and degenerative.
PRIVATE: St. Joseph's Private Hospital, Harding Avenue, Malpas, Newport, South Wales NP9 6ZE. Tel: 01633 820338 Fax: 01633 821487

Surrey

Mr Simon Bridle FRCS FRCS(Orth)
NHS POST: Consultant Orthopaedic Surgeon, St. George's Hospital.
SPECIAL INTEREST: Hip and knee replacement; revision surgery; sports injuries.
PRIVATE: St. Anthony's Hospital, London Road, North Cheam, Surrey, SM3 9DW. Tel: 0181 337 6691. Private secretary-0181 947 9524. Fax: 0181 947 0490

Mr Adrian C Fairbank MA FRCS FRCS(Orth)
YEAR QUALIFIED: 1986
NHS POST: Consultant Orthopaedic Surgeon, St. George's Hospital, Blackshaw Road, London SW17 0QT.
SPECIAL INTEREST: General orthopaedics with a special interest in hip and knee surgery.
PRIVATE: St. Anthony's Hospital, London Road, North Cheam, Surrey, SM3 9DW. Tel: 0181 337 6691 Fax: 0181 971 5096

Mr Richard Field PhD FRCS(Orth)
YEAR QUALIFIED: 1980
NHS POST: Consultant Orthopaedic Surgeon, St Helier NHS Trust.
SPECIAL INTEREST: Lower limb joint replacement surgery; revision hip and knee surgery; hip/knee/ankle arthroscopy; hip dysplasia; hip prosthesis design.
PRIVATE: St. Anthony's Hospital, London Road, North Cheam, Surrey, SM3 9DW. Tel: 0181 337 6691 ext 2205, 0181 335 0730 -direct Fax: 01737 812599

Orthopaedics. Surrey

Mr John Miller MB BS FRCS
- YEAR QUALIFIED: 1963
- NHS POST: Consultant Orthopaedic Surgeon, Mayday University Hospital, Croydon, Tel: 0181 401 3193 Fax: 0181 401 3100.
- SPECIAL INTEREST: Major joint replacement; revision hip surgery; general orthopaedic surgery.
- PRIVATE: Shirley Oaks Hospital, Poprey Lane, Croydon, Tel: 0181 401 3193
  North Downs Hospital, 46 Tupwood Lane, Caterham, Surrey CR3 6DP. Tel: 01883 348 981 Fax: 01883 341 163

Mr Michael A S Mowbray MSc MB MS LRCP FRCS(Ed) FRCS
- YEAR QUALIFIED: 1969
- NHS POST: Consultant Orthopaedic Surgeon, Mayday University Hospital.
- SPECIAL INTEREST: Arthroscopic knee surgery; acute & chronic knee ligament reconstruction; general orthopaedics.
- PRIVATE: Shirley Oaks Hospital, Poppy Lane, Shirley Oaks Village, Surrey, CR9 8AB. Tel: 0181 655 2255 Fax: 0181 656 2868

Mr Barrie Parker MB BS(Lond) FRCS(Eng)
- NHS POST: Consultant Trauma & Orthopaedic Surgeon Kingston NHS Trust
- SPECIAL INTEREST: Joint arthroplasty; hip and knee surgery; foot surgery; trauma and reconstructive surgery.
- PRIVATE: New Victoria Hospital, 184 Coombe Lane West, Kingston Upon Thames, Surrey, KT2 7EG. Tel: 0181 949 9000 Fax: 0181 949 9099
  Coombe Wing Private Patients Unit, Kingston Hospital, Galsworthy Road, Kingston Upon Thames, Surrey, KT2 7QB. Tel: 0181 546 6677 Fax: 0181 541 5613

Mr Marc Patterson FRCS AKC
- YEAR QUALIFIED: 1977
- NHS POST: Consultant In Orthopaedics And Trauma Princess Royal Hospital (Mid Sussex NHS Trust)
- SPECIAL INTEREST: Joint replacement; spinal surgery.
- PRIVATE: Gatwick Park Hospital, Povey Cross Road, Horley, Surrey RH6 0BB. Tel: 01293 785511 Fax: 01293 774883

Mr Rowan Pool MB ChB FRCS
- YEAR QUALIFIED: 1974
- NHS POST: Consultant Orthopaedic Surgeon, Ashford and St Peter's Hospital (NHS) Trust, Surrey.
- SPECIAL INTEREST: Hip reconstruction including hip replacement and revision; paediatrics and limb reconstruction (Ilizarov surgery) particularly in respect of congenital deformities.
- PRIVATE: The Woking Nuffield Hospital, Shores Road, Woking, Surrey GU21 4BY. Tel: 01483 730795 Fax: 01483 730795

Orthopaedics. Surrey

Mr David A Ward FRCSOrth FRCS(Ed)
YEAR QUALIFIED: 1985
NHS POST: Consultant Orthopaedic & Trauma Surgeon, Queen Mary's University Hospital, Roehampton and Kingston Hospital. NHS sec. Tel: 0181 546 7711 ext 3240.
SPECIAL INTEREST: Lower limb joint replacement and revision surgery; trauma and reconstructive surgery; foot surgery; amputation surgery.
PRIVATE: New Victoria Hospital, 184 Coombe Lane West, Kingston Upon Thames, Surrey, KT2 7EG. Tel: 0181 949 9000 Fax: 0181 949 9099 Private Secretary, Tel. & Fax:01932 336 676.
Coombe Wing Private Patients Unit, Kingston Hospital, Galsworthy Road, Kingston Upon Thames, Surrey, KT2 7QB. Tel: 0181 546 6677 Fax: 0181 541 5613 Private Secretary, Tel. & Fax:01932 336 676.

Tayside

Mr Alexander J G Swanson MB ChB FRCSEd
YEAR QUALIFIED: 1966
NHS POST: Consultant Orthopaedic Surgeon, Ninewells Hospital, Dundee.
SPECIAL INTEREST: General orthopaedics (joint replacement) and paediatric; orthopaedics.
PRIVATE: Fernbrae Hospital, 329 Perth Road, Dundee, Tayside DD2 1LJ. Tel: 01382 667203 Fax: 01382 660155

West Sussex

Mr Marc Patterson FRCS AKC
YEAR QUALIFIED: 1977
NHS POST: Consultant In Orthopaedics And Trauma Princess Royal Hospital (Mid Sussex NHS Trust)
SPECIAL INTEREST: Joint replacement; spinal surgery.
PRIVATE: Ashdown Hospital, Burrell Road, Haywards Heath, West Sussex RH16 1UD. Tel: 01444 456999 Fax: 01444 454111

West Yorkshire

Mr Keith Jepson MB FRCSE
YEAR QUALIFIED: 1965
NHS POST: Consultant Orthopaedic Surgeon, Royal Infirmary, Yorkshire.
SPECIAL INTEREST: Primary and revision total hip and knee replacement.
PRIVATE: Yorkshire Clinic, Bradford Road, Bingley, West Yorkshire BD16 1TW. Tel: 01274 560311 Fax: 01274 551247
Mid-Yorkshire, Nuffield Hospital, Outwood Lane, Horsforth, Leeds, West Yorkshire LS18 4HP. Tel: 0113 258 8756 Fax: 0113 258 3108
BUPA Hospital Elland, Elland Lane, Elland, Halifax, West Yorkshire HX5 9EB. Tel: 01422 375577
York Suite, Bradford Royal Infirmary, Duckworth Lane, Bradford, West Yorkshire BD9 6RJ. Tel: 01274 364668 Fax: 01274 366972

Orthopaedics.

Mr David A MacDonald MB BS FRCS
- YEAR QUALIFIED: 1982
- NHS POST: Consultant Orthopaedic Surgeon, St James University Hospital, Leeds.
- SPECIAL INTEREST: Lower limb arthroplasty including revision hip and revision knee replacement; arthroscopic knee surgery; trauma.
- PRIVATE: BUPA Hospital Leeds, Roundhay Hall, Jackson Avenue, Leeds, West Yorkshire LS8 1NT. Tel: 0113 269 3939 Fax: 0113 294 7896 E-mail: hamish_kirsty@msn.com

Mr Akos Bela Nevelos MD PhD LMSSA FRCSEd FRCSE
- YEAR QUALIFIED: 1967
- NHS POST: Consultant Arthopaedic Surgeon, Bradford NHS Trust.
- SPECIAL INTEREST: Paediatric orthopaedics; hip and knee replacement/reconstruction especially in the young.
- PRIVATE: Mornington Clinic, Cottingle Manor, Cottingley, West Yorkshire BD16 1TZ.

Wirral

Mr Jeremy Kaye MBBS FRCS
- YEAR QUALIFIED: 1977
- NHS POST: Consultant Orthopaedic Surgeon, Arrowe Park Hospital, Wirral.
- SPECIAL INTEREST: Shoulder surgery including sports injuries, arthroscopic surgery and joint replacement. Hip, primary and revision surgery.
- PRIVATE: Murrayfield Hospital, Holmwood Drive, Thingwall, Wirral, Tel: 0151 648 7000; 929 5180 Fax: 0151 648 4094

Worcestershire

Mr David Derek Robinson MA MB BS FRCS(Orth)
- NHS POST: Consultant Orthopaedic Surgeon, Worcester Royal Infirmary.
- SPECIAL INTEREST: Knee and shoulder surgery.
- PRIVATE: Droitwich Knee Clinic, St Andrew's Road, Droitwich, Worcestershire WR9 8YX. Tel: 01905 794858 Fax: 01905 795916

Mr Ebrahim Rouholamin MD FRCS
- YEAR QUALIFIED: 1969
- NHS POST: Consultant Orthopaedic Surgeon, Worcester Royal Infirmary.
- SPECIAL INTEREST: Arthroscopic surgery of the knee; ligament reconstruction; total knee replacement.
- PRIVATE: BUPA South Bank Hospital, 139 Bath Road, Worcester WR5 3YB. Tel: 01905 350003 Fax: 01905 357765

Orthopaedics - Hand Surgery

Berkshire

Mr David M Evans MBBS FRCS
YEAR QUALIFIED: 1965
NHS POST: Consultant Hand Surgeon, Royal National Orthopaedic Hospital, & St. Thomas' Hospital, London.
SPECIAL INTEREST: Hand surgery and rehabilitation. Surgery for congenital malformations of the hand, trauma and rheumatoid arthritis. Disorders of the wrist, Dupuytren's contracture, and peripheral nerve injury and compression.
PRIVATE: The Hand Clinic, Oakley Green, Windsor, Berks SL4 4LH.
Tel: 01753 831 333 Fax: 01753 832 109

Cheshire

Dr Jeremy M Auchincloss MB ChB FRCS (Eng & Ed) FRCSEd (Orth)
YEAR QUALIFIED: 1969
NHS POST: Consultant Orthopaedic and Hand Surgeon, Macclesfield District General Hospital. Secretary: 01625 661315.
SPECIAL INTEREST: Cubital and carpal tunnel surgery; Dupuytren's disease and rheumatoid hand and wrist surgery; day stay surgery for miscellaneous hand conditions.
PRIVATE: The BUPA Regency Hospital, West Street, Macclesfield, Cheshire SK11 8DW.
Tel: 01625 501150, Secretary: 01625 267839 Fax: 01625 501800

Glasgow

Mr Timothy E J Hems MA BM BCh DM FRCS(Eng) FRCSEd(Orth)
YEAR QUALIFIED: 1985
NHS POST: Consultant Hand and Orthopaedic Surgeon, The Victoria Infirmary, Glasgow.
SPECIAL INTEREST: Hand surgery, elective and trauma; surgical disorders of peripheral nerves including nerve injuries, brachial plexus surgery; shoulder surgery. European Diploma in Hand Surgery.
PRIVATE: Bon Secours Hospital, 36 Mansionhouse Road, Glasgow G41 3DW.
Tel: 0141 632 9231 Fax: 0141 636 5066

London

Mr Thomas P Carlstedt MD PhD Assc Prof FRCS(Ed Eng)
YEAR QUALIFIED: 1979
NHS POST: Consultant Orthopaedic and Hand Surgeon, The Royal National Orthopaedic Hospital.
SPECIAL INTEREST: Peripheral nerve, Brachial-Lumbosacral plexus injuries and nerve tumours, hand surgery and hand movement disorders after stroke and cerebral palsy.
PRIVATE: Princess Grace Hospital, 42-52 Nottingham Place, London, W1M 3FD.
Tel: 0171 224 3830 Fax: 0171 224 3831

Orthopaedics - Hand Surgery. London

Mr Brian Cohen MD FRCS FRCS(Orth)
YEAR QUALIFIED: 1982
NHS POST: Consultant Orthopaedic Surgeon, The Middlesex Hospital and University College Hospital, London.
SPECIAL INTEREST: Surgery of the shoulder, elbow wrist and hand.
PRIVATE: The Princess Grace Hospital, 42-52 Nottingham Place, London W1M 3FD.
Tel: 0171 486 2349 Fax: 0171 486 2349

Assoc. Professor B Povlsen MD PhD
YEAR QUALIFIED: 1984
NHS POST: Consultant, Guy's and St Thomas' Hospital: St. Thomas' Hospital, Lambeth Palace Road, London SE1 7EH.
Tel: 0171 928 9292. Guy's Hospital, St. Thomas Street, London SE1 9RT.
Tel: 0171 955 5000.
SPECIAL INTEREST: Endoscopic surgery of hands, elbows and shoulders. Joint replacement of hands, elbows and shoulders. Endoscopic surgery for excessive hand sweat. Nerve surgery.
PRIVATE: Churchill Clinic, 80 Lambeth Road, London, SE1 7PW.
Tel: 0171 620 1590 Fax: 0171 928 1702   E-mail: bo@povlsen.u-net.com

Orthopaedics - Knee Surgery

London

Mr Angus E Strover FRCS
- YEAR QUALIFIED: 1979
- NHS POST: Droitwich Spa Hospital, BUPA South Bank Hospital, London Bridge Hospital, The Wellington Hospital.
- SPECIAL INTEREST: Knee surgery including ligament, reconstruction and joint replacement.
- PRIVATE: The London Knee Clinic, 126 Harley Street, London W1N 1AH.
  Tel: 01905 794858 Fax: 01905 795916

Mr Glen Vardi FCS(Orth)SA
- YEAR QUALIFIED: 1994
- SPECIAL INTEREST: Knee surgery including ligament, reconstruction and joint replacement.
- PRIVATE: The London Knee Clinic, 126 Harley Street, London W1N 1AH.
  Tel: 01905 794858 Fax: 01905 795916

Worcestershire

Mr Angus E Strover FRCS
- YEAR QUALIFIED: 1979
- NHS POST: Droitwich Spa Hospital, BUPA South Bank Hospital, London Bridge Hospital, The Wellington Hospital.
- SPECIAL INTEREST: Knee surgery including ligament, reconstruction and joint replacement.
- PRIVATE: Droitwich Knee Clinic, St Andrew's Road, Droitwich, Worcestershire WR9 8YX.
  Tel: 01905 794558 Fax: 01905 795916

Mr Peter J Turner FCS SA Orth
- YEAR QUALIFIED: 1988
- SPECIAL INTEREST: Knee surgery including ligament reconstruction and joint replacement.
- PRIVATE: Droitwich Knee Clinic, St Andrew's Road, Droitwich, Worcestershire WR9 8YX.
  Tel: 01905 794858 Fax: 01905 795916

Mr Glen Vardi FCS(Orth)SA
- YEAR QUALIFIED: 1994
- SPECIAL INTEREST: Knee surgery including ligament, reconstruction and joint replacement.
- PRIVATE: Droitwich Knee Clinic, St Andrew's Road, Droitwich, Worcestershire WR9 8YX.
  Tel: 01905 794558 Fax: 01905 795916

Orthopaedics - Spinal Surgery

London

Mr Henry V Crock AO MD MS FRCS FRACS
NHS POST: Formerly Honorary Consultant, Royal Post-Graduate Medical School & Hammersmith Hospital
SPECIAL INTEREST: Spinal Surgery - excluding scoliosis
PRIVATE: Spinal Disorders Unit, Cromwell Hospital, Cromwell Road, London SW5 0TU. Tel: 0171 460 5646 Fax: 0171 460 5648

Mr M A Edgar MChir FRCS
YEAR QUALIFIED: 1963
NHS POST: Consultant Orthopaedic & Spinal Surgeon The Middlesex & University College London Hospitals Trust
SPECIAL INTEREST: Spinal Deformities & Other Spinal Conditions
PRIVATE: The London Clinic, 149 Harley Street, London, W1N 2DE. Tel: 0171 935 4444 Fax: 0171 486 3782

Suffolk

Mr David John Sharp MD FRCS
YEAR QUALIFIED: 1972
NHS POST: Consultant Orthropaedic and Spinal Surgeon, The Ipswich Hospital.
SPECIAL INTEREST: Neck and low back pain and spinal surgery.
PRIVATE: Suffolk Spinal Centre, Christchurch Park Hospital, 57-61 Fonnereau Road, Ipswich, Suffolk IP1 3JN. Tel: 01473 221031 Fax: 01473 219526

Paediatric Surgery

Devon

Mr Denis Charles Wilkins MB ChB FRCS MD
- YEAR QUALIFIED: 1966
- NHS POST: Consultant General and Vascular Surgeon, Derriford Hospital, Plymouth.
- SPECIAL INTEREST: General surgery; hernia; endocrine; thyroid; hyperhydrosis; medico-legal; arterial surgery; carotid disease; peripheral vascular disease; aneurysms; varicose veins; aortic surgery; vibratory white finger; parathyroid; cholecystectomy.
- PRIVATE: Nuffield Hospital, Derriford Road, Plymouth, Devon PL6 8BG. Tel: 01752 778892 Fax: 01752 778421

London

Mr C Martin Bailey BSc FRCS
- YEAR QUALIFIED: 1973
- NHS POST: Consultant E.N.T. Surgeon, Great Ormond Street Hospital For Children.
- SPECIAL INTEREST: Paediatric otolaryngology.
- PRIVATE: 55 Harley Street, London W1N 1DD. Tel: 0171 580 2426 Fax: 0171 436 1645

Mr David Paul Drake MA MB BChir FRCS DCH
- YEAR QUALIFIED: 1969
- NHS POST: Consulting Paediatric Surgeon, Great Ormond Street Children's Hospital Trust.
- SPECIAL INTEREST: Gastro-intestinal surgery; neonatal surgery; general paediatric surgery.
- PRIVATE: 34 Gt. Ormond Street, London WC1N 3JH. Tel: 0171 829 8632 Fax: 0171 829 8650

Mr Patrick G Duffy MB BCh BAO FRCS(I)
- YEAR QUALIFIED: 1973
- NHS POST: Consultant Paediatric Urologist, Great Ormond Street Hospital for Children NHS Trust.
- SPECIAL INTEREST: Paediatric urology; reconstruction urinary tract; undescended testicles; hypospadias.
- PRIVATE: Private Consulting Rooms, 234 Great Portland Street, London W1N 5PH. Tel: 0171 390 8322 Fax: 0171 390 8324

Mr Martin Elliott MBBS MD FRCS
- NHS POST: Consultant Cardiothoracic Surgeon Great Ormond Street Hospital for Children NHS Trust
- SPECIAL INTEREST: Correction of congenital heart & thoracic defects.
- PRIVATE: Great Ormond Street Hospital for Children NHS Trust, Great Ormond Street, London WC1N 3JH. Tel: 0171 829 8853 Fax: 0171 813 8262

Paediatric Surgery. London

Mr Keith Holmes ChM DCH FRCS
- NHS POST: Consultant Paediatric Surgeon, St. George's Hospital, London, Tel/Fax: 0181 725 2926 and Queen Mary's Hospital for Children, Carshalton SM5 1AA, Tel: 0181 296 3043.
- SPECIAL INTEREST: General Paediatric Surgery, Gastro-enterology, Oncology.
- PRIVATE: 17 Wimpole Street, London W1M 7AD.
Tel: 0171 323 1535 Fax: 0171 323 9126
Parkside Hospital, 53 Parkside, Wimbledon, London, SW19 5NX.
Tel: 0181 971 8000 Fax: 0181 971 8002

Mr Edward M Kiely FRCSI FRCS
- NHS POST: NHS Post: Hospital for Sick Children
- SPECIAL INTEREST: Paediatrics
- PRIVATE: 234 Great Portland Street, London W1N 5PH.
Tel: 0171 390 8332 Fax: 0171 813 8428

Merseyside

Mr Richard Turnock MBChB FRCS (Paediatric)
- YEAR QUALIFIED: 1977
- NHS POST: Consultant Paediatric Surgeon, Royal Liverpool Children's Hospital, Alderhey.
- SPECIAL INTEREST: General paediatric surgery; laparoscopy for undescended and impalpable testes; reconstruction of ano-rectal and associated malformations.
- PRIVATE: Department of Paediatric Surgery, Royal Liverpool Children's Hospital Alderhey, Eaton Road, Liverpool, Merseyside L12 2AP.
Tel: 0151 252 5750 Fax: 0151 252 5362

Surrey

Mr Keith Holmes ChM DCH FRCS
- NHS POST: Consultant Paediatric Surgeon, St. George's Hospital, London, Tel/Fax: 0181 725 2926 and Queen Mary's Hospital for Children, Carshalton SM5 1AA, Tel: 0181 296 3043.
- SPECIAL INTEREST: General Paediatric Surgery, Gastro-enterology, Oncology.
- PRIVATE: St. Anthony's Hospital, London Road, North Cheam, Surrey, SM3 9DW.
Tel: 0181 337 6691 Fax: 0181 337 0816

Paediatrics

Essex

Dr Alan Franklin FRCP FRCPCH DCH DRCOG
YEAR QUALIFIED: 1960
SPECIAL INTEREST: Hyperactivity (ADD) and chronic fatigue syndromes in children.
PRIVATE: Essex Nuffield Hospital, Shenfield Road, Brentwood, Essex, CM15 8EH.
Tel: 01277 263263 Fax: 01277 261924
Springfield Hospital, Lawn Lane, Springfield, Chelmsford, Essex CM1 7GU.
Tel: 01245 461 777 Fax: 01245 450317

Hertfordshire

Dr John Zia Heckmatt MB ChB MD FRCP
YEAR QUALIFIED: 1970
NHS POST: Consultant Paediatrician, Watford General Hospital.
SPECIAL INTEREST: Developmental problems in pre-school children; medical aspects of problems at school including language delay, autism, neurological disorders, neuromuscular problems.
PRIVATE: BUPA Hospital Bushey, Heathbourne Rd, Bushey, Watford, Hertfordshire WD2 1RD.
Tel: 0181 950 9090 ext 231

Lancashire

Dr Bratati Bose-Haider MBBS FRCP(L) FRCPCH DCH(L) DCCH (Warwick)
YEAR QUALIFIED: 1974
NHS POST: Consultant Paediatrician, Fairfield Hospital, Bury.
SPECIAL INTEREST: Developmental paediatrics and attention deficit disorder, see children with general paediatric problems.
PRIVATE: Fairfield Hospital, Bury, Lancashire BL9 7TD.
Tel: 0161 705 3867 Fax: 0870 055 7871

Dr Alastair Campbell MB BS FRCP FRCPCH
YEAR QUALIFIED: 1974
NHS POST: Consultant Paediatrician, Royal Preston Hospital.
SPECIAL INTEREST: General and neonatal paediatrics.
PRIVATE: Fulwood Hall Hospital, Midgery Lane, Fulwood, Preston, Lancashire PR2 9SZ.
Tel: 01772 704111 Fax: 01772 795131

London

Professor Charles G D Brook MA MD FRCP FRCPCH
YEAR QUALIFIED: 1964
NHS POST: Consultant Paediatric Endocrinologist, Great Ormond Street Hospital For Children and Middlesex Hospital.
SPECIAL INTEREST: Growth disorders; endocrine problems; physical development; puberty disorders.
PRIVATE: Middlesex Hospital, Mortimer Street, London, W1N 8AA.
Tel: 0181 521 0553 Fax: 0181 521 0553

Dr Elizabeth Bryan MD FRCP FRCPCH
YEAR QUALIFIED: 1966
NHS POST: Consultant, Queen Charlotte's & Chelsea Hospital.
SPECIAL INTEREST: Twins and Higher Multiple Births. Parental Advice, Paediatric Development, Behaviour and Bereavement.
PRIVATE: The Multiple Births Foundation, Queen Charlotte's & Chelsea Hospital, Goldhawk Road, London, W6 0XG. Tel: 0181 383 3519 Fax: 0181 383 3041
E-mail: ebryan@thefree.net

Dr Charles R Buchanan BSc MB(Hons) MRCP(UK) FRCPCH
YEAR QUALIFIED: 1979
NHS POST: Consultant in Paediatric Endocrinology, King's College Hospital.
SPECIAL INTEREST: Disorders of growth & puberty, thyroid, pituitary & adrenal glands etc; diabetes.
PRIVATE: King's College Hospital, Denmark Hill, London, SE5 9RS.
Tel: 0171 346 3431(sec) Fax: 0171 346 3643

Dr Marion Crouchman FRCP DCH FRCPCH
YEAR QUALIFIED: 1967
NHS POST: Consultant Neuro-Developmental Paediatrician, King's College Hospital.
SPECIAL INTEREST: Acquired brain injury: Causation, assessment, management, rehabilitation. Botulinum toxin treatment in cerebral palsy. Fluent in French.
PRIVATE: BMI Portland Hospital for Women & Children, 205-209 Great Portland Street, London, W1N 6AH. Tel: 0171 580 4400 Fax: 0171 610 5553
E-mail: marioncrouchman@rowanroad.demon.co.uk
Variety Club Children's Hospital, King's College Hospital, Denmark Hill, London, SE5 9RS. Tel: 0171 346 3690 Fax: 0171 610 5553

Professor John Deanfield MA MB BChir FRCP
NHS POST: Consultant Cardiologist, Great Ormond Street Hospital for Children NHS Trust and University College London Hospitals.
SPECIAL INTEREST: Paediatric cardiology; coronary disease and coronary risk factor management.
PRIVATE: Harley Street Clinic, 35 Weymouth Street, London, W1N 4BJ.
Tel: 0171 404 5094 Fax: 0171 813 8263

Paediatrics. London

Dr Ian Hann MD FRCP FRCP(Glas) FRCPath
- NHS POST: Consultant Paediatric Haematologist, Great Ormond Street Childrens Hospital
- SPECIAL INTEREST: Paediatric haematology and oncology; childhood leukaemia and lymphoma; childhood blood and bleeding disorders; haemophilia.
- PRIVATE: Great Ormond Street Hospital for Children NHS Trust, Great Ormond Street, London WC1N 3JH. Tel: 0171 829 8831 Fax: 0171 813 8410 E-mail: Ian.Hann@gosh-tr.nthames.nhs.uk

Dr Gwilym Hosking MBBS FRCP FRCPCH FFPM
- YEAR QUALIFIED: 1969
- NHS POST: Honorary Consultant Paediatric Neurologist, Hospital For Sick Children, Great Ormond Street, Charing Cross Hospital & Southend NHS Trust.
- SPECIAL INTEREST: Child neurology; epilepsy; cerebral palsy; head injury; neuro metabolic disorders; attention deficit disorder. Medico-legal practice.
- PRIVATE: Portland Neurocare Ltd. (Child Neurology &, Neurodisability Services), 234 Great Portland Street, London W1N 5PH. Tel: 0171 390 8286 Fax: 0171 390 8287 E-mail: admin@portlandneurocare.com Web: www.portlandneurocare.com

Dr Claus G H Newman MB BS FRCP DCH FRCPCH
- YEAR QUALIFIED: 1953
- NHS POST: Formerly - Director, Leon Gillis Unit - Queen Mary's University Hosp., Roehampton (now, Emeritus) Formerly - Consultant Paediatrician/Paediatric Cardiologist, Chelsea & Westminster Hospital (now, Emeritus)
- SPECIAL INTEREST: Congenital limb deficiency; paediatric handicapping conditions; heart murmurs; pre-school problems.
- PRIVATE: Cromwell Hospital, Cromwell Road, London SW5 OTU. Tel: 0181 886 4383 Fax: 0181 340 1457
BMI Portland Hospital for Women & Children, 209 Great Portland Street, London, W1N 6AH. Tel: 0181 886 4383 Fax: 0181 340 1457

Dr Vas Novelli MBBS FRCP FRACP FRCPCH
- YEAR QUALIFIED: 1974
- NHS POST: Consultant in Paediatric Infectious Diseases Great Ormond Street Hospital for Children NHS Trust
- SPECIAL INTEREST: Infectious Diseases and HIV
- PRIVATE: Great Ormond Street Hospital for Children NHS Trust, Great Ormond Street, London WC1N 3JH. Tel: 0171 405 9200 ext 5946 Fax: 0171 813 8266 E-mail: vnovelli@compuserve.com

Dr Shakeel Ahmed Qureshi MBChB FRCP
- YEAR QUALIFIED: 1976
- NHS POST: Consultant Paediatric Cardiologist, Guy's Hospital, London.
- SPECIAL INTEREST: Babies and children born with congenital heart disease; non surgical treatment of some specific congenital heart defects in children and adults.
- PRIVATE: Guy's Hospital, St Thomas Street, London, SE1 9RT. Tel: 0171 955 5000 ext 8772 Fax: 0171 955 4614 E-mail:s.a.qureshi@umds.ac.uk

Paediatrics. London

Dr Ricky Richardson BSc MBBS FRCP FRCPCH DCH DTM&H
YEAR QUALIFIED: 1973
NHS POST: Honorary Consultant Paediatrician, Great Ormond Street Hospital for Children NHS Trust and the Portland Hospital for Women and Children.
SPECIAL INTEREST: General paediatrics with specific interest in children with learning difficulties; tropical infectious diseases and psycho social paediatrics. Recognised authority on information technology in healthcare (Telemedicine).
PRIVATE: Richardson Consulting, 7 Emlyn Road, London W12 9TF.
Tel: 0181 749 4411 Fax: 0181 749 4422 E-mail: rjrichardson@compuserve.com

Dr Michael Rigby MD FRCP
NHS POST: Consultant Paediatric Cardiologist Royal Brompton Hospital
SPECIAL INTEREST: Paediatric cardiology.
PRIVATE: Private Outpatient Clinic, Royal Brompton Hospital, Sydney Street, London SW3 6NP.
Tel: 0171 351 8542 Fax: 0171 351 8547 E-mail: m.rigby@rbh.nthames.nhs.uk

Dr Mark Rosenthal MD MRCP BSc MBChB(Hons) FRCPCH
YEAR QUALIFIED: 1981
NHS POST: Consultant Paediatric Respiratory Physician Royal Brompton Hospital
SPECIAL INTEREST: Paediatric Respiratory Disease / Allergy
PRIVATE: Royal Brompton Hospital, Sydney Street, London SW3 6NP.
Tel: 0171 351 8754 Fax: 0171 351 8763
Portland Hospital for Women & Children, 205-209 Gt. Portland Street, London W1N 6AH. Tel: 0171 580 4400

Dr Elliot Shinebourne MD FRCP FRCPCH
NHS POST: Consultant Paediatric Cardiologist Royal Brompton Hospital/National Heart & Lung Institute
SPECIAL INTEREST: Congenital heart disease - diagnosis, investigation and management in infants, children, adolescents and young adults. Cardiac arrhythmias in children.
PRIVATE: Royal Brompton Hospital, Sydney Street, London SW3 6NP.
Tel: 0171 351 8541 Fax: 0171 351 8544

Dr Richard Stanhope BSc MD DCH FRCP
NHS POST: Consultant Paediatric Endocrinologist Great Ormond Street Hospital for Children NHS Trust & The Middlesex Hospital (UCLH)
SPECIAL INTEREST: Adolescent and Paediatric Endocrinology especially disorders of puberty and growth
PRIVATE: The Portland Hospital, 205-209 Great Portland Street, London W1N 6AH.
Tel: Appts - 0181 670 1957 Fax: 0181 670 1957
Private Consulting Rooms, Great Ormond Street Hospital for Children NHS Trust, Great Ormond Street, London WC1N 3JH. Tel: (44) 171 9052139, 0181 6701957-appts Fax: (44) 171 8138496, 0181 6701957- appts.

Dr John Stroobant MBBS FRCP DCH
NHS POST: Consultant Paediatrician Lewisham Hospital
SPECIAL INTEREST: Respiratory disease.
PRIVATE: BMI Blackheath Hospital, 40-42 Lee Terrace, London, SE3 9UD.
Tel: 0181 318 7722 Fax: 0181 318 2542

Paediatrics. London

Dr Sam Michael Tucker MBBCh FRCP FRCPE FRCPCH DCH
- YEAR QUALIFIED: 1953
- NHS POST: Consultant Paediatrician (Honorary) Hillingdon Hospital Post Graduate Research Centre
- SPECIAL INTEREST: Paediatric audiology and learning disorders/neonatology; general paediatrics.
- PRIVATE: Consulting Rooms, 152 Harley Street, London, W1N 1HH.
  Tel: 0171 935 1858/0181 959 0500(phone-fax) Fax: 0171 224 2574
  E-mail: sammtucker@aol.com.

Dr Robert M R Tulloh BM BCh MA MRCP FRCPCH
- NHS POST: Consultant Paediatric Cardiologist Guy's & St. Thomas' NHS Trust
- SPECIAL INTEREST: Paediatric cardiology; diagnosis and interventional treatment of children's heart disease.
- PRIVATE: Guy's Hospital, St Thomas Street, London, SE1 9RT.
  Tel: 0171 955 4616 Fax: 0171 955 4614 E-mail:r.tulloh@umds.ac.uk

Dr Peter Elton Walker MB B Chir FRCP FRCPCH DCH
- YEAR QUALIFIED: 1960
- NHS POST: Consultant Paediatrician (Emeritus), Frimley Park Hospital
- SPECIAL INTEREST: Behavioural and emotional problems of children, young children and adolescents; sleep disorders; psychosomatic disorders, including fatigue syndromes; enuresis and encopresis; pre-school problems; school difficulties; attention deficit disorders.
- PRIVATE: Portland Hospital for Women & Children, 234 Great Portland Street, London W1N 5PH. Tel: 0171 390 8312 Fax: 0171 390 8311

Middlesex

Dr Rodney Franklin MBBS MD FRCP FRCPCH
- YEAR QUALIFIED: 1979
- NHS POST: Consultant Paediatric Cardiologist, Royal Brompton and Harefield Hospital.
- SPECIAL INTEREST: Paediatric cardiology: particularly echo cardiology and fetal echo cardiography; paediatric cardiology intensive care, pre and post-operative.
- PRIVATE: Royal Brompton and Harefield Hospital, Harefield, Middlesex, UB9 6JH.
  Tel: 01895 828554 Fax: 01895 828554

Surrey

Dr Claus G H Newman MB BS FRCP DCH FRCPCH
- YEAR QUALIFIED: 1953
- NHS POST: Formerly - Director, Leon Gillis Unit - Queen Mary's University Hosp., Roehampton (now, Emeritus) Formerly - Consultant Paediatrician/Paediatric Cardiologist, Chelsea & Westminster Hospital (now, Emeritus)
- SPECIAL INTEREST: Congenital limb deficiency; paediatric handicapping conditions; heart murmurs; pre-school problems.
- PRIVATE: New Victoria Hospital, 184 Coombe Lane West, Kingston Upon Thames, Surrey, KT2 7EG. Tel: 0181 949 1661 Fax: 0181 949 6392
  New Victoria Hospital, 184 Coombe Lane West, Kingston Upon Thames, Surrey, KT2 7EG. Tel: 0181 949 9020 Fax: 0181 340 1457

Paediatrics. Surrey

Dr Mark Rosenthal MD MRCP BSc MBChB(Hons) FRCPCH
- YEAR QUALIFIED: 1981
- NHS POST: Consultant Paediatric Respiratory Physician Royal Brompton Hospital
- SPECIAL INTEREST: Paediatric Respiratory Disease / Allergy
- PRIVATE: Queen Mary's Childrens Hospital St. Helier NHS Trust, Wrythe Lane, Surrey SM5 1AA. Tel: 0181 296 3067

Dr Peter Elton Walker MB B Chir FRCP FRCPCH DCH
- YEAR QUALIFIED: 1960
- NHS POST: Consultant Paediatrician (Emeritus), Frimley Park Hospital
- SPECIAL INTEREST: Behavioural and emotional problems of children, young children and adolescents; sleep disorders; psychosomatic disorders, including fatigue syndromes; enuresis and encopresis; pre-school problems; school difficulties; attention deficit disorders.
- PRIVATE: Merrydown Clinic, 86 Broomleaf Road, Farnham, Surrey Tel: 01252 737 107 Fax: 01252 737 107

Pain Relief

Berkshire

Dr Richard Fell MB BS FFARCS DA
YEAR QUALIFIED: 1961
NHS POST: Consultant Anaesthetist Wexham Park Hospital
SPECIAL INTEREST: Migraine; complex regional pain syndrome; idiopathic upper quadrant abdominal pain; pelvic pain.
PRIVATE: The Thames Valley Nuffield Hospital, Wexham Street, Slough, Buckinghamshire SL3 6NH. Tel: 01753 662 241 Fax: 01753 662 129

Essex

Dr Charles A Gauci MD FRCA
YEAR QUALIFIED: 1971
NHS POST: Consultant in Pain Relief Therapy, Whipps Cross Hospital, London. King George Hospital, Redbridge.
SPECIAL INTEREST: Back pain, head & neck pain and sciatica.
PRIVATE: Holly House Hospital, High Road, Buckhurst Hill, Essex, IG9 5HX. Tel: 0181 505 3311. Private Sec. Tel/Fax: 0181 504 4816 Fax: 0181 502 9735 E-mail:cagauci@compuserve.com
BUPA Roding Hospital, Roding Lane South, Redbridge, Ilford, Essex IG4 5PZ. Tel: 0181 551 1100. Private Sec. Tel/Fax: 0181 504 4816 Fax: 0181 551 9452 E-mail: cagauci@compuserve.com

Dr Alan Thorogood MRCS LRCP FRCA DA
YEAR QUALIFIED: 1951
NHS POST: Consultant Anaesthetist/Pain Clinic, Colchester Hospitals.
SPECIAL INTEREST: Back pain/sciatica; shoulder pain; caudal epidurals as out-patient or domiciliary procedure; intra-articular shoulder injections.
PRIVATE: Colchester Oaks Hospital, Oaks Place, Mile End Road, Colchester, Essex CO4 5XR. Tel: 01206 575915

Hertfordshire

Dr Charles A Gauci MD FRCA
YEAR QUALIFIED: 1971
NHS POST: Consultant in Pain Relief Therapy, Whipps Cross Hospital, London. King George Hospital, Redbridge.
SPECIAL INTEREST: Back pain, head & neck pain and sciatica.
PRIVATE: The Rivers Hospital, High Wych Road, Sawbridgeworth, Hertfordshire CM21 6HH. Tel: 01279 600 282. Private Sec. Tel/Fax: 0181 504 4816 Fax: 01279 600 212 E-mail: cagauci@compuserve.com

Kent

Dr Charles A Gauci MD FRCA
- YEAR QUALIFIED: 1971
- NHS POST: Consultant in Pain Relief Therapy, Whipps Cross Hospital, London. King George Hospital, Redbridge.
- SPECIAL INTEREST: Back pain, head & neck pain and sciatica.
- PRIVATE: Chelsfield Park Hospital, Bucks Cross Road, Chelsfield, Kent, BR6 7RG.
Tel: 01689 877 855. Private Sec. Tel/Fax: 0181 504 4816 Fax: 01689 837 439
E-mail: cagauci@compuserve.com

London

Dr Nadia Coote MB BCh FFA DA
- YEAR QUALIFIED: 1960
- NHS POST: Consultant in Anaesthetics & Pain Relief, Greenwich District Hospital (Retired).
- SPECIAL INTEREST: Acupuncture for pain relief.
- PRIVATE: BMI Blackheath Hospital, 40-42 Lee Terrace, London, SE3 9UD.
Tel: 0181 318 7722

Dr David Denison Davies Ph.D MRCS LRCP FRCA DA
- NHS POST: Consultant in Anaesthetics/Pain Management, Central Middlesex Hospital, Acton Lane, London NW10 7NS, Tel: 0181 453 2160.
- SPECIAL INTEREST: Pain Management (in intractable pain).
- PRIVATE: Churchill Clinic, 80 Lambeth Road, London, SE1 7PW.
Tel: 0171 928 5633 ext 209

Dr Abina C O'Callaghan MBBS LRCP MRCS FRCA
- YEAR QUALIFIED: 1977
- SPECIAL INTEREST: Pain management - acute and chronic; anaesthesia.
- PRIVATE: Cromwell Hospital, Cromwell Road, London SW5 OTU.
Tel: 0171 460 5700 Fax: 0181 991 8198
The Wellington Hospital, Wellington Place, London, NW8 9LE.
Tel: 0171 586 3213 Fax: 0171 483 0297

Middlesex

Dr Laurie Allan MRCS LRCP MBBS FRCA
- NHS POST: Director Chronic Pain Services, Northwick Park & St. Mark's NHS Trust
- SPECIAL INTEREST: Pain management, especially spinal pain.
- PRIVATE: Consulting Rooms, Clementine Churchill Hospital, Sudbury Hill, Harrow, Middlesex, HA1 3RX. Tel: Secretary-0181 869 3976. Hospital-0181 872 3872. Fax: 0181 869 3976
E-mail: l.allan@ic.ac.uk

Pain Relief. Middlesex

Dr Abina C O'Callaghan MBBS LRCP MRCS FRCA
YEAR QUALIFIED: 1977
SPECIAL INTEREST: Pain management - acute and chronic; anaesthesia.
PRIVATE: Clementine Churchill Hospital, Sudbury Hill, Harrow, Middlesex, HA1 3RX.
Tel: 0181 872 3939 Fax: 0181 872 3836

Norfolk

Dr Jonathan M J Valentine MBChB FRCA MRCP(UK)
YEAR QUALIFIED: 1986
NHS POST: Consultant in Anaesthetics/Pain Management, Norfolk and Norwich Healthcare NHS Trust.
SPECIAL INTEREST: Chronic pain management; back pain/sciatica; neck pain/whiplash etc.
PRIVATE: Norfolk and Norwich Hospital, St Stephen's Road, Norwich, Norfolk NR1 3SE.
Tel: 01603 660585 Fax: 01603 767527

Oxfordshire

Dr Christopher J Glynn MA MB DCH FRCA MSc
NHS POST: Consultant Anaesthetist Churchill Hospital
SPECIAL INTEREST:
PRIVATE: Oxford Regional Pain Relief Unit, Oxford Radcliffe Hospital The Churchill, Old Road, Headington, Oxford OX3 7LJ. Tel: 01865 226 193 Fax: 01865 226 160

Surrey

Dr John Fozard MB FRCA
YEAR QUALIFIED: 1970
NHS POST: Consultant in Anaesthetics & Pain Relief, Royal Surrey County Hospital.
SPECIAL INTEREST: Pain relief.
PRIVATE: Mount Alvernia Hospital, Harvey Road, Guildford, Surrey GU1 3LX.
Tel: 01483 570 122/01252 782 164 Secretary: 01483 406616

Dr Peter Houlton MBBS LRCP MRCS FRCA
YEAR QUALIFIED: 1971
NHS POST: Consultant in Pain Relief, St. Peter's Hospital Chertsey - 01932 872 000 ext 2599.
SPECIAL INTEREST: Pain Management: backpain - acute backpain management.
PRIVATE: Ottermead, Castle Road, Woking, Surrey GU21 4ES.
Tel: 01483 729992 Fax: 01483 729992
Runnymede Hospital, Guildford Road, Ottershaw, Surrey, KT16 0RQ.
Tel: 01483 729 992, 01932 872007 Fax: 01483 729 992
Woking Nuffield Hospital, Shores Road, Woking, Surrey, GU21 4BY.
Tel: 01483 763 511 / 729 992 Fax: 01483 729 992

Warwickshire

Dr Shelton Nethisinghe MD LMSSA FFARCSI
YEAR QUALIFIED: 1970
NHS POST: Consultant Anaesthetist, Hospital of St Cross, Rugby.
SPECIAL INTEREST: Relief of chronic pain (musculoskeletal) using nerve blocks, epidural, acupuncture and laser treatments.
PRIVATE: Wennel Ways, Southam Road, Dunchurch, Rugby, Warwickshire CV22 6NW.
Tel: 01788 545207   Fax: 01788 545267   E-mail: nethisinghe@thefree.net

Pathology

Kent

Dr Yvette I Lolin MD PhD FRCPath
YEAR QUALIFIED: 1978
NHS POST: Consultant in Chemical Pathology and Metabolic Medicine, Kent and Sussex Hospital.
SPECIAL INTEREST: Hyperlipidaemia, hyperhomocysteinaemia and other risk factors for coronary heart disease; lead poisoning; metabolic bone disease and /or hypercalcaemia; renal stones; endocrine disorders: particularly thyroid, pituitary and adrenal; fluid and electrolyte imbalance.
PRIVATE: Kent and Sussex Hospital, Mount Ephraim, Tunbridge Wells, Kent TN4 8AT.
Tel: 01892 526111 ext 2366 Fax: 01892 516698

London

Dr Stuart Blackie MB ChB BSc FRCPath
YEAR QUALIFIED: 1976
SPECIAL INTEREST: General histopathology and cytology.
PRIVATE: 43A Wimpole Street, London W1M 7AF.
Tel: 0171 486 5091 Fax: 07070 608 925 E-mail: RASBlackie@aol.com

Professor Tom Robin Caine Boyde MB BS MD FRCPath
YEAR QUALIFIED: 1955
SPECIAL INTEREST: Chemical pathology.
PRIVATE: 21D Devonshire Place, London W1N 1PD. Tel: 0171 487 2926 Fax: 0171 487 2926

Dr Gilbert Igboaka MB BS FRCPath DMJ
YEAR QUALIFIED: 1975
NHS POST: Consultant Histopathologist and Cytopathologist, Central Middlesex Hospital, London NW10 7NS Tel: 0181 453 2174; Fax: 0181 453 2532.
SPECIAL INTEREST: General and Diagnostic Histopathology; Gynaecological and Non-Gynaecological Cytology including Breast Screening; Medico-Legal Autopsies.
PRIVATE: 91 Brownlow Road, New Southgate, London N11 2BN.
Tel: 0181 539 5522/888 0482 Fax: 0181 889 5600
E-mail: gilbert.igboaka@cmh-tr.nthames.nhs.uk

West Midlands

Dr Christopher Edwards MD FRCPath
YEAR QUALIFIED: 1963
NHS POST: Consultant Histopathologist, Formerly Birmingham Heartlands Hospital.
SPECIAL INTEREST: Pulmonary and thoracic histopathology; histopathology of industrial lung and pleural disease.
PRIVATE: 30 Lovelace Avenue, Solihull, West Midlands B91 3JR. Tel: 0121 705 0709

Psychiatry

Berkshire

Dr Galal A Badrawy MBBCh MRCPsych
SPECIAL INTEREST: Psychiatry
PRIVATE: Cardinal Clinic, Oakley Green, Windsor, Berkshire SL4 5LU.
Tel: 01753 869 755 Fax: 01753 842 852

Dr Bryan Lask MBBS MPhil FRCPsych FRCPCH
YEAR QUALIFIED: 1966
SPECIAL INTEREST: Eating disorders in young people.
PRIVATE: Huntercombe Manor Hospital, Huntercombe Lane South, Taplow, Maidenhead, Berkshire SL6 0PQ. Tel: 01628 667881 Fax: 01628 666989
E-mail:lask-wise@dial.pipex.com

Dr Peter D Maddocks MB MRCP FRCPsych
NHS POST: Consultant Psychiatrist, Wexham Park Hospital.
SPECIAL INTEREST: General adult psychiatry.
PRIVATE: 47 Alma Road, Windsor, Berkshire SL4 3HH.
Tel: 01753 851 551
Cardinal Clinic Bishops Lodge Ltd, Oakley Green, Windsor, Berkshire SL4 5UL.
Tel: 01753 869 755

Dr Mark Tattersall MB BS MRCPsych
YEAR QUALIFIED: 1981
NHS POST: Honorary Consultant Psychiatrist, Eating Disorders Service, Pathfinder Mental Health Services NHS Trust and St George's Hospital Medical School.
SPECIAL INTEREST: Eating disorders (in children and adults) general and medico-legal psychiatry.
PRIVATE: Huntercombe Manor Hospital, Huntercombe Lane South, Taplow, Maidenhead, Berkshire SL6 0PQ. Tel: 01628 667881 Fax: 01628 666989

Buckinghamshire

Dr William Walsh MBBS MRCPsych FRANZCP
YEAR QUALIFIED: 1968
NHS POST: Consultant Psychiatrist Aylesburyvale NHS Trust
SPECIAL INTEREST: Adult general psychiatry.
PRIVATE: The Paddocks Hospital, Aylesbury Road, Princes Risborough, Buckinghamshire HP27 0JS. Tel: 01844 346 951 Fax: 01844 344 521

Cambridgeshire

Dr Richard O'Flynn MB BS MRCPsych
YEAR QUALIFIED: 1981
NHS POST: Consultant Psychiatrist, West Suffolk Hospital.
SPECIAL INTEREST: General psychiatry; management of depression and anxiety; stress and occupational psychiatry; post traumatic stress and medico-legal aspects of psychiatry; drug and alcohol abuse.
PRIVATE: The Evelyn Hospital, 4 Trumpington Road, Cambridge, Cambridgeshire CB2 2AF. Tel: 01223 303336

Cheshire

Dr Thomas Carnwath MA FRCPsych MRCGP
YEAR QUALIFIED: 1974
NHS POST: Consultant Addiction Psychiatrist, Trafford General Hospital.
SPECIAL INTEREST: General adult psychiatry/addictions particularly illicit drugs (heroin, cocaine, cannabis, amphetamine etc).
PRIVATE: Actrincham Priory Hospital, Rappax Road, Hale, Actrincham, Cheshire WA15 0NX. Tel: 0161 904 0050 Fax: 0161 980 4322

Dr Brendan Thomas Monteiro MBBS LRCP MRCS MRCPsych
YEAR QUALIFIED: 1978
NHS POST: Consultant Psychiatrist, National Centre for Mental Health and Deafness.
SPECIAL INTEREST: General adult psychiatry mainly mental health and deafness and eating disorders. Provision of out-patient assessments, day-patient, in-patient care. I direct the Eating Disorder Programme at Altrincham Priory Hospital.
PRIVATE: Staff Consultant Psychiatrist, Director of Eating Disorder Programme Altrincham Priory Hospital, Hale, Cheshire WA15 0NX. Tel: 0161 904 0050 Fax: 0161 980 4322
E-mail: goabtm@aol.com

Dr Claire Sillince MB ChB MRCP(UK) FRCPsych
YEAR QUALIFIED: 1975
SPECIAL INTEREST: I have a pragmatic/eclectic approach and see myself very much as a generalist. I have particular experience in treating doctors and other health professionals.
PRIVATE: Russell House, Cheadle Royal Healthcare, 100 Wilmslow Road, Cheadle, Cheshire SK8 3DG. Tel: 0161 428 9511 Fax: 0161 491 1501

Cleveland

Dr Sikandar Hayat Kamlana MBBS DPM FRCPsych Dip. Psychother Dip. Psychopharm
YEAR QUALIFIED: 1970
NHS POST: Consultant Psychiatrist / Psychotherapist, North Tees General Hospital.
SPECIAL INTEREST: Psychotherapy and psychopharmacology; have diplomas in both major treatment modalities. Apply integrated approach to mental disorders both major and minor illnesses including eating disorders, sexual disorders and addiction disorders.
PRIVATE: Mental Health Department, North Tees General Hospital, Hardwick, Stockton-on-Tees, Cleveland TS19 8PE. Tel: 01642 617517 Fax: 01642 642089

Dorset

Dr Michael Ford MBBS DCH MRCP FRCPsych
- YEAR QUALIFIED: 1977
- NHS POST: Consultant Psychiatrist, Alderney Hospital, Dorset.
- SPECIAL INTEREST: Adult psychiatry; eating disorders; psychosomatic illness; psychological assessment.
- PRIVATE: 19 Wellington Road, Parkstone, Poole, Dorset NH14 9LF. Tel: 01202 734241

East Sussex

Dr Hartmut Steffen State Exam Med 1965 Heidelberg
- YEAR QUALIFIED: 1965
- SPECIAL INTEREST: Child adolescent family psychiatry; psychosomatic illness; behavior disorder; post traumatic stress disorder; ADHD; childhood autism; family crisis: assessment, holistic therapy, family therapy; medico-legal work; male-female team with Cornelia Steffen M.A.
- PRIVATE: Young Persons Unit Outpatient Clinic, Ticehurst House Hospital, Ticehurst, Wadhurst, East Sussex, TN5 7HU. Tel: 01580 202226 Fax: 01580 201006

Essex

Dr Colin Brewer MBBS MRCS LRCP DPM MRCPsych
- YEAR QUALIFIED: 1963
- SPECIAL INTEREST: Alcohol and drug abuse.
- PRIVATE: The Stapleford Unit, London Road, Stapleford Tawney, Essex RM4 1SR. Tel: 01708 688 328

Dr Richard O'Flynn MB BS MRCPsych
- YEAR QUALIFIED: 1981
- NHS POST: Consultant Psychiatrist, West Suffolk Hospital.
- SPECIAL INTEREST: General psychiatry; management of depression and anxiety; stress and occupational psychiatry; post traumatic stress and medico-legal aspects of psychiatry; drug and alcohol abuse.
- PRIVATE: Dukes Priory Hospital, Stump Lane, Springfield Green, Springfield, Chelmsford Essex CM1 5SJ. Tel: 01245 345345

Professor Brice Pitt MD BS FRCPsych
- NHS POST: Professor of Psychiatry of Old Age Hammersmith Hospital
- SPECIAL INTEREST: Old Age Psychiatry, Perinatal Psychiatry, Depression, Memory Disorders
- PRIVATE: Palmers House, Maltings Drive, Epping, Essex CM16 6SG. Tel: 01992 574748 Fax: 01992 575471

Psychiatry. Essex

Dr Jason Taylor MBBS MRCPsych MSc(Econ)
- YEAR QUALIFIED: 1976
- NHS POST: Consultant Psychiatrist, Warley Hospital, Essex.
- SPECIAL INTEREST: Depressive disorders; anxiety; schizophrenia and related disorders.
- PRIVATE: BUPA Hartswood Hospital, Eagle Way, Brentwood, Essex, CM13 3LE. Tel: 01277 232 525 E-mail:100015.3000@compuserve.com

Dr Gillian Waldron MB ChB MRCPsych
- SPECIAL INTEREST: Psychiatric disorders in women.
- PRIVATE: Holly House Hospital, High Road, Buckhurst Hill, Essex, IG9 5HX. Tel: 0181 505 3311 Fax: 0181 506 1013

Glasgow

Dr Alan A Fraser BSc MB ChB MRCPsych
- YEAR QUALIFIED: 1979
- NHS POST: Consultant Psychiatrist, Southern General Hospital, Glasgow.
- SPECIAL INTEREST: General psychiatry; alcohol and drug misuse; post-traumatic stress disorder; legal and forensic aspects of psychiatry.
- PRIVATE: Langside Priory Hospital, 38 Mansionhouse Road, Glasgow G41 3DW. Tel: 0141 636 6116 Fax: 0141 636 5151

Greater Manchester

Dr Maurice Silverman MD FRCPsych DPM
- YEAR QUALIFIED: 1943
- NHS POST: Formerly Consultant, Ribble Valley Hospital Trust.
- SPECIAL INTEREST: Neuroses and other conditions requiring relaxation techniques or hypnotherapy. I am a member of the British Society of Medical and Dental Hypnosis.
- PRIVATE: The Fir Trees, 2 Ringley Drive, Whitefield, Greater Manchester M45 7LF. Tel: 0161 766 3576

Hampshire

Dr Morgan Ross O'Connell MB BCh BAO DPM FRCPsych
- YEAR QUALIFIED: 1968
- NHS POST: St Joseph's Centre, Holy Cross Hospital, Haslemebe.
- SPECIAL INTEREST: Post traumatic stress disorder (PTSD) and substance abuse; the needs of ex-servicemen and women.
- PRIVATE: Marchwood Priory Hospital, Hythe Road, Marchwood, Southampton, Hampshire SO40 4WU. Tel: 01703 840044 Fax: 01703 207554
  Sprint Associates Wickham House, Wickham, Hampshire PO17 5JU. Tel: 01329 834512 Fax: 01329 835150

Dr Mark Slaney MA MB BS DRCOG MRCPsych
YEAR QUALIFIED: 1983
NHS POST: Consultant Psychiatrist, Loddon NHS Trust, Parklands Hospital, Basingstoke.
SPECIAL INTEREST: General adult psychiatry.
PRIVATE: Mulfords Hill Centre, 37-39 Mulfords Hill, Tadley, Hampshire RG26 3HX. Tel: 0118 940 9701 Fax: 0118 982 0233

Dr Alan Nicholas Wear BSc MB BS MRCPsych
YEAR QUALIFIED: 1980
SPECIAL INTEREST: Liaison psychiatry; eating disorders; somatisation disorders; psychological approaches to common psychiatric conditions including chronic fatigue syndrome.
PRIVATE: Marchwood Priory Hospital, Hythe Road, Marchwood, Southampton, Hampshire SO40 4WU. Tel: 01703 840044 Fax: 01703 207554

Hertfordshire

Dr Jerome Hart MBBS DRCOG MRCPsych
YEAR QUALIFIED: 1979
SPECIAL INTEREST: Adult psychiatry.
PRIVATE: BUPA Hospital Harpenden, Ambrose Lane, Harpenden, Herts, AL5 4BP. Tel: 01582 763191 Fax: 01582 712312

Dr George Mathew MBBS DPM MRCPsych
YEAR QUALIFIED: 1973
NHS POST: Consultant Psychiatrist Queen Elizabeth II Hospital, Welwyn Garden City, Hertfordshire.
SPECIAL INTEREST: General psychiatry; depression and affective disorders; organic psychiatry.
PRIVATE: BUPA Hospital Harpenden, Ambrose Lane, Harpenden, Herts, AL5 4BP. Tel: 01582 763191 Fax: 01582 761358

Kent

Dr Julian Bird MA MB BChir FRCP FRCPsych
NHS POST: NHS Post: Portnall's Unit Farnborough Hospital
SPECIAL INTEREST: Psychiatry
PRIVATE: Hayes Grove Priory Hospital, Prestons Road, Hayes, Bromley, Kent BR2 7AS. Tel: 0181 462 7722

Lancashire

Dr Brendan Thomas Monteiro MBBS LRCP MRCS MRCPsych
YEAR QUALIFIED: 1978
NHS POST: Consultant Psychiatrist, National Centre for Mental Health and Deafness.
SPECIAL INTEREST: General adult psychiatry mainly mental health and deafness and eating disorders. I direct the Eating Disorder Programme at Altrincham Priory Hospital.
PRIVATE: Lancashire Priory Hospital, Rosemary Lane, Bartle, Preston, Lancashire PR4 0HB. Tel: 01772 691122 Fax: 01772 691246 E-mail: goabtm@aol.com

London

Dr Bernard Adams MSc MB FRCP FRCPsych DPM
- NHS POST: Emeritus Consultant, University College Hospital.
- SPECIAL INTEREST: General psychiatry; psycho pharmacology.
- PRIVATE: 7 Wimpole Street, London W1M 7AB.
  Tel: 0171 436 6346 Fax: 0181 340 9879

Dr Galal A Badrawy MBBCh MRCPsych
- SPECIAL INTEREST: Psychiatry
- PRIVATE: 121 Harley Street, London, W1N 1DH.
  Tel: 0171 935 6875

Dr Harold Behr MB BCh FRCPsych DPM MInstGA
- YEAR QUALIFIED: 1963
- NHS POST: Formerly Consultant Child Psychiatrist, Central Middlesex Hospital.
- SPECIAL INTEREST: Group psychotherapy and family therapy.
- PRIVATE: North London Centre For Group Therapy, 138 Bramley Road, Oakwood, London N14 4HU. Tel: 0181 440 1451 Fax: 0181 440 1451

Dr Arnon Bentovim MBBS FRCPsych FRCPCH DPM
- YEAR QUALIFIED: 1959
- NHS POST: Honorary Consultant Psychiatrist, Great Ormond Street Hospital for Children and the Tavistock Clinic.
- SPECIAL INTEREST: Child and adolescent psychiatry; emotional and behavioural problems of childhood and adolescence; family relational problems; individual and family therapy; medico-legal practice.
- PRIVATE: London Child & Family Consultation Service, 234 Great Portland Street, London W1N 5PH. Tel: 0171 390 8377 Fax: 0171 390 8287; Secretary: 0171 831 4489

Dr Colin Brewer MBBS MRCS LRCP DPM MRCPsych
- YEAR QUALIFIED: 1963
- SPECIAL INTEREST: Alcohol and drug abuse.
- PRIVATE: The Stapleford Centre, 25A Eccleston Street, London SW1W 9NP.
  Tel: 0171 823 6840 Fax: 0171 730 3409

Dr Paul Bridges TD MD PhD MRCS FRCPsych DPM
- YEAR QUALIFIED: 1956
- NHS POST: Consultant Psychiatrist, Guy's & Maudsley Hospitals.
- SPECIAL INTEREST: Medico-legal cases.
- PRIVATE: Keats House, Guy's Hospital, 24-26 St. Thomas Street, London SE1 9RT.
  Tel: 0171 378 9464 / 955 5000 ext 5569 Fax: 0171 378 0931

Dr Lachlan Campbell MBBS MRCPsych
- YEAR QUALIFIED: 1972
- NHS POST: Consultant Psychiatrist, Bethlem Royal and Maudsley Hospitals.
- SPECIAL INTEREST: Medico-legal assessments for civil and criminal proceedings including personal injury claims, stress related disorders, parental assessment for child care and mental health review tribunals.
- PRIVATE: Guthrie Clinic Consulting Rooms, King's College Hospital, Denmark Hill, London, SE5 9RS. Tel: 0171 362 0100 Fax: 0973 583 065 E-mail: info@medexpert.co.uk

Dr Jeremy Christie-Brown BM FRCP FRCPsych DPM
- SPECIAL INTEREST: General psychiatry.
- PRIVATE: 127 Harley Street, London W1N 1DJ. Tel: 0171 486 3631 Fax: 0181 265 2026

Dr Lewis J Clein MD FRCPsych MRCP DPM
- YEAR QUALIFIED: 1949
- SPECIAL INTEREST: Adult psychiatry; neuroses; addictive disorders; depression; psychotic illnesses.
- PRIVATE: 80 Harley Street, London W1N 1AE. Tel: 0171 935 4647

Dr Jan Falkowski BSc MBBS MRCPsych MBA TD
- YEAR QUALIFIED: 1984
- NHS POST: Consultant Psychiatrist, The Royal London Hospital.
- SPECIAL INTEREST: General adult psychiatry including drug and alcohol problems.
- PRIVATE: The Churchill Priory, Churchill Clinic, 80 Lambeth Road, London, SE1 7PW. Tel: 01713 777 960

Dr Paul Flower MA(Cantab) MSc MBBS MRCPsych
- SPECIAL INTEREST: Eating disorders in young people; psychotherapy.
- PRIVATE: Rhodes Farm Clinic, The Ridgeway, London NW7 1RH. Tel: 0181 906 0885 Fax: 0181 906 3155

  91 South Hill Park, London NW3 2SP. Tel: 0171 794 4398 Fax: 0171 794 4398

Dr Stephen Frank TD MRCP FRCPsych DPM
- NHS POST: Consultant Psychiatrist, Gordon Hospital.
- SPECIAL INTEREST: General adult psychiatry; liaison psychiatry; medicolegal work.
- PRIVATE: 14 Devonshire Place, London, W1N 1PB. Tel: 0171 935 0640

  Out patient Dept. 2nd Floor, Lister Hospital, Chelsea Bridge Road, London, SW1W 8RH. Tel: 0171 730 8298

Psychiatry. London

Dr Anthony H Fry MB MRCPsych MPhil DPM
- YEAR QUALIFIED: 1967
- NHS POST: Formerly consultant, Guy's Hospital. Examiner, Royal College of Psychiatry. Teacher, University of London.
- SPECIAL INTEREST: General psychiatry; neurotic disorders; post traumatic stress disorder; reactive depression, cognitive behavioural therapy; stress management; psychotherapeutic counselling, brief focal counselling; medico-legal assessments.
- PRIVATE: Emblem House London Bridge Hospital, 27 Tooley Street, London, SE1 2PR.
Tel: 0171 607 3937 Fax: 0171 607 3815 E-mail: anthony@frydoc.demon.co.uk
14 Devonshire Place, London, W1N 1PB.
Tel: 0171 607 3937 Fax: 0171 607 3815 E-mail: anthony@frydoc.demon.co.uk

Dr Maurice Greenberg BSc Mphil FRCP FRCPsych
- NHS POST: Consultant Psychiatrist, Psychotherapist and Head of Student Counselling Service, University College London Hospital
- SPECIAL INTEREST: Somatization and Stress Disorders, General Psychiatry, Psychotherapy (individual & group), Young Adults.
- PRIVATE: Private Patients Wing, University College London Hospitals, 25 Grafton Way, London WC1E 6AU. Tel: 0171 383 7911 / 0171 935 3103 Fax: 0171 380 9816 / 0171 935 1397
E-mail:m.greenberg@ucl.ac.uk

Dr Jerome Hart MBBS DRCOG MRCPsych
- YEAR QUALIFIED: 1979
- SPECIAL INTEREST: Adult psychiatry.
- PRIVATE: The Garden Hospital, 46-50 Sunny Gardens Road, Hendon, London, NW4 1RX.
Tel: 0181 203 6832 Fax: 0181 203 4343

Dr Roger B Howells BSc (Hons) MBBChir MRCPsych
- YEAR QUALIFIED: 1980
- NHS POST: Consultant Psychiatrist, Maudsley Hospital.
- SPECIAL INTEREST: General psychiatry; child and adolescent emotional and behavioural problems; family problems; alcohol dependence; occupational psychiatry.
- PRIVATE: The Consulting Rooms, 7 Radnor Walk, Chelsea, London SW3 4PB.
Cromwell Hospital, Cromwell Road, London SW5 0TU.
Tel: Appointments: 0171 731 7889 Fax: 0171 731 7889
Information: http://homepages.which.net/~roger.howells/

Dr George Ikkos BSc LMSSA MRCPsych MInstGA
- YEAR QUALIFIED: 1981
- NHS POST: Consultant Psychiatrist, Barnet Healthcare Trust and Royal National Orthopaedic Hospital.
- SPECIAL INTEREST: General psychiatry; stress secondary to injury and illness; psychiatric aspects of spinal injury; body image disorder; mental health of parents of abused children; interpersonal psychotherapy; Greek.
- PRIVATE: Grovelands Priory Hospital, The Bourne, Southgate, London, N14 6RA.
Tel: 01426 917 231 Fax: 0181 444 1203
London Child & Family Consultation Service, 234 Great Portland Street, London W1N 5PH. Tel: 01426 917 231 Fax: 0181 444 1203

Dr Bryan Lask MBBS MPhil FRCPsych FRCPCH
- YEAR QUALIFIED: 1966
- SPECIAL INTEREST: Eating disorders in young people.
- PRIVATE: St George's Child & Adolescent Eating Disorders Service, Harewood House Springfield University Hospital, 61 Glenburnie Road, London SW17 7DJ.
Tel: 0181 682 6751 Fax: 0181 682 6724 E-mail: lask-wise@dial.pipex.com
Department of Psychiatry, Jenner Wing St George's Hospital Medical School, Cranmer Terrace, London SW17 0RE. Tel: 0181 725 5514 Fax: 0181 725 5514
E-mail: lask-wise@dial.pipex.com

Dr Gerald Libby FRCPsych
- NHS POST: Consultant and Honorary Senior Lecturer St. Bartholomew's Hospital
- SPECIAL INTEREST: General Psychiatry And Psychosomatic Disorders. Member of British Society of Gastroenterology. Functional Gastrointestinal Disorders And Pain.
- PRIVATE: The Princess Grace Hospital, 42-52 Nottingham Place, London W1M 3FD.
Tel: 0171 486 1234
17 Harley Street, London W1N 1DA.
Tel: 0171 636 7916 Fax: 0171 637 2373

Dr Bron Lipkin MB BS FRCPsych DPM
- SPECIAL INTEREST: General adult psychiatry; assessment for psychotherapy both psychodynamic and cognitive behavioural; second opinion assessments.
- PRIVATE: Grovelands Priory Hospital, The Bourne, Southgate, London, N14 6RA.
Tel: 0181 882 8191 xt 374 Fax: 0181 447 8138
Charter Nightingale Hospital, 11-19 Lisson Grove, London, NW1 6SH.
Tel: 0181 882 8191(c/o Grovelands Hospital). Fax: 0181 447 8138

Dr George Mathew MBBS DPM MRCPsych
- YEAR QUALIFIED: 1973
- NHS POST: Consultant Psychiatrist Queen Elizabeth II Hospital, Welwyn Garden City, Hertfordshire.
- SPECIAL INTEREST: General psychiatry; depression and affective disorders; organic psychiatry.
- PRIVATE: St. Andrew's At Harrow, Bowden House Clinic, London Road, Harrow on the Hill, Middlesex HA1 3JL. Tel: 0181 966 7000 Fax: 0181 864 6092

Dr Peter George Mellett MBBS FRCPsych DPM
- SPECIAL INTEREST: General adult and adolescent psychiatry; psychotherapy (including hypno-psychotherapy); psychosomatics; post traumatic stress disorder; sequelae of childhood abuse; panic; hyperventilation; phobias (including flying); expert legal reports (civil and criminal).
- PRIVATE: 7 Wimpole Street, London W1M 7AB.
Tel: 0171 580 1584, Private secretary-01372 275161/276161.
Fax: Private secretary-01372 277494.

Psychiatry. London

Dr Donald H Montgomery MB ChB FRCPsych FRANZCP
- YEAR QUALIFIED: 1966
- NHS POST: Consultant Psychiatrist & Psychotherapist, Charing Cross Hospital and Tolworth Hospital.
- SPECIAL INTEREST: Member of Institute of Group Analysis; psychosexual medicine, especially gender identity disorders and gender dysphoria.
- PRIVATE: Charing Cross Hospital, Fulham Palace Road, London, W6 8RF.
  Tel: 0181 846 1516/1148
  Group Analytic Practice, 88 Montagu Mansions, London W1H 1LF.
  Tel: 0171 935 3103/935 3085 Fax: 0171 935 1397

Dr Morgan Ross O'Connell MB BCh BAO DPM FRCPsych
- YEAR QUALIFIED: 1968
- NHS POST: St Joseph's Centre, Holy Cross Hospital, Haslemebe.
- SPECIAL INTEREST: Post traumatic stress disorder (PTSD) and substance abuse; the needs of ex-servicemen and women.
- PRIVATE: 14 Devonshire Place, London, W1N 1PB.
  Tel: 0171 935 0640 Fax: 0171 224 6256

Dr Raj Persaud MRCPsych MPhil MSc BSc MB BS
- YEAR QUALIFIED: 1986
- NHS POST: Consultant Psychiatrist, Maudsley Hospital.
- SPECIAL INTEREST: Treatment and prevention of all mental illness including anxiety disorders, depression and psychosis.
- PRIVATE: Westways, 49 St. James Road, West Croydon, London CR9 2RR.
  Tel: 0181 700 8512 Fax: 0181 700 8504

Dr Jeremy M Pfeffer BSc MBBS FRCP FRCPsych
- NHS POST: Consultant Psychiatrist & Honorary Senior Lecturer, The Royal Brompton Hospital.
- SPECIAL INTEREST: Psychosomatic disorders; marital therapy.
- PRIVATE: 97 Harley Street, London, W1N 1DF.
  Tel: 0171 935 3878 Fax: 0171 935 3865
  Charter Nightingale Hospital, 11-19 Lisson Grove, London, NW1 6SH.
  Tel: 0171 258 3828 Fax: 0171 724 8294
  Grovelands Priory Hospital, The Bourne, Southgate, London, N14 6RA.
  Tel: 0181 882 8191
  Cromwell Hospital, Cromwell Road, London SW5 0TU.
  Tel: 0171 370 4233 Fax: 0171 460 5555

Dr Lester Sireling MB BS LRCP MRCS MRCPsych
- YEAR QUALIFIED: 1974
- NHS POST: Consultant Psychiatrist Barnet General Hospital
- SPECIAL INTEREST:
- PRIVATE: Grovelands Priory Hospital, The Bourne, Southgate, London, N14 6RA.
  Tel: 0181 731 9004 Fax: 0181 731 9004 E-mail: sireling@msn.com

Psychiatry. London

Dr Vera E Sutton MB ChB
- YEAR QUALIFIED: 1957
- NHS POST: Honorary Consultant Friern Hospital
- SPECIAL INTEREST: Psychiatry
- PRIVATE: 40 Holne Chase, Hampstead Garden Suburb, London N2 0QQ.
  Tel: 0181 455 0825 Fax: 0181 458 7188

Dr David Veale MD BSc MRCPsych MPhil Dip CACP
- SPECIAL INTEREST: Obsessive compulsive disorder; phobias; depression; body dysmorphic disorder; eating disorders and their treatment by cognitive behaviour therapy.
- PRIVATE: Grovelands Priory Hospital, The Bourne, Southgate, London, N14 6RA.
  Tel: 0181 882 8191 Fax: 0181 447 8138
  E-mail: david@veale.co.uk. Web site: http://www.veale.co.uk
  Church Crescent, Muswell Hill, London N10.
  Tel: 0181 882 8191 Fax: 0181 447 8138
  E-mail: david@veale.co.uk. Web site: http://www.veale.co.uk

Dr Gillian Waldron MB ChB MRCPsych
- SPECIAL INTEREST: Psychiatric disorders in women.
- PRIVATE: Grovelands Priory Hospital, The Bourne, Southgate, London, N14 6RA.
  Tel: 0181 882 8191 xt 217 Fax: 0181 447 8138

Dr Peter Elton Walker MB B Chir FRCP FRCPCH DCH
- YEAR QUALIFIED: 1960
- NHS POST: Consultant Paediatrician (Emeritus), Frimley Park Hospital
- SPECIAL INTEREST: Behavioural and emotional problems of children, young children and adolescents; sleep disorders; psychosomatic disorders, including fatigue syndromes; enuresis and encopresis; pre-school problems; school difficulties; attention deficit disorders.
- PRIVATE: Portland Hospital for Women & Children, 234 Great Portland Street, London W1N 5PH. Tel: 0171 390 8312 Fax: 0171 390 8311

Dr David Wood MB BS MRCPsych DRCOG M.Inst.Group.Analysis.
- YEAR QUALIFIED: 1975
- SPECIAL INTEREST: Eating disorders in children and adolescents.
- PRIVATE: Rhodes Farm Clinic, The Ridgeway, Mill Hill, London NW7 1RH.
  Tel: 0181 906 0885 Fax: 0181 906 3155 E-mail: rhodesfarm@messages.co.uk

Dr Felicity I S de Zulueta BSc MA(Cantab) MBChB MRCPsych
- NHS POST: Honorary Consultant Psychiatrist / Psychotherapist, Maudsley Hospital, Traumatic Stress Service.
- SPECIAL INTEREST: Post traumatic stress disorder assessment and treatment of patients suffering from the effects of childhood or adult trauma and associated depression and panic/phobias. Medico legal reports for patients suffering from PTSD.
- PRIVATE: Traumatic Stress Service, Maudsley Hospital, Denmark Hill, London, SE5 8AZ.
  Tel: 0171 919 2969 Fax: 0171 919 3573 E-mail: f.dezulueta@iop.bpmf.ac.uk

Merseyside

Dr Brendan Thomas Monteiro MBBS LRCP MRCS MRCPsych
YEAR QUALIFIED: 1978
NHS POST: Consultant Psychiatrist, National Centre for Mental Health and Deafness.
SPECIAL INTEREST: General adult psychiatry mainly mental health and deafness and eating disorders. I direct the Eating Disorder Programme at Altrincham Priory Hospital.
PRIVATE: BUPA Murrayfield Hospital, Holmwood Drive, Thingwall, Wirral, Merseyside L61 1AU. Tel: 0151 648 7000 Fax: 0151 648 7684 E-mail: goabtm@aol.com

Dr Nagalingam Murugananthan MBBS FRCPsych DPM
YEAR QUALIFIED: 1965
NHS POST: Consultant Psychiatrist, Whiston Hospital, Prescot.
SPECIAL INTEREST: Adult mental illness; medico-legal work; mental health tribunal.
PRIVATE: Fairfield Independent Hospital, Crank, St. Helens, WA11 7RS. Tel: 01744 739311 Fax: 01744 453358

Middlesex

Dr Jerome Hart MBBS DRCOG MRCPsych
YEAR QUALIFIED: 1979
SPECIAL INTEREST: Adult psychiatry.
PRIVATE: St. Andrew's At Harrow (Bowden House), London Road, Harrow On The Hill, Middlesex HA1 3JL. Tel: 0181 966 7000 Fax: 0181 864 6092

Dr David Veale MD BSc MRCPsych MPhil Dip CACP
SPECIAL INTEREST: Obsessive compulsive disorder; phobias; depression; body dysmorphic disorder; eating disorders and their treatment by cognitive behaviour therapy.
PRIVATE: Clementine Churchill Hospital, Sudbury Hill, Harrow, Middlesex, HA1 3RX. Tel: 0181 882 8191 Fax: 0181 447 8138
E-mail: david@veale.co.uk. Web site: http://www.veale.co.uk

Dr William Walsh MBBS MRCPsych FRANZCP
YEAR QUALIFIED: 1968
NHS POST: Consultant Psychiatrist Aylesburyvale NHS Trust
SPECIAL INTEREST: Adult general psychiatry.
PRIVATE: St. Andrew's At Harrow, Bowden House Clinic, London Road, Harrow on the Hill, Middlesex HA1 3JL. Tel: 0181 966 7000 Fax: 0181 864 6092

Nottinghamshire

Dr David Anthony Toms MB BS MRCP FRCPsych DCH DRCOG DPM
YEAR QUALIFIED: 1960
NHS POST: Emeritus Consultant Psychiatrist, Mapperley Hospital, Nottingham Health Authority.
SPECIAL INTEREST: General adult psychiatry; psychotherapy and supervision; forensic reports; eating disorders and medically related problems.
PRIVATE: 2 Regent Street, Nottingham, Nottinghamshire NG1 5BQ.
Tel: 0115 947 4755 Fax: 0115 958 7098

Oxfordshire

Dr Peter Amies MB BS MSc MRCPsych
YEAR QUALIFIED: 1973
NHS POST: Consultant Psychotherapist, Kingshill House, Swindon, Warneford Hospital, Oxford (Honorary).
SPECIAL INTEREST: Specialise in the integrated psychological/pharmacological management of all non-psychotic disorders.
PRIVATE: 77 Victoria Road, Summertown, Oxford, Oxfordshire OX2 7QG.
Tel: 01565 556322 Fax: 01793 491047

Suffolk

Dr Richard O'Flynn MB BS MRCPsych
YEAR QUALIFIED: 1981
NHS POST: Consultant Psychiatrist, West Suffolk Hospital.
SPECIAL INTEREST: General psychiatry; management of depression and anxiety; stress and occupational psychiatry; post traumatic stress and medico-legal aspects of psychiatry; drug and alcohol abuse.
PRIVATE: West Suffolk Hospital, Hardwick Lane, Bury Street, Edmunds, Suffolk IP33 2QZ.
Tel: 01284 713390 Fax: 01284 713694
Suffolk Nuffield Hospital, Foxhall Road, Ipswich, Suffolk
Tel: 01473 279100 Fax: 01473 279101

Surrey

Dr Anthony Baker MBBS MRCPsych
YEAR QUALIFIED: 1974
SPECIAL INTEREST: Therapeutic Assessment And Therapy After Childhood Abuse (Children & Adults). Also 'Asperger's Syndrome' And Attention Deficit Hyperactivity Disorder (ADHD). Medico-legal childcare and family assessments.
PRIVATE: Baker & Duncan Ashwood Centre, Stonemason's Court, Cemetery Pales, Brookwood, Surrey GU24 0BL. Tel: 01483 487979 Fax: 01483 486464

Psychiatry. Surrey

Dr Tim G A Cantopher BSc MBBS FRCPsych
- YEAR QUALIFIED: 1979
- SPECIAL INTEREST: Depression.
- PRIVATE: Sturt Priory Hospital, Sturt's Lane, Walton-on-the-Hill, Surrey, KT20 7RQ. Tel: 0173 781 4488 Fax: 0173 781 3926

Dr Peter George Mellett MBBS FRCPsych DPM
- SPECIAL INTEREST: General adult and adolescent psychiatry; psychotherapy (including hypno-psychotherapy); psychosomatics; post traumatic stress disorder; sequelae of childhood abuse; panic; hyperventilation; phobias (including flying); expert legal reports (civil and criminal).
- PRIVATE: Ashtead Hospital, The Warren, Ashtead, Surrey KT21 2SB. Tel: Private secretary-01372 275161/276161. Fax: Private secretary-01372 277494.

Dr Michael Rowlands MB ChB MRCPsych
- YEAR QUALIFIED: 1979
- SPECIAL INTEREST: Eating disorders; depression; post traumatic stress disorder.
- PRIVATE: Sturt Priory Hospital, Sturt's Lane, Walton On The Hill, Surrey KT20 7RQ. Tel: 01737 814488 Fax: 01737 813926
  BUPA Gatwick Park Hospital, Povey Cross Road, Horley, Surrey RH6 0BB. Tel: 01293 785511 Fax: 01293 774883

Dr Richard Stern MD FRCPsych DPM
- YEAR QUALIFIED: 1967
- NHS POST: Consultant St. George's & St Helier Hospitals
- SPECIAL INTEREST: Treatment of depression; obsessive-compulsive disorder; phobic disorders; post traumatic stress disorder; psychosomatic disorders. Behavioural and cognitive psychotherapy. Medico-legal reporting, and acting as expert witness.
- PRIVATE: St. Anthony's Hospital, London Road, North Cheam, Surrey, SM3 9DW. Tel: 0181 337 6691 Fax: 0181 335 3325

West Yorkshire

Dr Christopher M Taylor MA MB BChir MRCPsych
- YEAR QUALIFIED: 1976
- NHS POST: Consultant Psychiatrist and Senior Clinical Lecturer, St James's University Hospital, Leeds.
- SPECIAL INTEREST: Adult psychiatry; severe mental illness; recurrent depression; childhood sexual abuse; panic disorder; obsessional compulsive disorder; behavioural problems; narcolepsy; chronic fatigue syndrome; post-traumatic stress disorder and alcohol dependence.
- PRIVATE: BUPA Hospital Leeds, Roundhay Hall, Jackson Avenue, Leeds, West Yorkshire LS8 1NT. Tel: 0113 269 3939 Fax: 0113 268 1340
  42 The Drive, Adel, Leeds, West Yorkshire LS16 6BQ. Tel: 0113 226 4463 Fax: 0113 226 4463

Psychotherapy

Cleveland

Dr Sikandar Hayat Kamlana MBBS DPM FRCPsych Dip. Psychother Dip. Psychopharm
- YEAR QUALIFIED: 1970
- NHS POST: Consultant Psychiatrist / Psychotherapist, North Tees General Hospital.
- SPECIAL INTEREST: Psychotherapy and psychopharmacology; have diplomas in both major treatment modalities. Apply integrated approach to mental disorders both major and minor illnesses including eating disorders, sexual disorders and addiction disorders.
- PRIVATE: Mental Health Department, North Tees General Hospital, Hardwick, Stockton-on-Tees, Cleveland TS19 8PE. Tel: 01642 617617 Fax: 01642 642089

Hertfordshire

Dr Joan Farewell MB BS MRCPsych DPM
- YEAR QUALIFIED: 1961
- SPECIAL INTEREST: Short term hypnotherapy, treating phobias and psychosomatic and habit disorders.
- PRIVATE: 27 Canons Close, Radlett, Hertfordshire WD7 7ER.
  Tel: 01923 857388

Kent

Dr Ruth Margaret Hirons MB ChB MRCPsych Mem. Brit. Assc. Psychotherapists
- YEAR QUALIFIED: 1969
- NHS POST: Consultant Psychotherapist, Invicta Trust, Maidstone, Kent.
  Tel: 01622 776355
- SPECIAL INTEREST: Psychodynamic psychotherapy with: 1) Health care professionals; 2) borderline personality disorders; 3) sexual deviations. Prefer longer term work with more disturbed patients. Supervision and teaching.
- PRIVATE: 1 Lavender Bank, Beesfield Lane, Farningham, Kent DA4 0DA.
  Tel: 01322 862629

London

Dr Margaret Christie-Brown MBBS MBAPsychotherapy
- NHS POST: Formerly - Consultant Psychotherapist, Quenn Charlottes & Chelsea Hospital for Women.
- SPECIAL INTEREST: Psychosexual and psychosomatic problems. Analytical psychotherapy for anxiety and relationship problems.
- PRIVATE: 127 Harley Street, London W1N 1DJ.
  Tel: 0181 670 1071 Fax: 0181 265 2026

Dr Maureen Gledhill MD ChB MRCPsych DCH
- YEAR QUALIFIED: 1957
- SPECIAL INTEREST: Anxiety; depression; stress disorders; relationship problems; child and family problems; psychosomatic disorders in women.
- PRIVATE: 528 Finchley Road, London NW11 8DD.
  Tel: 0171 731 8642

Dr Maurice Greenberg BSc Mphil FRCP FRCPsych
- NHS POST: Consultant Psychiatrist, Psychotherapist and Head of Student Counselling Service, University College London Hospital
- SPECIAL INTEREST: Somatization and Stress Disorders, General Psychiatry, Psychotherapy (individual & group), Young Adults.
- PRIVATE: Group Analytic Practice, 88 Montagu Mansions, London W1H 1LF.
  Tel: 0171 935 3103 / 0171 383 7911 Fax: 0171 935 1397 / 0171 380 9816
  E-mail:m.greenberg@ucl.ac.uk

Dr Edward Richard Herst MA MD FRCPsych
- YEAR QUALIFIED: 1952
- SPECIAL INTEREST: Psychotherapy in primary care and psychiatric settings, analytical psychology.
- PRIVATE: 9 Fitzroy Road, London NW1 8TU.
  Tel: 0171 722 1661

Dr Eric Ledermann FRCPsych
- SPECIAL INTEREST: A true-self psychotherapy, explained in published books and articles, based on acceptance of patients' conscience
- PRIVATE: 121 Harley Street, London, W1N 1DH.

Dr Donald H Montgomery MB ChB FRCPsych FRANZCP
- YEAR QUALIFIED: 1966
- NHS POST: Consultant Psychiatrist & Psychotherapist, Charing Cross Hospital and Tolworth Hospital.
- SPECIAL INTEREST: Member of Institute of Group Analysis; psychosexual medicine, especially gender identity disorders and gender dysphoria. Group and individual psychoanalytic psychotherapy.
- PRIVATE: Group Analytic Practice, 88 Montagu Mansions, London W1H 1LF.
  Tel: 0171 935 3103/935 3085 Fax: 0171 935 1397

Dr Michael R. Pokorny MB ChB DPM FRCPsych
- YEAR QUALIFIED: 1961
- SPECIAL INTEREST: Conjoint marital psychotherapy
- PRIVATE: 167 Sumatra Road, West Hampstead, London NW6 1PN.
  Tel: 0171 431 4693 Fax: 0171 435 5712

Dr Felicity I S de Zulueta BSc MA(Cantab) MBChB MRCPsych
- NHS POST: Honorary Consultant Psychiatrist / Psychotherapist, Maudsley Hospital, Traumatic Stress Service.
- SPECIAL INTEREST: Post traumatic stress disorder assessment and treatment of patients suffering from the effects of childhood or adult trauma and associated depression and panic/phobias. Medico legal reports for patients suffering from PTSD.
- PRIVATE: Traumatic Stress Service, Maudsley Hospital, Denmark Hill, London, SE5 8AZ.
  Tel: 0171 919 2969 Fax: 0171 919 3573 E-mail: f.dezulueta@iop.bpmf.ac.uk

Strathclyde

Dr Robert Whyte MB ChB FRCPsych DPM
- YEAR QUALIFIED: 1966
- NHS POST: Consultant Psychotherapist, Parkhead Hospital, Glasgow.
- SPECIAL INTEREST: Treatment of people with relationship problems in individual; psychodynamic; psychotherapy.
- PRIVATE: 3 Fitzroy Place, Glasgow, Strathclyde G3 7RH.
Tel: 0141 248 5451

West Midlands

Dr Helen Lloyd MB BCh MRCPsych UKCP Reg.
- YEAR QUALIFIED: 1958
- NHS POST: Formerly Consultant Child and Adolescent Psychiatrist, Dudley Priority Trust.
- SPECIAL INTEREST: Psycho-analytic; psychotherapy - individual adult and family therapy.
- PRIVATE: 65 Blakedown Road, Halesowen, West Midlands B63 4NG.
Tel: 0121 501 3194 Fax: 0121 501 3194

Radiology

Bedfordshire

Dr Martin John Warren MB BS BSc MRCP FRCR
- YEAR QUALIFIED: 1978
- NHS POST: Consultant Radiologist, Luton and Dunstable.
- SPECIAL INTEREST: General abdominal and pelvic ultrasound; musculoskeletal imaging and ENT using ultrasound, MRI, CT and nuclear medicine.
- PRIVATE: Diagnostic Imaging, Luton and Dunstable Hospital, Lewsey Road, Luton, Bedfordshire, LU4 0DZ. Tel: 01582 497059 Fax: 01582 497418
E-mail: martin.warren@ldh-tr.anglox.nhs.uk

Buckinghamshire

Dr Martin John Warren MB BS BSc MRCP FRCR
- YEAR QUALIFIED: 1978
- NHS POST: Consultant Radiologist, Luton and Dunstable.
- SPECIAL INTEREST: General abdominal and pelvic ultrasound; musculoskeletal imaging and ENT using ultrasound, MRI, CT and nuclear medicine.
- PRIVATE: The Paddocks Hospital, Aylesbury Road, Princes Risborough, Buckinghamshire HP27 0JS. Tel: 01844 346951 Fax: 01844 344521

Durham

Dr Terence Featherstone MB BS DMRD FRCR
- YEAR QUALIFIED: 1982
- NHS POST: Consultant Radiologist, Sunderland Royal Hospital.
- SPECIAL INTEREST: Magnetic resonance imaging and all aspects of musculoskeletal radiology including medico-legal and sports injury work.
- PRIVATE: Darlington MRI Centre, Hollyhurst Road, Darlington, Durham DL3 6UA. Tel: 01325 369696 Fax: 01325 361754

Hampshire

Dr Nigel Hacking BSc MBBS MRCP FRCR
- YEAR QUALIFIED: 1980
- NHS POST: Consultant Radiologist, Southampton University Hospitals.
- SPECIAL INTEREST: Hepatobiliary; urological; vascular; gynaecological imaging and intervention; fibroid embolisation; x-ray; ultrasound; CT; MR and angiography.
- PRIVATE: X-Ray Department, BUPA Chalybeate Hospital, Chalybeate Close, Tremona Road, Southampton, Hampshire SO16 6UY.
Tel: 01703 775544 Fax: 01703 704804
Department of Clinical Imaging, Wessex Nuffield Hospital, Winchester Road, Chandler's Ford, Eastleigh, Hampshire SO53 2DW.
Tel: 01703 266377 Fax: 01703 258410

Hertfordshire

Dr Martin John Warren MB BS BSc MRCP FRCR
YEAR QUALIFIED: 1978
NHS POST: Consultant Radiologist, Luton and Dunstable.
SPECIAL INTEREST: General abdominal and pelvic ultrasound; musculoskeletal imaging and ENT using ultrasound, MRI, CT and nuclear medicine.
PRIVATE: BUPA Hospital Harpenden, Ambrose Lane, Harpenden, Herts, AL5 4BP.
Tel: 01582 763191 Fax: 01582 763246
BUPA Hospital Bushey, Heathbourne Rd, Bushey, Watford, Hertfordshire WD2 1RD.
Tel: 0181 901 5566 Fax: 0181 420 4913

London

Dr John B Bingham MA MSC FRCP FRCR
YEAR QUALIFIED: 1969
NHS POST: Consultant and Senior Lecturer, Guy's and St. Thomas' Trust.
SPECIAL INTEREST: Magnetic resonance.
PRIVATE: BMI Blackheath Hospital, 40-42 Lee Terrace, London, SE3 9UD.
Tel: 0181 318 4405 Fax: 0181 318 2542
The London Bridge Hospital, 27 Tooley Street, London, SE1 2PR.
Tel: 0171 403 4911 Fax: 0171 403 2185
Cromwell Hospital, Cromwell Road, London SW5 OTU.
Tel: 0171 460 2000 Fax: 0171 370 7700

Dr Paul Cannon FRCR MB BCh BAO
NHS POST: Consultant Radiologist, St. Bartholomew's Hospital.
SPECIAL INTEREST: Ultrasound.
PRIVATE: The London Imaging Centre, Lister House, 11 Wimpole Street, London, W1M 7AB.
Tel: 0171 467 8800 Fax: 0171 631 1604

Dr Neil Wardlaw Garvie MA MSc MRCP FRCR
NHS POST: Consultant in Radiology and Nuclear Medicine, Royal London Hospital.
SPECIAL INTEREST: Nuclear medicine.
PRIVATE: The London Imaging Centre, Lister House, 11 Wimpole Street, London, W1M 7AB.
Tel: 0171 467 8800 Fax: 0171 631 1604
The London MRI Centre, 110 Harley Street, London W1N 1AF.
Tel: 0171 935 3563 Fax: 0171 224 2302

Dr Allan Irvine MBBS DMRD MRCP FRCR
YEAR QUALIFIED: 1977
NHS POST: Consultant Radiologist, St. Thomas' Hospital.
SPECIAL INTEREST: Cross-sectional imaging; including body CT, abdominal ultrasound and musculoskeletal MRI; interventional radiology-CT; invasive procedures and angiography.
PRIVATE: The London Imaging Centre, Lister House, 11 Wimpole Street, London, W1M 7AB.
Tel: 0171 637 0632 Fax: 0171 631 1604
The London MRI Centre, 110 Harley Street, London W1N 1AF.
Tel: 0171 935 3563 Fax: 0171 224 2302

Radiology. London

Dr Lesley MacDonald MB BS FRCR
NHS POST: Consultant Radiologist, St. Thomas' Hospital.
SPECIAL INTEREST: Ultrasound including obstetrics, gynaecology and vascular studies; paediatrics.
PRIVATE: The London Imaging Centre, Lister House, 11 Wimpole Street, London, W1M 7AB.
Tel: 0171 467 8800 Fax: 0171 631 1604

Dr Ingeborg Nockler MB ChB FRCR
YEAR QUALIFIED: 1971
NHS POST: Consultant Radiologist Central Middlesex Hospital
SPECIAL INTEREST: Breast imaging; interventional uroradiology; angiography; ultrasound and general radiology.
PRIVATE: The London Clinic, 20 Devonshire Place, London, W1N 2DH.
Tel: 0171 935 4444 ext 3353
Princess Grace Hospital, 42-52 Nottingham Place, London, W1M 3FD.
Tel: 0171 486 7401

Dr Chandra Thakkar MD DMRD FRCR MBBS DMRE
NHS POST: Consultant Neuro-Radiologist, Royal London Hospital & St Bartholomew's Hospital.
SPECIAL INTEREST: Neuro-radiology.
PRIVATE: The London MRI Centre, 110 Harley Street, London W1N 1AF.
Tel: 0171 935 3563 Fax: 0171 224 2302
The London Imaging Centre, Lister House, 11 Wimpole Street, London, W1M 7AB.
Tel: 0171 467 8800 Fax: 0171 631 1604

Dr Keith Tonge BSc MBBS FRCR
NHS POST: Consultant Radiologist, Guy's & St. Thomas' Hospital.
SPECIAL INTEREST: Neuro radiology - Ophthalmological - MRI
PRIVATE: The London MRI Centre, 110 Harley Street, London W1N 1AF.
Tel: 0171 935 3563 Fax: 0171 224 2302
The London Imaging Centre, Lister House, 11 Wimpole Street, London, W1M 7AB.
Tel: 0171 467 8800 Fax: 0171 631 1604

Norfolk

Dr John Bannerman Latham MB ChB FRCR
YEAR QUALIFIED: 1966
NHS POST: Consultant Radiologist, Norfolk and Norwich.
SPECIAL INTEREST: General radiology including CT, MRI, ultrasound and mammography.
PRIVATE: X-Ray Department, Norfolk & Norwich Hospital, Brunswick Road, Norwich, Norfolk NR1 3SR. Tel: 01603 286087 Fax: 01603 286088

Renal Medicine

London

Dr Laurence R I Baker MA MD FRCP FRCPE
YEAR QUALIFIED: 1963
NHS POST: Consultant Physician and Nephrologist, St. Bartholomew's Hospital / Royal London Hospital, London.
SPECIAL INTEREST: Nephrology
PRIVATE: The London Clinic, 20 Devonshire Place, London, W1N 2DH.
Tel: 0171 224 5234 Fax: 0171 486 8706

Dr Richard W E Watts MD DSc PhD FRCP
NHS POST: Honorary Consultant Physician Hammersmith Hospital
SPECIAL INTEREST: Endocrinology; metabolism; diabetes; renal medicine; general medicine.
PRIVATE: Harley Street Clinic, 35 Weymouth Street, London, W1N 4BJ.
Tel: 0171 935 7700, Appointments: 0171 586 5959 ext 2572
Hammersmith Hospital, Du Cane Road, London, W12 OHS.
Tel: Appts.-0171 586 5959 xt 2572. 0181 743 2030 Fax: 0181 746 2410 Aircall- 01459 126538
Sainsbury Wing, Hammersmith Hospital, Du Cane Road, London, W12 OHS.
Tel: 0171 586 5959 ext.2572. Fax: 0171 483 0297 E-mail: info@wellingtonchc.demon.co.uk

Respiratory Medicine

London

Dr Malcolm Green BM BCh BSc BA MA DM FRCP
YEAR QUALIFIED: 1967
NHS POST: Consultant Physician, Royal Brompton Hospital, London SW3 6NP.
SPECIAL INTEREST: Pulmonary infections; asthma.
PRIVATE: Lister Hospital, Chelsea Bridge Road, London, SW1W 8RH.
Tel: 0171 376 4985 Fax: 0171 351 8939

Rheumatology

Cheshire

Dr Dianne Bulgen MB, BS FRCP
YEAR QUALIFIED: 1968
NHS POST: Consultant Rheumatologist, Countess of Chester Hospital NHS Trust.
SPECIAL INTEREST: Inflammatory joint disease, soft tissue rheumatism.
PRIVATE: Grosvenor Nuffield Hospital, Wrexham Road, Chester, Cheshire CH4 7QP.
Tel: 01244 680444 Fax: 01244 680812

Conwy

Dr Wyn Williams FRCP
YEAR QUALIFIED: 1967
NHS POST: Consultant Rheumatologist, Glan Clwynd Hospital NHS Trust.
SPECIAL INTEREST: General rheumatology; osteoporosis.
PRIVATE: North Wales Medical Centre, Queens Road, Llandudno, Conwy LL30 1UD.
Tel: 01492 879031 Fax: 01492 876754

Essex

Dr Kuntal Chakravarty FRCP(Lond) MRCP(Irel) FACP(USA)
YEAR QUALIFIED: 1981
NHS POST: Consultant Rheumatologist, Haroldwood Hospital, Essex.
SPECIAL INTEREST: Inflammatory arthritides, connective tissue disease, vasculitis and metabolic bone disease (osteoporosis and Paget's disease of bone).
PRIVATE: BUPA Hartswood Hospital, Eagle Way, Brentwood, Essex, CM13 3LE.
Tel: 01277 232525

Dr Douglas Golding MA MD FRCP DPhys Med
YEAR QUALIFIED: 1954
SPECIAL INTEREST: Back pain; arthritis; soft tissue rheumatism.
PRIVATE: Holly House Hospital, High Road, Buckhurst Hill, Essex, IG9 5HX.
Tel: 0181 505 3311
BUPA Roding Hospital, Roding Lane South, Redbridge, Ilford, Essex IG4 5PZ.
Tel: 0181 551 1100

Hertfordshire

Dr Douglas Golding MA MD FRCP DPhys Med
YEAR QUALIFIED: 1954
SPECIAL INTEREST: Back pain; arthritis; soft tissue rheumatism.
PRIVATE: The Rivers Hospital, High Wych Road, Sawbridgeworth, Hertfordshire CM21 6HH.
Tel: 01279 600 282 Fax: 01279 600 212

Kent

Dr Thomas Richard Price BSc PhD MBBS FRCP
NHS POST: Consultant Rheumatologist Greenwich District Hospital
SPECIAL INTEREST: Rheumatology & Paediatric rheumatology
PRIVATE: Chelsfield Park Hospital, Bucks Cross Road, Chelsfield, Kent, BR6 7RG.
Tel: 01689 877 855 Fax: 01689 837 439

Dr Michael Wright FRCP
YEAR QUALIFIED: 1963
NHS POST: Consultant Rheumatologist Newham & Royal London Hospitals
SPECIAL INTEREST: Spinal problems.
PRIVATE: 12 Den Close, Beckenham, Kent, BR3 6RP.
Tel: 0181 658 3201 Fax: 0181 658 3201

Lancashire

Dr Michael J Burke BA MBCHB FRCP
YEAR QUALIFIED: 1970
NHS POST: Consultant Rheumatologist, Burnley General Hospital.
SPECIAL INTEREST: Osteoporosis and paget's disease.
PRIVATE: Higher Small Hazels, Woodplumpton Road, Habergham Eaves, Burnley, Lancashire BB11 3RS.
Tel: 01282 438974 Fax: 01282 474434

Leicestershire

Dr Roger Oldham BSc MB FRCP FRCP(E)
YEAR QUALIFIED: 1969
NHS POST: Consultant Rheumatologist, Leicester General Hospital.
SPECIAL INTEREST: Spinal disorders; soft tissue rheumatism; arthritis and connective tissue disorders.
PRIVATE: BUPA Hospital Leicester, Gartree Road, Oadby, Leicester, Leicestershire LE2 2FF.
Tel: 0116 265 3655 Fax: 0116 272 0566
Nuffield Hospital Leicester, Scraptoft Lane, Leicester, Leicestershire LE5 1HY.
Tel: 0116 276 9401 Fax: 0116 246 1076

London

Dr Simon Allard BSc MBBS MD FRCP
YEAR QUALIFIED: 1979
NHS POST: Consultant Physician and Rheumatologist, West Middlesex University Hospital.
SPECIAL INTEREST: General physician with an interest in rheumatology. Specific interests: inflammatory connective tissue disorders, regional musculoskeletal disorders.
PRIVATE: 149 Harley Street, London W1N 2DE. Tel: 0171 616 7693 Fax: 0171 616 7633
Cromwell Hospital, Cromwell Road, London SW5 0TU.
Tel: 0171 460 2000 Fax: 0171 460 5555

Rheumatology. London

Dr Colin G Barnes BSc MB BS FRCP
- YEAR QUALIFIED: 1961
- NHS POST: Honorary Consulting Rheumatologist, The Royal London Hospital.
- SPECIAL INTEREST: Clinical Rheumatology.
- PRIVATE: The London Independent Hospital, 1 Beaumont Square, Stepney Green, London E1 4NL. Tel: 0171 790 0990
  96 Harley Street, London W1N 1AF. Tel: 0171 486 0967 Fax: 0171 935 1107

Dr Hedley Berry MA DM FRCP
- YEAR QUALIFIED: 1967
- NHS POST: Consultant Rheumatologist, King's College Hospital.
- SPECIAL INTEREST: Inflammatory joint disease; back pain; soft tissue rheumatic diseases; osteoporosis.
- PRIVATE: 96 Harley Street, London W1N 1AF.
  Tel: 0171 486 0967 or 0181 952 5557 Fax: 0171 935 1107 Portable: 0793 0371 391

Professor John Elfed Davies MRCS D.Phys.Med Dip.SportsMed PM Rehab (EU)
- NHS POST: Consultant Physician In Sports Medicine, Physical Medicine And Rehabilitation Guy's Hospital, London
- SPECIAL INTEREST: Rehabilitation of low back pain and diagnosis of musculo-skeletal sports injuries; treatment of fibro myalgia and chronic fatigue syndrome; foot problems; bio-mechanics and surgery.
- PRIVATE: The Harley Street Rheumatism Clinic, Devonshire Hospital, Devonshire Street, London, W1. Tel: 0171 486 2494 Fax: 0171 486 0090

Dr Timothy F W Dilke MA FRCP
- YEAR QUALIFIED: 1964
- NHS POST: Consultant Rheumatologist, Queen Mary's and Queen Elizabeth Hospital.
- SPECIAL INTEREST: Rheumatology
- PRIVATE: BMI Blackheath Hospital, 40-42 Lee Terrace, Blackheath, London SE3 9UD.
  Tel: 0181 318 7722 Fax: 0181 318 2542
  152 Harley Street, London W1N 1HH.
  Tel: 0171 935 0444 Fax: 0171 224 2574

Professor Rodney Grahame MD FRCP FACP
- YEAR QUALIFIED: 1955
- NHS POST: Consultant Rheumatologist, UCL Hospitals.
- SPECIAL INTEREST: Rheumatology including back pain, soft tissue lesions and hypermobility.
- PRIVATE: Hospital of St. John & St. Elizabeth, 60 Grove End Road, St Johns Wood, London, NW8 9NH. Tel: 0171 286 3126 Fax: 0171 266 2316

Dr Charles Mackworth-Young MA MD FRCP
- YEAR QUALIFIED: 1978
- NHS POST: Consultant Physician, Charing Cross Hospital.
- SPECIAL INTEREST: Inflammatory rheumatic disorders; connective tissue disease; soft tissue rheumatism.
- PRIVATE: Cromwell Hospital, Cromwell Road, London SW5 OTU.
  Tel: 0171 460 5700 Fax: 0171 460 5555
  Lister Hospital, Chelsea Bridge Road, London, SW1W 8RH.
  Tel: 0171 730 8298 Fax: 0171 259 9218
  134 Harley Street, London W1N 1AH.
  Tel: 0171 486 3846

Rheumatology. London

Dr Vivian M Martin MBBS MRCP
- SPECIAL INTEREST: Rheumatology.
- PRIVATE: 8 Upper Wimpole Street, London, W1M 7TD.
  Tel: 0171 486 2365 Fax: 0171 224 0034
  Cromwell Hospital, Cromwell Road, London SW5 0TU.
  Tel: 0171 460 2000 Fax: 0171 460 5555

Dr John Martin Outhwaite MA(oxon) BM BCh FRCP
- YEAR QUALIFIED: 1978
- NHS POST: Consultant Physician Orthopaedic Rehabilitation, Nuffield Orthopaedic Centre.
- SPECIAL INTEREST: Musculo skeletal rehabilitation of low back pain; whiplash injury; RSI; assistive technology for severe disability.
- PRIVATE: Cromwell Hospital, Cromwell Road, London SW5 0TU.
  Tel: 0171 460 2000. Secretary-01793 821 082 Fax: 01865 227460

Professor Gabriel Panayi ScD MD FRCP
- NHS POST: Professor Guy's Hospital
- SPECIAL INTEREST: Inflammatory arthritic diseases and rheumatoid arthritis; connective tissue disease; back pain and soft tissue rheumatism.
- PRIVATE: Guy's Hospital, St Thomas Street, London, SE1 9RT.
  Tel: 0171 955 4394 Fax: 0171 955 2472 E-mail: g.panayi@umds.ac.uk

Dr J David Perry FRCP MB
- YEAR QUALIFIED: 1969
- NHS POST: Consultant Rheumatologist Royal London Hospital, Mile End.
- SPECIAL INTEREST: Rheumatology and sports medicine.
- PRIVATE: London Independent Hospital, 1 Beaumont Square, Stepney Green, London E1 4NL.
  Tel: 0171 791 1688

Dr Thomas Richard Price BSc PhD MBBS FRCP
- NHS POST: Consultant Rheumatologist Greenwich District Hospital
- SPECIAL INTEREST: Rheumatology & Paediatric rheumatology
- PRIVATE: BMI Blackheath Hospital, 40-42 Lee Terrace, London, SE3 9UD.
  Tel: 0181 312 7722 Fax: 0181 318 2542

Dr Richard G Rees MB FRCP
- NHS POST: Consultant Rheumatologist, St. Mary's Hospital
- SPECIAL INTEREST: General rheumatology; inflammatory arthritis; soft tissue rheumatism; pain relief.
- PRIVATE: Lindo Wing, St. Mary's Hospital, Praed Street, Paddington, London, W2 1NY.
  Tel: 0171 886 1046 Fax: 0171 886 6083
  Parkside Hospital, 53 Parkside, Wimbledon, London, SW19 5NX.
  Tel: 0181 946 4202 ext. 3223 / 3335 Fax: 0181 946 7775

Dr Tim Spector MBBS MD MSc FRCP
- YEAR QUALIFIED: 1982
- NHS POST: Consultant Rheumatologist, St. Thomas' Hospital
- SPECIAL INTEREST: Osteoporosis and general rheumatology including osteoarthritis, rheumatoid arthritis and other inflammatory conditions.
- PRIVATE: York House Consulting Rooms, 199 Westminster Bridge Road, London SE1 7UT.
  Tel: 0171 928 5485 Fax: 0171 928 3748

Dr Anthony White MB ChB FRCP DPhysMed
NHS POST: Consultant Rheumatologist, The Royal Free Hospital and Whittington Hospital.
SPECIAL INTEREST: Inflammatory arthritis particularly psoriatic arthropathy and spondylosis; spinal disorders and electromyography/nerve conduction tests.
PRIVATE: 152 Harley Street, London W1N 1HH.
Tel: 0171 935 8868 Fax: 0171 224 2574

Professor Patricia Woo BSc MBBS PhD FRCP
NHS POST: Hon Consultant Rheumatologist Great Ormond Street Hospital, Middlesex Hospital
SPECIAL INTEREST: Paediatric rheumatology.
PRIVATE: Great Ormond Street Hospital for Children NHS Trust, Great Ormond Street, London WC1N 3JH. Tel: 0171 504 9148 Fax: 0171 436 0783

Dr Michael Wright FRCP
YEAR QUALIFIED: 1963
NHS POST: Consultant Rheumatologist Newham & Royal London Hospitals
SPECIAL INTEREST: Spinal problems.
PRIVATE: 10 Harley Street, London W1N 1AA.
Tel: 0171 467 8345 Fax: 0171 467 8312
London Independent Hospital, 1 Beaumont Square, Stepney Green, London E1 4NL.
Tel: 0171 790 0990 Fax: 0171 265 9032

Middlesex

Dr Hedley Berry MA DM FRCP
YEAR QUALIFIED: 1967
NHS POST: Consultant Rheumatologist, King's College Hospital.
SPECIAL INTEREST: Inflammatory joint disease; back pain; soft tissue rheumatic diseases; osteoporosis.
PRIVATE: Clementine Churchill Hospital, Sudbury Hill, Harrow, Middlesex, HA1 3RX.
Tel: 0181 872 3872/3939 or 0181 952 5557 Fax: 0181 872 3871 Portable: 0793 0371 391

Dr Richard G Rees MB FRCP
NHS POST: Consultant Rheumatologist, St. Mary's Hospital
SPECIAL INTEREST: General rheumatology; inflammatory arthritis; soft tissue rheumatism; pain relief.
PRIVATE: The Clementine Churchill Hospital, Sudbury Hill, Harrow, Middlesex, HA1 3RX.
Tel: 0181 872 3939 Fax: 0181 872 3871

Nottinghamshire

Dr Chris Deighton MD BmedSci FRCP
YEAR QUALIFIED: 1984
NHS POST: Consultant Rheumatologist, Nottingham City Hospital.
SPECIAL INTEREST: Inflammatory arthritis, medico-legal work.
PRIVATE: Park Hospital, Sherwood Lodge Drive, Arnold, Nottingham NG5 8RX.
Tel: 0115 967 0670 Fax: 0115 926 0905
Nuffield Hospital, 748 Mansfield Road, Nottingham NG5 3FZ.
Tel: 0115 920 9209 Fax: 0115 967 3005

Surrey

Dr Rodney Hughes MD MA MRCP
- YEAR QUALIFIED: 1982
- NHS POST: Consultant Rheumatologist & General Physician, St Peter Hospital NHS Trust.
- SPECIAL INTEREST: General rheumatology; inflammatory joint disease; osteoporosis.
- PRIVATE: Runnymede Hospital, Guildford Road, Ottershaw, Surrey, KT16 0RQ. Tel: 01932 872 007 for Secretary and Appointments.

Tyne & Wear

Professor Terence John Daymond MB ChB FRCP(London) FRCP(Edin) Dip. Phys Med
- YEAR QUALIFIED: 1967
- NHS POST: Consultant Rheumatology and Rehabilitation, Royal Hospital Sunderland.
- SPECIAL INTEREST: Rheumatoid arthritis osteoarthritis; osteoporosis; back pain; chronic fatigue syndrome.
- PRIVATE: BUPA Hospital Washington, Picktree Lane, Rickleton, Washington, Tyne & Wear NE38 9JZ. Tel: 0191 415 1272

Dr Kishin Hingorani FRCP
- YEAR QUALIFIED: 1953
- SPECIAL INTEREST: Back pain; neck pain.
- PRIVATE: The Old Granary North Brunton Farm, Gosforth, Newcastle Upon Tyne, NE3 5HD. Tel: 0191 236 6442 Fax: 0191 236 6442

SURGERY - Breast

East Sussex

Mr Brian J Stoodley MA MChir FRCS
- NHS POST: Consultant Surgeon Eastbourne District General & Uckfield Hospitals
- SPECIAL INTEREST: Colorectal and gastrointestinal/breast/varicose vein surgery.
- PRIVATE: Consulting Rooms, 21 Lushington Road, Eastbourne, East Sussex BN26 5UX.
  Tel: 01323 410 441 Fax: 01323 410 978

Mr Andrew Yelland MB BS FRCS(Ed) MS
- YEAR QUALIFIED: 1986
- NHS POST: Lead Consultant in Breast Surgery, Royal Sussex County Hospital, Brighton.
- SPECIAL INTEREST: Surgical oncology of the breast; breast reconstruction, reduction and augmentation.
- PRIVATE: Hove Nuffield Hospital, 55 New Church Road, Hove, East Sussex BN3 4BG.
  Tel: 01273 627044

Essex

Mr James Wellwood MA MChir(Camb) FRCS(Eng)
- NHS POST: Consultant Surgeon - Director Of Surgery Whipps Cross Hospital, Leytonstone
- SPECIAL INTEREST: Laparoscopic abdominal surgery; breast disease; gastro intestinal/colorectal surgery.
- PRIVATE: Holly House Hospital, High Road, Buckhurst Hill, Essex, IG9 5HX.
  Tel: 0181 505 6423 Fax: 0181 502 9735
  BUPA Roding Hospital, Roding Lane South, Redbridge, Ilford, Essex IG4 5PZ.
  Tel: 0181 551 1100 Fax: 0181 551 9452

Hertfordshire

Mr Simon J Cox MBBS FRCS
- YEAR QUALIFIED: 1965
- SPECIAL INTEREST: Breast surgery; general surgery.
- PRIVATE: BUPA Hospital Bushey, Heathbourne Rd, Bushey, Watford, Hertfordshire WD2 1RD.
  Tel: 0181 950 9090/0181 386 5115 Fax: 0181 420 8514/0181 386 5775

Kent

Mr David B Jackson BSc MB FRCS
- NHS POST: Consultant Surgeon, Kent & Canterbury Hospital.
- SPECIAL INTEREST: Surgical oncology specialising in breast reconstruction and major pelvic surgery; ileo-anal pouch surgery and laparoscopic procedures.
- PRIVATE: Winters Farm, Nackington Road, Canterbury, Kent CT4 7AY.
  Tel: 01227 472 581 Fax: 01227 472 581 E-mail: davidjackson@uk-consultants.co.uk

SURGERY - Breast. Kent

Mr Michael Parker BSc MS FRCS FRCS(Ed)
- NHS POST: Consultant General Surgeon Joyce Green Hospital
- SPECIAL INTEREST: Breast Cancer; colorectal cancer and laparoscopic surgery.
- PRIVATE: Chelsfield Park Hospital, Bucks Cross Road, Chelsfield, Kent, BR6 7RG.
Tel: 01689 877 855 / 01474 879 987 Fax: 01689 837 439
Fawkham Manor Hospital, Manor Lane, Fawkham, Longfield, Kent DA3 8ND.
Tel: 01474 879 987 Fax: 01474 872 585

London

Mr Tim Davidson ChM MRCP FRCS
- NHS POST: Consultant Breast and General Surgeon, Royal Free Hospital, Hampstead, London NW3 2QG. Secretary Tel: 0171 830 2794. Fax: 0171 830 2194.
- SPECIAL INTEREST: Breast surgery including breast reconstruction; thyroid and general surgery; salivary gland and parotid surgery; skin and soft tissue tumours.
- PRIVATE: The London Clinic, 149 Harley Street, London, W1N 2DE.
Tel: 0171 616 7693 Fax: 0171 616 7633
Portland Hospital for Women & Children, 205-209 Gt. Portland Street, London W1N 6AH. Tel: 0171 390 8083 Fax: 0171 390 8266

Sir Arnold Elton MS(Lond) FRCS(Eng) FICS
- NHS POST: Honorary Consulting Surgeon, Northwick Park Hospital.
- SPECIAL INTEREST: Breast surgery. Founder Officer Of British Association Of Surgical Oncology. Member European Society Of Surgical Oncology. Member Council and International Advisor World Federation of Surgery Oncology Societies. Member, Government Committee on National Breast Screening.
- PRIVATE: The Consulting Rooms, Wellington Hospital,, Wellington Place, St John's Wood, London NW8 9LE. Tel: 0171 935 4101 Fax: 0171 483 0297
Web site: www.medicalnet.co.uk/sir.arnold.elton

Mr Jerry Gilmore MS FRCS FRCS(Ed)
- YEAR QUALIFIED: 1966
- SPECIAL INTEREST: Breast surgery; assessment, diagnosis and treatment of all benign and malignant breast disease.
- PRIVATE: The London Breast Clinic, 108 Harley Street, London W1N 2ET.
Tel: 0171 637 8820 Fax: 0171 935 3901

Mr John Lynn MS FRCS
- YEAR QUALIFIED: 1964
- NHS POST: Consultant Endocrine Surgeon, Hammersmith Hospital, London.
- SPECIAL INTEREST: Surgical endocrinology of thyroid, pancreas, parathyroid and adrenal. Surgery of breast diseases.
- PRIVATE: Cromwell Hospital, Cromwell Road, London SW5 OTU.
Tel: 0836 285832 Fax: 0181 566 6402

SURGERY - Breast. London

Mr Harvey Minasian MS(London) FRCS
- YEAR QUALIFIED: 1969
- SPECIAL INTEREST: Breast surgery; surgical oncology; gastroenterology and minimally invasive surgery.
- PRIVATE: Cromwell Hospital, Cromwell Road, London SW5 0TU.
  Tel: 0171 460 5700 / 0181 997 5026 Fax: 0171 460 5555 / 0181 810 4783

Mr Nigel P M Sacks MS FRCS FRACS
- NHS POST: Consultant Surgeon, The Royal Marsden Hospital and St. George's Hospital
- SPECIAL INTEREST: Breast and endocrine surgery.
- PRIVATE: Lister Hospital, Chelsea Bridge Road, London, SW1W 8RH.
  Tel: 0171 730 4647 Fax: 0171 730 2567
  Parkside Hospital, 53 Parkside, Wimbledon, London, SW19 5NX.
  Tel: 0171 730 4647 Fax: 0171 730 2567
  The Royal Marsden Hospital, Fulham Road, London, SW3 6JJ.
  Tel: 0171 352 8171 ext.2782

Mr David Skidmore OBE MA MD FRCS(Ed) (Eng)
- YEAR QUALIFIED: 1964
- NHS POST: Honorary Senior Lecturer, University College London Hospital.
- SPECIAL INTEREST: Surgical Oncology - Breast and Colo-rectal Surgery
- PRIVATE: Private Patient Unit, Middlesex Hospital, Mortimer Street, London, W1N 8AA.
  Tel: 0181 318 6923 Fax: 0181 852 6919
  BMI Blackheath Hospital, 40-42 Lee Terrace, London, SE3 9UD.
  Tel: 0181 318 6923 Fax: 0181 852 6919

Professor Irving Taylor MB ChB MD ChM FRCS
- YEAR QUALIFIED: 1968
- NHS POST: University College London Hospital Trust
- SPECIAL INTEREST: Surgical oncology which includes breast disease. Colorectal cancer and liver malignancy.
- PRIVATE: Woolavington Wing, Middlesex Hospital, Mortimer Street, London, W1N 8AA.
  Tel: 0171 504 9312 Fax: 0171 636 5176 E-mail: j.stumcke@ucl.ac.uk

Manchester

Mr Lester Barr MBChB (Hons) ChM FRCS
- YEAR QUALIFIED: 1978
- NHS POST: Consultant Surgeon, Withington and Christie Hospitals, Manchester.
- SPECIAL INTEREST: Surgeon to the specialist breast unit and the sarcoma unit at the Nightingale Centre and Christie Hospital.
- PRIVATE: BUPA Hospital Manchester, Russell Road, Manchester M16 8AJ.
  Tel: 0161 232 2574 Fax: 0161 226 1187

Staffordshire

Mr Timothy Eric Bucknall MS FRCS
YEAR QUALIFIED: 1974
NHS POST: Consultant Surgeon, Queens Hospital, Burton Upon Trent.
SPECIAL INTEREST: General surgeon with special interest in breast disease including rapid diagnosis, genetic screening and reconstruction.
PRIVATE: 1 Tutbury Road, Burton upon Trent, Staffordshire DE13 0NU.
Tel: 01283 566333 Fax: 01283 593014

Mr Terence J Duffy MA BM BCh FRCS
YEAR QUALIFIED: 1972
NHS POST: Consultant Surgeon (Lead), North Staffordshire Hospital Trust.
SPECIAL INTEREST: Breast surgery (benign and malignant), diagnosis and management breast disease, breast screening.
PRIVATE: North Staffordshire Nuffield Hospital, Clayton Road, Newcastle-under-Lyme, Staffordshire ST5 4DB. Tel: 01782 625431 Fax: 01782 712748

Surrey

Mr William Allum BSc MD FRCS
YEAR QUALIFIED: 1977
NHS POST: Consultant Surgeon, Epsom General Hospital.
SPECIAL INTEREST: Gastrointestinal and breast disease.
PRIVATE: Ashtead Hospital, The Warren, Ashtead, Surrey KT21 2SB.
Tel: 01372 275 161 Fax: 01372 277 494

SURGERY - Cardiothoracic

Cambridgeshire

Mr Samer A M Nashef BSc MB ChB FRCS
YEAR QUALIFIED: 1980
NHS POST: Consultant, Papworth
SPECIAL INTEREST: Coronary surgery; minimally invasive surgery; all adult cardiothoracic surgery.
PRIVATE: Papworth Hospital, Cambridge CB3 8RE.
Tel: 01480 364299 Fax: 01480 364334

Mr Francis Charles Wells MA(Cantab) MS FRCS MB BS
YEAR QUALIFIED: 1976
NHS POST: Consultant Cardiothoracic Surgeon, University Lecturer, Papworth.
SPECIAL INTEREST: Cardiac valve reconstruction; coronary artery surgery; surgical management; lung cancer and oesophageal cancer; benign oesophageal conditions.
PRIVATE: Papworth Hospital, Cambridge CB3 8RE.
Tel: 01480 364421 Fax: 01480 831442

London

Mr Martin Elliott MBBS MD FRCS
NHS POST: Consultant Cardiothoracic Surgeon Great Ormond Street Hospital for Children NHS Trust
SPECIAL INTEREST: Correction of congenital heart & thoracic defects.
PRIVATE: Great Ormond Street Hospital for Children NHS Trust, Great Ormond Street, London WC1N 3JH. Tel: 0171 829 8853 Fax: 0171 813 8262

Mr Charles William Pattison MB ChB FRCS FRCS(Ed)
YEAR QUALIFIED: 1980
NHS POST: Consultant Cardiothoracic Surgeon, Middlesex And University College Hospital
SPECIAL INTEREST: Adult cardiac surgery; coronary artery and valve surgery; redo-procedures and surgery of the aorta.
PRIVATE: 42 Wimpole Street, London W1M 7AF.
Tel: 0171 486 7416 Fax: 0171 487 2569

Mr Richard Sayer MBBS FRCS
YEAR QUALIFIED: 1969
NHS POST: Consultant Thoracic Surgeon, St. George's Hospital.
SPECIAL INTEREST: All aspects of non-cardiac thoracic surgery with particular interest in lung and oesophageal cancer and minimally invasive thoracic surgery. Laparoscopic surgery for benign oesophageal disease.
PRIVATE: Cromwell Hospital, Cromwell Road, London SW5 OTU.
Tel: 0171 460 2000. Secretary 0181 337 6691 Fax: 0171 460 5555
E-mail: richard.sayer@ccmail.stgh-tr.sthames.nhs.uk

SURGERY - Cardiothoracic. London

Mr Peter Smith MBBS FRCP FRCS
YEAR QUALIFIED: 1975
NHS POST: Consultant Cardiothoracic Surgeon Hammersmith and Charing Cross Hospitals
SPECIAL INTEREST: Coronary artery bypass graft surgery, redo cardiac surgery and surgery for lung cancer.
PRIVATE: The Heart Hospital, 16-18 Westmoreland Street, London W1M 8PH.
Tel: 0171 573 8888 Fax: 0171 573 8801
Sainsbury Private Patients Wing, Hammersmith Hospital, Du Cane Road, London, W12 OHS. Tel: 0181 383 3198 Fax: 0181 746 1127 / 0181 383 2034
Harley Street Clinic, 35 Weymouth Street, London, W1N 4BJ.
Tel: 0171 935 7700 Fax: 0171 487 4415
Cromwell Hospital, Cromwell Road, London SW5 OTU.
Tel: 0171 370 4233 Fax: 0171 370 4063

Mr Rakesh Uppal BSc MBChB FRCS FRCS(CTh)
NHS POST: Consultant Cardiothoracic Surgeon, London Chest Hospital and St. Bartholomew's Hospital
SPECIAL INTEREST: Myocardial revascularization; aortic surgery.
PRIVATE: 149 Harley Street, London W1N 2DE.
Tel: 0171 935 6397

Mr Graham Venn MS FRCS FICS FETCS
YEAR QUALIFIED: 1977
NHS POST: Consultant Cardiothoracic Surgeon, Cardiothoracic Surgery Guy's & St. Thomas' Hospitals
SPECIAL INTEREST: Adult cardiothoracic surgery.
PRIVATE: Suite 203, Emblem House London Bridge Hospital, 27 Tooley Street, London, SE1 2PR.
Tel: 0171 378 6566 Fax: 0171 378 8156

Merseyside

Mr Brian M Fabri MD FRCS(Ed)
YEAR QUALIFIED: 1975
NHS POST: Consultant Cardiac Surgeon, The Cardiothoracic Centre, Liverpool.
SPECIAL INTEREST: All adult cardiac surgery with special interest in: Surgery for ischaemic heart disease including transmyocardial laser revascularisation and mitral valve repair.
PRIVATE: Audrey Leigh Private Patient's Wing, The Cardiothoracic Centre, Thomas Drive, Liverpool, Merseyside L18 0HE. Tel: 0151 228 1616 Fax: 0151 220 8573
E-mail: bfabri@ccl-tr.nwest.nhs.uk

Plymouth

Mr Terence Lewis MBBS FRCS
YEAR QUALIFIED: 1968
NHS POST: Consultant Cardiac Surgeon.
SPECIAL INTEREST: Adult cardiac surgery.
PRIVATE: South West Cardiothoracic Centre, The Meavy Clinic Private Rooms, Level 5, Derriford Hospital, Plymouth, PL6 8DH. Tel: 01752 763537 Fax: 01752 763538

Surrey

Mr Richard Sayer MBBS FRCS
YEAR QUALIFIED: 1969
NHS POST: Consultant Thoracic Surgeon, St. George's Hospital.
SPECIAL INTEREST: All aspects of non-cardiac thoracic surgery with particular interest in lung and oesophageal cancer and minimally invasive thoracic surgery. Laparoscopic surgery for benign oesophageal disease.
PRIVATE: St. Anthony's Hospital, London Road, North Cheam, Surrey, SM3 9DW.
Tel: 0181 337 6691 Fax: 0181 337 0816 E-mail: richard.sayer@ccmail.stgh-tr.sthames.nhs.uk

SURGERY - Colorectal & Gastrointestinal

Cheshire

Mr George Foster MD FRCS
YEAR QUALIFIED: 1968
NHS POST: Consultant General Surgeon and Coloproctologist, Countess of Chester Hospital.
SPECIAL INTEREST: General surgery; surgery for colorectal cancer and inflammatory bowel disease; minimal access surgery; thyroid surgery.
PRIVATE: Grosvenor Nuffield Hospital, Wrexham Road, Chester, Cheshire CH4 7QP.
Tel: 01244 680444 Fax: 01244 680812

Conwy

Mr David John Hay FRCS FACS
YEAR QUALIFIED: 1969
NHS POST: Consultant Surgeon, Glan Clwyd Hospital NHS Trust.
SPECIAL INTEREST: General surgery with interest in coloproctology and laparoscopic surgery; colorectal cancer and sphincter preservation is a major interest.
PRIVATE: Glan Clwyd Hospital NHS Trust, Plas Craig, Marine Drive, Llandudno, Conwy LL30 2QZ. Tel: 01492 878247 Fax: 01492 878247 E-mail: djhay@glanclwyd-tr.wales.nhs.uk
North Wales Medical Centre, Queens Road, Llandudno, Conwy LL30 1UD.
Tel: 01492 879031 Fax: 01492 876754

East Sussex

Mr Brian J Stoodley MA MChir FRCS
NHS POST: Consultant Surgeon Eastbourne District General & Uckfield Hospitals
SPECIAL INTEREST: Colorectal and gastrointestinal/breast/varicose vein surgery.
PRIVATE: Consulting Rooms, 21 Lushington Road, Eastbourne, East Sussex BN26 5UX.
Tel: 01323 410441 Fax: 01323 410 978

Enfield Middlesex

Mr David Melville MA MB BS DM FRCS FRCS(Ed)
NHS POST: Consultant General Surgeon, North Middlesex Hospital.
SPECIAL INTEREST: Colorectal surgery; paediatric surgery; general surgery including hernias, varicose veins and emergency abdominal surgery.
PRIVATE: King's Oak Hospital, Chase Farm, Enfield, Middlesex EN2 8SD.
Tel: 0181 364 5520

SURGERY - Colorectal & Gastrointestinal. Enfield Middlesex

Mr David L Stoker MD FRCS FRCSE
YEAR QUALIFIED: 1979
NHS POST: Consultant General Surgeon North Middlesex Hospital
SPECIAL INTEREST: Gastrointestinal surgery, including gastroscopy and ERCP. Laparoscopic surgery with interest in gallstones and hernias.
PRIVATE: North London Nuffield Hospital, Cavell Drive, Uplands Park Road, Enfield, EN2 7PR.
Tel: 0181 366 2122 Fax: 0181 367 8032
The King's Oak Hospital, Chase Farm Hospital (North Side), The Ridgeway, Enfield, Middlesex EN2 8SD. Tel: 0181 370 9500 Fax: 0181 370 9551

Essex

Mr James Wellwood MA MChir(Camb) FRCS(Eng)
NHS POST: Consultant Surgeon - Director Of Surgery Whipps Cross Hospital, Leytonstone
SPECIAL INTEREST: Laparoscopic abdominal surgery; breast disease; gastro intestinal/colorectal surgery.
PRIVATE: Holly House Hospital, High Road, Buckhurst Hill, Essex, IG9 5HX.
Tel: 0181 505 6423 Fax: 0181 502 9735
BUPA Roding Hospital, Roding Lane South, Redbridge, Ilford, Essex IG4 5PZ.
Tel: 0181 551 1100 Fax: 0181 551 9452

Hertfordshire

Mr Rodney Hallan MA MS FRCS
YEAR QUALIFIED: 1979
NHS POST: Consultant Surgeon, St Albans and Hemel Hempstead NHS Trust.
SPECIAL INTEREST: General surgery with a special interest in coloproctology and minimally invasive surgery.
PRIVATE: BUPA Hospital Harpenden, Ambrose Lane, Harpenden, Herts, AL5 4BP.
Tel: 01582 763 191 / 769 067 - direct line Fax: 01582 761 358

Kent

Mr David B Jackson BSc MB FRCS
NHS POST: Consultant Surgeon, Kent & Canterbury Hospital.
SPECIAL INTEREST: Surgical oncology specialising in breast reconstruction and major pelvic surgery; ileo-anal pouch surgery and laparoscopic procedures.
PRIVATE: Winters Farm, Nackington Road, Canterbury, Kent CT4 7AY.
Tel: 01227 472 581 Fax: 01227 472 581 E-mail: davidjackson@uk-consultants.co.uk

Mr Michael Parker BSc MS FRCS FRCS(Ed)
NHS POST: Consultant General Surgeon Joyce Green Hospital
SPECIAL INTEREST: Breast Cancer; colorectal cancer and laparoscopic surgery.
PRIVATE: Fawkham Manor Hospital, Manor Lane, Fawkham, Longfield, Kent DA3 8ND.
Tel: 01474 879 987 Fax: 01474 872 585
Chelsfield Park Hospital, Bucks Cross Road, Chelsfield, Kent, BR6 7RG.
Tel: 01689 877 855 / 01474 879 987 Fax: 01689 837 439

Lancashire

Mr D Andrew Evans MB BS FRCS MD
- YEAR QUALIFIED: 1980
- NHS POST: Consultant General Surgeon, Blackburn Royal Infirmary, Lancashire.
- SPECIAL INTEREST: Coloproctology.
- PRIVATE: Beardwood Hospital, Preston New Road, Blackburn, Lancashire BB2 7AE. Tel: 01254 56421 Fax: 01254 695032
Gisburne Park Private Hospital, Gisburn, Lancashire BB7 4HX. Tel: 01200 445693 Fax: 01200 445688

Mr John Holland Hobbiss MD FRCS MRCP
- YEAR QUALIFIED: 1974
- NHS POST: Consultant Surgeon, Royal Bolton Hospital.
- SPECIAL INTEREST: The management of colo-rectal cancer; laparoscopic cholecystectomy; inguinal hernia surgery.
- PRIVATE: Beaumont Hospital, Old Hall Clough, Chorley New Road, Lostock, Bolton, Lancashire BL6 4LA. Tel: 01204 404404

Liverpool

Mr Michael Hershman MSc MS FRCS(Eng, Ed, Glas and Irel) FICS
- YEAR QUALIFIED: 1980
- NHS POST: Consultant Surgeon, Royal Liverpool University Hospital.
- SPECIAL INTEREST: General surgery with particular interests in colorectal and minimal access surgery.
- PRIVATE: Lourdes Hospital, 57 Greenbank Road, Liverpool, L18 1HQ. Tel: 0151 733 7123 Fax: 0151 735 0446

London

Professor Timothy G Allen-Mersh MD FRCS
- YEAR QUALIFIED: 1973
- NHS POST: Consultant Surgeon & Professor of Gastrointestinal Surgery, Chelsea and Westminster Hospital.
- SPECIAL INTEREST: Colorectal surgery.
- PRIVATE: Lister Hospital, Chelsea Bridge Road, London, SW1W 8RH. Tel: 0181 746 8468 Fax: 0181 746 8231 E-mail: tallen-mersh@ic.ac.uk
Cromwell Hospital, Cromwell Road, London SW5 0TU. Tel: 0181 746 8468 Fax: 0181 746 8231 E-mail: tallen-mersh@ic.ac.uk

Professor A Darzi MD FRCS FRCSI FACS
- NHS POST: Professor of Surgery, St. Mary's Hospital.
- SPECIAL INTEREST: Colorectal & Laparoscopic Surgery, Minimal Access Surgery
- PRIVATE: Lindo Wing, St. Mary's Hospital, Praed Street, Paddington, London, W2 1NY. Tel: 0171 886 6487 Fax: 0171 886 6486

SURGERY - Colorectal & Gastrointestinal. London

Mr Peter R Hawley MS FRCS
- YEAR QUALIFIED: 1956
- SPECIAL INTEREST: Colorectal and gastrointestinal surgery.
- PRIVATE: King Edward VII Hospital, Beaumont Street, London, W1N 2AA.
  Tel: 0171 935 4444 ext 4003. 0171 935 2825-direct. Fax: 0171 486 1406
  The London Clinic, 149 Harley Street, London, W1N 2DE.
  Tel: 0171 935 4444 ext 4003. 0171 935 2825-direct. Fax: 0171 486 1406

Mr John Squire Kirkham MA MChir FRCS FRCS Ed
- YEAR QUALIFIED: 1960
- SPECIAL INTEREST: Colorectal and gastrointestinal surgery; general surgery; hepatobiliary surgery; oncological surgery; varicose vein surgery; upper GI and colorectal cancer; gastro-oesophageal reflux disease; endoscopy; anorectal problems.
- PRIVATE: 149 Harley Street, London W1N 2DE.
  Tel: 0171 935 4444 Fax: 0171 935 3690
  Parkside Hospital, 53 Parkside, Wimbledon, London, SW19 5NX.
  Tel: 0181 971 8000 Fax: 0181 971 8002

Mr M Russell Lock MB BS FRCS
- NHS POST: Consultant Surgeon Whittington Hospital
- SPECIAL INTEREST: General surgery, Colorectal surgery
- PRIVATE: Woolaston House, 25 Southwood Lane, London N6 5ED.
  Tel: 0181 348 6990 Fax: 0181 340 1376 E-mail: woolastonhouse@btinternet.com

Mr John D Maynard MS FRCS
- SPECIAL INTEREST: Thyroid & salivary gland (parotid) surgery.
- PRIVATE: 97 Harley Street, London W1N 1DF.
  Tel: 0171 935 4988 Fax: 0171 935 6617

Mr David Melville MA MB BS DM FRCS FRCS(Ed)
- NHS POST: Consultant General Surgeon, North Middlesex Hospital.
- SPECIAL INTEREST: Colorectal surgery; paediatric surgery; general surgery including hernias, varicose veins and emergency abdominal surgery.
- PRIVATE: 148 Harley Street, London W1N 1AH.
  Tel: 0171 935 1207 Fax: 0171 935 7362 E-mail: MELVILLE_FAMILY@msn.com

Mr Harvey Minasian MS(London) FRCS
- YEAR QUALIFIED: 1969
- SPECIAL INTEREST: Breast surgery; surgical oncology; gastroenterology and minimally invasive surgery.
- PRIVATE: Cromwell Hospital, Cromwell Road, London SW5 OTU.
  Tel: 0171 460 5700 / 0181 997 5026 Fax: 0171 460 5555 / 0181 810 4783

Professor R John Nicholls MChir FRCS(Eng) FRCS(Glas)
- YEAR QUALIFIED: 1967
- NHS POST: Consultant Surgeon St. Mark's Hospital
- SPECIAL INTEREST: Colorectal surgery.
- PRIVATE: (Clinic Tuesdays), The London Clinic, 149 Harley Street, London, W1N 2DE.
  Tel: 0171 935 4444

SURGERY - Colorectal & Gastrointestinal. London

Mr John Northover MS FRCS
- YEAR QUALIFIED: 1970
- NHS POST: Consultant Surgeon, St. Mark's Hospital, Northwick Park, Harrow.
- SPECIAL INTEREST: All aspects of colorectal and intestinal surgery.
- PRIVATE: The London Clinic, 149 Harley Street, London, W1N 2DE.
  Tel: 0171 486 1008 Fax: 0171 486 0665

Mr John Rogers MBBS(Lond) MD(Lond) FRCS(Eng)
- YEAR QUALIFIED: 1979
- NHS POST: Consultant Surgeon And Senior Lecturer, Royal London Hospital.
- SPECIAL INTEREST: 1) Gastro-oesophageal reflux disease and laparoscopic antireflux surgery (Director of GORD Centre). 2) Gastro-intestinal surgery - oesophago-gastric and colorectal surgery. 3) Laparoscopic surgery. 4) Laparoscopic anti-obesity surgery.
- PRIVATE: The Wellington Hospital, Wellington Place, London, NW8 9LE.
  Tel: 0171 483 5151, 0171 486 1515-Appointments. Fax: 0171 935 4984 E-mail: jrogers@gordcentre.org
  The Princess Grace Hospital, 42-52 Nottingham Place, London W1M 3FD.
  Tel: 0171 483 5151, 0171 486 1515-Appointments. Fax: 0171 935 4984 E-mail: jrogers@gordcentre.org
  The London Independent Hospital, 1 Beaumont Square, Stepney Green, London E1 4NL. Tel: 0171 790 0990-Reservations Fax: 0171 935 4984
  E-mail: jrogers@gordcentre.org
  The Lister Hospital, Chelsea Bridge Road, London, SW1W 8RH.
  Tel: 0171 483 5151, 0171 486 1515-Appointments. Fax: 0171 935 4984
  E-mail: jrogers@gordcentre.org
  Referrals: By letter to:, 32 Nottingham Place, London, W1M 3FD
  Tel: 0171 486 1515-For enquiries. Fax: 0171 935 4984-For referrals and enquiries.
  E-mail:referrals@gordcentre.org E-mail:enquiries@gordcentre.org

Mr R Christopher G Russell MS FRCS
- NHS POST: Consultant Surgeon UCL Hospitals, Middlesex Hospital
- SPECIAL INTEREST: Biliary and pancreatic surgery.
- PRIVATE: The London Clinic, 149 Harley Street, London, W1N 2DE.
  Tel: 0171 486 1164 Fax: 0171 487 5997

Mr Donal Shanahan MBBS FRCS MS
- NHS POST: Consultant Surgeon, Homerton Hospital. Senior Lecturer, St. Bartholomew's Hospital
- SPECIAL INTEREST: Gastroenterology; laparoscopic surgery; colorectal surgery.
- PRIVATE: The London Clinic, 149 Harley Street, London, W1N 2DE.
  Tel: 0181 504 3465 Fax: 0171 486 3782

Mr David Skidmore OBE MA MD FRCS(Ed) (Eng)
- YEAR QUALIFIED: 1964
- NHS POST: Honorary Senior Lecturer, University College London Hospital.
- SPECIAL INTEREST: Surgical Oncology - Breast and Colo-rectal Surgery
- PRIVATE: Private Patient Unit, Middlesex Hospital, Mortimer Street, London, W1N 8AA.
  Tel: 0181 318 6923 Fax: 0181 852 6919

SURGERY - Colorectal & Gastrointestinal. London

Mr Roger G Springall ChM FRCS
- NHS POST: Charing Cross Hospital
- SPECIAL INTEREST: Oncology
- PRIVATE: The London Clinic, 20 Devonshire Place, London, W1N 2DH.
  Tel: 0171 935 4444

Professor Irving Taylor MB ChB MD ChM FRCS
- YEAR QUALIFIED: 1968
- NHS POST: University College London Hospital Trust
- SPECIAL INTEREST: Surgical oncology which includes breast disease. Colorectal cancer and liver malignancy.
- PRIVATE: Woolavington Wing, Middlesex Hospital, Mortimer Street, London, W1N 8AA.
  Tel: 0171 504 9312 Fax: 0171 636 5176 E-mail: j.stumcke@ucl.ac.uk

Professor Anthony Watson MD FRCS(Eng) FRCS(Ed) FRACS
- YEAR QUALIFIED: 1965
- NHS POST: Visiting Professor Of Surgery, Royal Free Hospital School Of Medicine
- SPECIAL INTEREST: Investigation and management of upper gastro-intestinal disease, with a special interest in the oesophagus, including laparoscopic anti-reflux surgery; hiatus hernia repair, endoscopy.
- PRIVATE: Consulting Rooms, Princess Grace Hospital, 42-52 Nottingham Place, London, W1M 3FD. Tel: 0171 487 4731 Fax: 0171 487 5731

Mr Farouk Younis MB ChB FRCS
- YEAR QUALIFIED: 1971
- SPECIAL INTEREST: Urology; laparoscopic surgery.
- PRIVATE: 129 Harley Street, London W1N 1DJ.
  Tel: 0171 487 4897 Fax: 0171 224 6398 Mobile: 0860 231 685;
  E-mail: fmyounis@aol.com

Middlesex

Professor A Darzi MD FRCS FRCSI FACS
- NHS POST: Professor of Surgery, St. Mary's Hospital.
- SPECIAL INTEREST: Colorectal & Laparoscopic Surgery, Minimal Access Surgery
- PRIVATE: Clementine Churchill Hospital, Sudbury Hill, Harrow, Middlesex, HA1 3RX.
  Tel: 0181 422 3464 Fax: 0181 864 1747

Mr Robin Phillips MS FRCS
- YEAR QUALIFIED: 1975
- NHS POST: Consultant Colorectal Surgeon, St. Mark's Hospital.
- SPECIAL INTEREST: Colorectal surgeon; director of polyposis registry (inherited cancer); Research and clinical interest in surgery of faecal incontinence and inflammatory bowel disease.
- PRIVATE: The Robert & Lisa Sainsbury Wing, St. Mark's Hospital, Watford Road, Harrow, Middlesex HA1 3UJ.
  Tel: 01923 827988/0181 869 3112 Fax: 01923 841330/0181 235 4277

Oxfordshire

Mr Neil James M Mortensen MB ChB MD FRCS
- YEAR QUALIFIED: 1973
- NHS POST: Consultant Surgeon, John Radcliffe Oxford.
- SPECIAL INTEREST: Colonoscopy; cancer of colon and rectum; inflammatory bowel disease; anal sphincter surgery; local excision techniques.
- PRIVATE: 23 Banbury Road, Oxford, Oxon OX2 6NX.
  Tel: 01565 220926 Fax: 01565 760390

South Wales

Mr Keith D Vellacott DM FRCS DCH
- YEAR QUALIFIED: 1972
- NHS POST: Consultant General Surgeon, Royal Gwent Hospital, Newport.
- SPECIAL INTEREST: General/laparoscopic and colorectal surgery including endoscopy.
- PRIVATE: Glasllwch House, 4 Glasllwch Crescent, Newport, South Wales N19 3SE.
  Tel: 01633 252303 Fax: 01633 223127

Staffordshire

Mr Roderic Hutchinson MBBS FRCS
- YEAR QUALIFIED: 1984
- NHS POST: Consultant Surgeon and Coloproctologist, Staffordshire General Hospital.
- SPECIAL INTEREST: General surgery with colorectal interest; special coloproctological interests in rapid diagnosis of rectal bleeding; colonoscopy; faecal incontinence and pelvic floor disorders; colorectal cancer and inflammatory bowel disease.
- PRIVATE: Rowley Hall Hospital, Rowley Park, Stafford, Staffs ST17 9AQ.
  Tel: 01785 223 203 Fax: 01785 249 532

Surrey

Mr William Allum BSc MD FRCS
- YEAR QUALIFIED: 1977
- NHS POST: Consultant Surgeon, Epsom General Hospital.
- SPECIAL INTEREST: Gastrointestinal and breast disease.
- PRIVATE: Ashtead Hospital, The Warren, Ashtead, Surrey KT21 2SB.
  Tel: 01372 275 161 Fax: 01372 277 494

West Midlands

Mr Frank Curran MBChB(Birm) FRCSEd FRCSEng MD
YEAR QUALIFIED: 1979
NHS POST: Consultant Surgeon, New Cross Hospital, Wolverhampton, West Midlands.
SPECIAL INTEREST: Gastrointestinal and colorectal oncology, laparoscopic surgery.
PRIVATE: The Consulting Rooms, 8 Summerfield Road, Wolverhampton, West Midlands WV1 4PR. Tel: 01902 429044 Fax: 01902 710290

Mr Adrian Savage MA MB BChir MChir FRCS
YEAR QUALIFIED: 1977
NHS POST: Consultant Surgeon, Russells Hall Hospital.
SPECIAL INTEREST: All aspects of coloproctology; laparoscopic; gall bladder surgery; diagnostic and therapeutic upper and lower gastrointestinal endoscopy; surgery for abdominal wall and inguinal hernia.
PRIVATE: West Midlands Hospital, Colman Hill, Halesowem, West Midlands B63 2AH. Tel: Appointments - 01384 560123, Secretary - 01384 244093

West Sussex

Mr Jay N L Simson MA MB MRCP FCS MChir FRCS
YEAR QUALIFIED: 1974
NHS POST: Consultant Surgeon, St. Richard's Hospital.
SPECIAL INTEREST: Screening; prevention and treatment of colorectal cancer by endoscopic, laparoscopic and microsurgical techniques.
PRIVATE: 24 West Street, Chichester, West Sussex PO19 1QP. Tel: 01243 789 630 Fax: 01243 536 591

Wrexham

Mr Michael K H Crumplin MB BS MRCS LRCP FRCS (Eng)
YEAR QUALIFIED: 1965
NHS POST: Consultant General Surgeon, Wrexham Maelor Hospital, Wrexham.
SPECIAL INTEREST: Upper gastrointestinal surgery; breast surgery; thyroid surgery.
PRIVATE: Wrexham Maelor Hospital, Croesnewydd Road, Wrexham LL13 7TD.

SURGERY - Endocrine

Devon

Mr Denis Charles Wilkins MB ChB FRCS MD
YEAR QUALIFIED: 1966
NHS POST: Consultant General and Vascular Surgeon, Derriford Hospital, Plymouth.
SPECIAL INTEREST: General surgery; hernia; endocrine; thyroid; hyperhydrosis; medico-legal; arterial surgery; carotid disease; peripheral vascular disease; aneurysms; varicose veins; aortic surgery; vibratory white finger; parathyroid; cholecystectomy.
PRIVATE: Nuffield Hospital, Derriford Road, Plymouth, Devon PL6 8BG.
Tel: 01752 778892 Fax: 01752 778421

Kent

Mrs Marie South MS FRCS
YEAR QUALIFIED: 1968
NHS POST: Consultant General Surgeon, Maidstone Hospital.
SPECIAL INTEREST: Vascular, laparoscopic, endocrine and paediatric surgery; minimally invasive procedures e.g. laparoscopic cholecystectomy, laparoscopic fundoplication, laparoscopic hernia repair and thoracoscopic cervical sympathectomy for hyperhydrosis.
PRIVATE: Somerfield Hospital, 63-77 London Road, Maidstone, Kent, ME16 0DU.
Tel: 01622 672829 Fax: 01622 672829

London

Mr John Lynn MS FRCS
YEAR QUALIFIED: 1964
NHS POST: Consultant Endocrine Surgeon, Hammersmith Hospital, London.
SPECIAL INTEREST: Surgical endocrinology of thyroid, pancreas, parathyroid and adrenal. Surgery of breast diseases.
PRIVATE: Cromwell Hospital, Cromwell Road, London SW5 0TU.
Tel: 0836 285832 Fax: 0181 566 6402

Mr Nigel P M Sacks MS FRCS FRACS
NHS POST: Consultant Surgeon, The Royal Marsden Hospital and St. George's Hospital
SPECIAL INTEREST: Breast and endocrine surgery.
PRIVATE: The Royal Marsden Hospital, Fulham Road, London, SW3 6JJ.
Tel: 0171 352 8171 ext.2782
Lister Hospital, Chelsea Bridge Road, London, SW1W 8RH.
Tel: 0171 730 4647 Fax: 0171 730 2567
Parkside Hospital, 53 Parkside, Wimbledon, London, SW19 5NX.
Tel: 0171 730 4647 Fax: 0171 730 2567

South Glamorgan

Professor Malcolm H Wheeler MD FRCS
YEAR QUALIFIED: 1965
NHS POST: Professor and Consultant Surgeon, University Hospital of Wales, Cardiff.
SPECIAL INTEREST: General surgery with specialisation in endocrine and gastroenterological surgery.
PRIVATE: Glamorgan House, BUPA Hospital, Pentwyn, Cardiff, South Glamorgan CF2 7XL. Tel: 01222 736011 Fax: 01222 549930

SURGERY - General

Bedfordshire

Mr Roberts J E Foley MBBS FRCS
- YEAR QUALIFIED: 1966
- NHS POST: Consultant General Surgeon, Bedford Hospital (South Wing).
- SPECIAL INTEREST: General surgery; upper GI and laparoscopic surgery including laparoscopic cholecystectomy and anti-reflux surgery and laparoscopic hernia repair.
- PRIVATE: 20 Park Avenue, Bedford MK40 2LB.
  Tel: 01234 341604 Fax: 01234 269190

Cheshire

Mr George Foster MD FRCS
- YEAR QUALIFIED: 1968
- NHS POST: Consultant General Surgeon and Coloproctologist, Countess of Chester Hospital.
- SPECIAL INTEREST: General surgery; surgery for colorectal cancer and inflammatory bowel disease; minimal access surgery; thyroid surgery.
- PRIVATE: Nuffield Hospital, Wrexham Road, Chester, Cheshire CH4 7QP.
  Tel: 01244 680444 Fax: 01244 680812

Devon

Mr Denis Charles Wilkins MB ChB FRCS MD
- YEAR QUALIFIED: 1966
- NHS POST: Consultant General and Vascular Surgeon, Derriford Hospital, Plymouth.
- SPECIAL INTEREST: General surgery; hernia; endocrine; thyroid; hyperhydrosis; medico-legal; arterial surgery; carotid disease; peripheral vascular disease; aneurysms; varicose veins; aortic surgery; vibratory white finger; parathyroid; cholecystectomy.
- PRIVATE: Nuffield Hospital, Derriford Road, Plymouth, Devon PL6 8BG.
  Tel: 01752 778892 Fax: 01752 778421 E-mail: denis.wilkins@phnt.swest.nhs.uk

East Sussex

Mr Brian J Stoodley MA MChir FRCS
- NHS POST: Consultant Surgeon Eastbourne District General & Uckfield Hospitals
- SPECIAL INTEREST: Colorectal and gastrointestinal/breast/varicose vein surgery.
- PRIVATE: Consulting Rooms, 21 Lushington Road, Eastbourne, East Sussex BN26 5UX.
  Tel: 01323 410 441 Fax: 01323 410 978

SURGERY - General. East Sussex

Mr Andrew Yelland MB BS FRCS(Ed) MS
YEAR QUALIFIED: 1986
NHS POST: Lead Consultant in Breast Surgery, Royal Sussex County Hospital, Brighton.
SPECIAL INTEREST: Surgical oncology of the breast; breast reconstruction, reduction and augmentation.
PRIVATE: Hove Nuffield Hospital, 55 New Church Road, Hove, East Sussex BN3 4BG.
Tel: 01273 627044

Enfield Middlesex

Mr David Melville MA MB BS DM FRCS FRCS(Ed)
NHS POST: Consultant General Surgeon, North Middlesex Hospital.
SPECIAL INTEREST: Colorectal surgery; paediatric surgery; general surgery including hernias, varicose veins and emergency abdominal surgery.
PRIVATE: North London Nuffield Hospital, Cavell Drive, Uplands Park Road, Enfield, EN2 7PR.
Tel: 0181 366 2122   Fax: 0181 367 8032

Mr David L Stoker MD FRCS FRCSE
YEAR QUALIFIED: 1979
NHS POST: Consultant General Surgeon North Middlesex Hospital
SPECIAL INTEREST: Gastrointestinal surgery, including gastroscopy and ERCP. Laparoscopic surgery with interest in gallstones and hernias.
PRIVATE: The King's Oak Hospital, Chase Farm Hospital (North Side), The Ridgeway, Enfield, Middlesex EN2 8SD.
Tel: 0181 366 2122
North London Nuffield Hospital, Cavell Drive, Uplands Park Road, Enfield, EN2 7PR.
Tel: 0181 366 2122   Fax: 0181 367 8032

Essex

Mr David St. John Collier MA MS FRCS
NHS POST: Consultant Surgeon, Basildon And Thurrock General Hospital.
SPECIAL INTEREST: Breast; upper gastrointestinal including laparoscopic surgery.
PRIVATE: BUPA Hartswood Hospital, Eagle Way, Brentwood, Essex, CM13 3LE.
Tel: 01277 232525

Glasgow

Mr Robert Paul Teenan MD FRCS
YEAR QUALIFIED: 1981
NHS POST: Consultant Surgeon, Stobhill NHS Trust, Glasgow.
SPECIAL INTEREST: General surgery with a major interest in vascular disease, both arterial and venous.
PRIVATE: Glasgow Nuffield Hospital, Beaconsfield Road, Glasgow G12 0PJ.
Tel: 0141 334 9441   Fax: 0141 339 1352

Hampshire

Mr Nicholas M Wilson MBBS BSc MS FRCS
- YEAR QUALIFIED: 1981
- NHS POST: Consultant Surgeon, Royal Hampshire County Hospital.
- SPECIAL INTEREST: General surgery, subspecialty vascular and varicose vein surgery.
- PRIVATE: Private Hospital, Sarum Road, Winchester, Hampshire SO22 5HA.
Tel: 01962 826105

Hertfordshire

Mr Rodney Hallan MA MS FRCS
- YEAR QUALIFIED: 1979
- NHS POST: Consultant Surgeon, St Albans and Hemel Hempstead NHS Trust.
- SPECIAL INTEREST: General surgery with a special interest in coloproctology and minimally invasive surgery.
- PRIVATE: BUPA Hospital Harpenden, Ambrose Lane, Harpenden, Herts, AL5 4BP.
Tel: 01582 763 191 / 769 067 - direct line Fax: 01582 761 358

Mr Geoffrey R Sagor MB ChB ChM FRCS
- YEAR QUALIFIED: 1967
- NHS POST: Consultant Surgeon, St. Albans & Hemel Hempstead NHS Trust
- SPECIAL INTEREST: Laparoscopic surgery; gastro intestinal & colorectal surgery; endoscopy; breast surgery; general surgery.
- PRIVATE: BUPA Hospital Harpenden, Ambrose Lane, Harpenden, Herts, AL5 4BP.
Tel: 01582 763191

Kent

Mr Ian Higton MB BS FRCS AKC
- NHS POST: Formerly Consultant Surgeon, Bromley, Farnborough And Beckenham Hospitals.
- SPECIAL INTEREST: Day surgery; hernia; coloproctology; laparoscopic cholecystectomy.
- PRIVATE: Sloane Hospital, 125 Albemarle Road, Beckenham, Kent BR3 5HS.
Tel: 0181 460 6998 Fax: 0181 313 9547
Chelsfield Park Hospital, Bucks Cross Road, Chelsfield, Kent, BR6 7RG.
Tel: 01689 877855 Fax: 01689 837439

Mr Ronald Hoile MS FRCS
- YEAR QUALIFIED: 1968
- NHS POST: Consultant Surgeon, Medway Hospital.
- SPECIAL INTEREST: Vascular surgery and gastrointestinal surgery.
- PRIVATE: BUPA Alexandra Hospital, Impton Lane, Walderslade, Chatham, Kent ME5 9PG.
Tel: 01634 400 677 - appts. via secretary Fax: 01634 377 070
Somerfield Hospital, 63-77 London Road, Maidstone, Kent ME16 0DU.
Tel: 01634 400 667 - appts. via secretary Fax: 01634 377 070

Mr David B Jackson BSc MB FRCS
NHS POST: Consultant Surgeon, Kent & Canterbury Hospital.
SPECIAL INTEREST: Surgical oncology specialising in breast reconstruction and major pelvic surgery; ileo-anal pouch surgery and laparoscopic procedures.
PRIVATE: Winters Farm, Nackington Road, Canterbury, Kent CT4 7AY.
Tel: 01227 472 581 Fax: 01227 472 581 E-mail: davidjackson@uk-consultants.co.uk

Mr Omar Khan MB MS FRCS
YEAR QUALIFIED: 1969
NHS POST: Medway NHS Trust, Medway Hospital.
PRIVATE: BUPA Alexandra Hospital, Impton Lane, Walderslade, Chatham, Kent ME5 9PG.
Tel: 0634 687166

Mr James L Lewis MS MRCP(UK) FRCS (Eng)
NHS POST: Consultant Urologist & General Surgeon, Kent & Sussex Hospital.
SPECIAL INTEREST: General urology; prostate and bladder cancer; minimal access surgery.
PRIVATE: BUPA Hospital Tunbridge Wells, Fordcombe Road, Fordcombe, Tunbridge Wells, Kent TN3 0RD. Tel: 01892 740037 Fax: 01892 740037

Mr Michael Parker BSc MS FRCS FRCS(Ed)
NHS POST: Consultant General Surgeon Joyce Green Hospital
SPECIAL INTEREST: Breast Cancer; colorectal cancer and laparoscopic surgery.
PRIVATE: Fawkham Manor Hospital, Manor Lane, Fawkham, Longfield, Kent DA3 8ND.
Tel: 01474 879 987 Fax: 01474 872 585
Chelsfield Park Hospital, Bucks Cross Road, Chelsfield, Kent, BR6 7RG.
Tel: 01689 877 855 / 01474 879 987 Fax: 01689 837 439

Mrs Marie South MS FRCS
YEAR QUALIFIED: 1968
NHS POST: Consultant General Surgeon, Maidstone Hospital.
SPECIAL INTEREST: Vascular, laparoscopic, endocrine and paediatric surgery; minimally invasive procedures e.g. laparoscopic cholecystectomy, laparoscopic fundoplication, laparoscopic hernia repair and thoracoscopic cervical sympathectomy for hyperhydrosis.
PRIVATE: Somerfield Hospital, 63-77 London Road, Maidstone, Kent, ME16 0DU.
Tel: 01622 672829 Fax: 01622 672829

Liverpool

Mr Michael Hershman MSc MS FRCS(Eng, Ed, Glas and Irel) FICS
YEAR QUALIFIED: 1980
NHS POST: Consultant Surgeon, Royal Liverpool University Hospital.
SPECIAL INTEREST: General surgery with particular interests in colorectal and minimal access surgery.
PRIVATE: Lourdes Hospital, 57 Greenbank Road, Liverpool, L18 1HQ.
Tel: 0151 733 7123 Fax: 0151 735 0446

London

Mr Christopher Bishop MChir FRCS
NHS POST: Consultant Surgeon, Middlesex Hospital.
SPECIAL INTEREST: General surgery; vascular and varicose vein surgery; carotid artery surgery; aneurysm surgery.
PRIVATE: 149 Harley Street, London W1N 2DE.
Tel: 0171 235 6086 Fax: 0171 730 2840
Lister Hospital, Chelsea Bridge Road, London, SW1W 8RH.
Tel: 0171 235 6086 Fax: 0171 730 2840
Cromwell Hospital, Cromwell Road, London SW5 0TU.
Tel: 0171 235 6086 Fax: 0171 730 2840
Humana Hospital Wellington, Wellington Place, St Johns Wood, London, NW8 9LE.
Tel: 0171 235 6086 Fax: 0171 730 2840

Professor Kevin Guiver Burnand MBBS FRCS MS
NHS POST: Honorary Consultant Surgeon, St. Thomas' Hospital.
SPECIAL INTEREST: Carotid, aortic and peripheral vascular disease; varicose veins, *** limb and lymphoedema.
PRIVATE: St. Thomas' Hospital, Lambeth Palace Road, London, SE1 7EH.
Tel: 0171 928 9292 xt 2428 Fax: 0171 928 8742 E-mail: k.burnand@unds.ac.uk

Mr Frank W Cross MB MS FRCS
YEAR QUALIFIED: 1975
NHS POST: Consultant Surgeon Royal London Hospital
SPECIAL INTEREST: Vascular surgery and varicose vein.
PRIVATE: The London Clinic, 149 Harley Street, London W1N 2HG.
Tel: 0171 935 4444 / 0171 486 4688 - direct line. Fax: 0171 487 5479
E-mail: f.cross@dial.pipex.com

Professor A Darzi MD FRCS FRCSI FACS
NHS POST: Professor of Surgery, St. Mary's Hospital.
SPECIAL INTEREST: Colorectal & Laparoscopic Surgery, Minimal Access Surgery
PRIVATE: Lindo Wing, St. Mary's Hospital, Praed Street, Paddington, London, W2 1NY.
Tel: 0171 886 6487 Fax: 0171 886 6486

Mr Tim Davidson ChM MRCP FRCS
NHS POST: Consultant Breast and General Surgeon, Royal Free Hospital, Hampstead, London NW3 2QG. Secretary
Tel: 0171 830 2794. Fax: 0171 830 2194.
SPECIAL INTEREST: Thyroid and general surgery; salivary gland and parotid surgery; skin and soft tissue tumours; venous access; breast surgery including breast reconstruction.
PRIVATE: Portland Hospital for Women & Children, 205-209 Gt. Portland Street, London W1N 6AH. Tel: 0171 390 8083 Fax: 0171 390 8266
The London Clinic, 149 Harley Street, London, W1N 2DE.
Tel: 0171 616 7693 Fax: 0171 616 7633

SURGERY - General. London

Mr Ellis S Field MA MB BChir FRCS
- YEAR QUALIFIED: 1962
- NHS POST: Consultant Surgeon, Greenwhich District Hospital.
- SPECIAL INTEREST: Medico-Legal (Abdominal).
- PRIVATE: BMI Blackheath Hospital, 40-42 Lee Terrace, London, SE3 9UD.
  Tel: 0181 318 7722

Mr Jerry Gilmore MS FRCS FRCS(Ed)
- YEAR QUALIFIED: 1966
- SPECIAL INTEREST: Breast surgery; assessment, diagnosis and treatment of all benign and malignant breast disease.
- PRIVATE: The Day Surgery Centre, 108 Harley Street, London W1N 2ET.
  Tel: 0171 637 8820 Fax: 0171 935 3901
  The Groin and Hernia Clinic, 108 Harley Street, London W1N 2ET.
  Tel: 0171 935 3707 Fax: 0171 935 3901

Mr Geoffrey Glazer MS FRCS FACS
- NHS POST: Consultant Surgeon, St. Mary's Hospital.
- SPECIAL INTEREST: General surgery; abdominal surgery; laparoscopic surgery; thyroid surgery.
- PRIVATE: The Wellington Hospital, Wellington Place, London, NW8 9LE.
  Tel: 0171 483 3020 Fax: 0171 483 3087
  Lindo Wing, St. Mary's Hospital, South Wharf Road, Paddington, London W2 1NY.
  Correspondence and appointments:, 84a St. John's Wood High Street, London NW8 7SH. Tel: 0171 483 3020 Fax: 0171 483 3087

Mr Michael James Knight MS FRCS
- NHS POST: Consultant Surgeon, St George's Hospital.
- SPECIAL INTEREST: Gallbladder; biliary tract; pancreas.
- PRIVATE: 135 Harley Street, London W1N 1DJ.
  Tel: 0171 487 3501 Fax: 0171 935 3148

Mr M Russell Lock MB BS FRCS
- NHS POST: Consultant Surgeon Whittington Hospital
- SPECIAL INTEREST: General surgery, Colorectal surgery
- PRIVATE: Woolaston House, 25 Southwood Lane, London N6 5ED.
  Tel: 0181 348 6990 Fax: 0181 340 1376 E-mail: woolastonhouse@btinternet.com

Mr John D Maynard MS FRCS
- SPECIAL INTEREST: Thyroid & salivary gland (parotid) surgery.
- PRIVATE: 97 Harley Street, London W1N 1DF.
  Tel: 0171 935 4988 Fax: 0171 935 6617

Mr Harvey Minasian MS(London) FRCS
- YEAR QUALIFIED: 1969
- SPECIAL INTEREST: Breast surgery; surgical oncology; gastroenterology and minimally invasive surgery.
- PRIVATE: Cromwell Hospital, Cromwell Road, London SW5 OTU.
  Tel: 0171 460 5700 / 0181 997 5026 Fax: 0171 460 5555 / 0181 810 4783

SURGERY - General. London

Mr David Negus MA DM MCh FRCS LRCP
- YEAR QUALIFIED: 1958
- NHS POST: Retired from NHS/Emeritus Consultants Surgeon.
- SPECIAL INTEREST: Recurrent varicose veins; venous ulcers; TUREAD veins.
- PRIVATE: Lister Hospital, Chelsea Bridge Road, London, SW1W 8RH.
  Tel: 0171 730 3417 Fax: 0171 257 9218
  BMI Blackheath Hospital, 40-42 Lee Terrace, London, SE3 9UD.
  Tel: 0181 318 7722

Mr David Nott BSc MD FRCS
- YEAR QUALIFIED: 1981
- NHS POST: Consultant Surgeon Chelsea & Westminster Hospital
- SPECIAL INTEREST: Laparoscopic surgery - all aspects of abdominal keyhole surgery.
- PRIVATE: Seretary at, Chelsea & Westminster Hospital, 396 Fulham Road, London SW10 9TH.
  Tel: 0181 746 8464
  Lister Hospital, Chelsea Bridge Road, London, SW1W 8RH.
  Tel: 0171 730 3417
  Cromwell Hospital, Cromwell Road, London SW5 OTU.
  Tel: 0171 370 4233
  King Edward VII Hospital, Beaumont Street, London, W1N 2AA.
  Tel: 0171 486 4411

Mr Markus Ornstein MB ChB FRCS
- YEAR QUALIFIED: 1969
- SPECIAL INTEREST: General surgery with an interest in urology and laparoscopic surgery. Endoscopic hernia repair; laparoscopic gall-bladder surgery; colorectal, prostatic and bladder disorders; renal calculi. Emergency patients especially welcome.
- PRIVATE: 118 Harley Street, London W1N 1AG.
  Tel: 0181 423 8236 Fax: 0181 423 3339
  The Garden Hospital, 46-50 Sunny Gardens Road, Hendon, London, NW4 1RX.
  Tel: 0181 423 8236 Fax: 0181 423 3339

Mr R David Rosin MS MB FRCS FRCS (Ed)
- YEAR QUALIFIED: 1966
- NHS POST: Consultant Surgeon, St. Mary's Hospital.
- SPECIAL INTEREST: Upper gastro-intestinal surgery with particular experience in oesophageal surgery. Hepato-biliary surgery; liver problems; bile duct problems; minimal access surgery; laparoscopic; hiatus hernia repair; surgical oncology especially soft tissue and skin malignancies.
- PRIVATE: 80 Harley Street, London W1N 1AE.
  Tel: 0171 631 3447 Fax: 0171 224 0645
  St. Mary's Hospital, Praed Street, Paddington, London, W2 1NY.
  Tel: 0171 886 6041 Fax: 0171 725 1571

SURGERY - General. London

Mr Nigel P M Sacks MS FRCS FRACS
- NHS POST: Consultant Surgeon, The Royal Marsden Hospital and St. George's Hospital
- SPECIAL INTEREST: Breast and endocrine surgery.
- PRIVATE: The Royal Marsden Hospital, Fulham Road, London, SW3 6JJ.
  Tel: 0171 352 8171 ext.2782
  Lister Hospital, Chelsea Bridge Road, London, SW1W 8RH.
  Tel: 0171 730 4647 Fax: 0171 730 2567
  Parkside Hospital, 53 Parkside, Wimbledon, London, SW19 5NX.
  Tel: 0171 730 4647 Fax: 0171 730 2567

Mr Jeremy Thompson MChir FRCS
- YEAR QUALIFIED: 1977
- NHS POST: Consultant Surgeon Chelsea & Westminster Hospital and Royal Marsden Hospital
- SPECIAL INTEREST: Biliary; pancreatic; gastric and oesophageal surgery; abdominal adhesions.
- PRIVATE: Royal Marsden Hospital, Fulham Road, London, SW3 6JJ.
  Tel: 0171 352 8171 ext 2781 Fax: 0171 352 3942
  Cromwell Hospital, Cromwell Road, London SW5 0TU.
  Tel: 0958 629 666 Fax: 0181 991 1077
  Lister Hospital, Chelsea Bridge Road, London, SW1W 8RH.
  Tel: 0958 629 666 Fax: 0181 991 1077

Professor Anthony Watson MD FRCS(Eng) FRCS(Ed) FRACS
- YEAR QUALIFIED: 1965
- NHS POST: Visiting Professor Of Surgery, Royal Free Hospital School Of Medicine
- SPECIAL INTEREST: Investigation and management of upper gastro-intestinal disease, with a special interest in the oesophagus, including laparoscopic anti-reflux surgery; hiatus hernia repair, endoscopy.
- PRIVATE: Consulting Rooms, Princess Grace Hospital, 42-52 Nottingham Place, London, W1M 3FD. Tel: 0171 487 4731 Fax: 0171 487 5731

Mr James Wellwood MA MChir(Camb) FRCS(Eng)
- NHS POST: Consultant Surgeon - Director Of Surgery Whipps Cross Hospital, Leytonstone
- SPECIAL INTEREST: Laparoscopic abdominal surgery; breast disease; gastro intestinal/colorectal surgery.
- PRIVATE: 134 Harley Street, London W1N 1AH.
  Tel: 0171 487 4212 Fax: 0171 486 1042

Manchester

Mr Lester Barr MBChB (Hons) ChM FRCS
- YEAR QUALIFIED: 1978
- NHS POST: Consultant Surgeon, Withington and Christie Hospitals, Manchester.
- SPECIAL INTEREST: Surgeon to the specialist breast unit and the sarcoma unit at the Nightingale Centre and Christie Hospital.
- PRIVATE: BUPA Hospital Manchester, Russell Road, Manchester M16 8AJ.
  Tel: 0161 232 2574 Fax: 0161 226 1187

Merseyside

Mr David Tempest Reilly MD FRCS
YEAR QUALIFIED: 1971
NHS POST: Consultant General and Vascular Surgeon, Wirral Hospital NHS Trust.
SPECIAL INTEREST: Full range of general surgery, including thyroid, parathyroid, biliary surgery and hernias; vascular surgery including carotid endarterectomy, aneurysm repair; bypass grafting and modern varicose vein management.
PRIVATE: BUPA Hospital Murrayfield, Holmwood Drive, Thingwall, Wirral, Merseyside L61 1AU.
Tel: 0151 648 7000; 929 5050 Fax: 0151 648 7684

Middlesex

Professor A Darzi MD FRCS FRCSI FACS
NHS POST: Professor of Surgery, St. Mary's Hospital.
SPECIAL INTEREST: Colorectal & Laparoscopic Surgery, Minimal Access Surgery
PRIVATE: Clementine Churchill Hospital, Sudbury Hill, Harrow, Middlesex, HA1 3RX.
Tel: 0181 422 3464 Fax: 0181 864 1747

Mr Peter McDonald MS FRCS
YEAR QUALIFIED: 1975
NHS POST: Consultant General Surgeon, Northwick Park & St Mark's NHS Trust.
SPECIAL INTEREST: General surgery with an interest in coloproctology.
PRIVATE: Clementine Churchill Hospital, Sudbury Hill, Harrow, Middlesex, HA1 3RX.
Tel: 0181 872 3872
Charles Kingsley Suite, Northwick Park Hospital, Watford Road, Harrow, Middlesex, HA1 3UJ. Tel: 0181 869 3390 / 2627-secretary

Oxfordshire

Mr Carl Lindsay Griffiths MB FRCS
YEAR QUALIFIED: 1975
NHS POST: Consultant Surgeon - Breast & GI, Horton Districs General Hospital, Radcliffe Trust.
SPECIAL INTEREST: Breast carcinoma and breast surgery; gastrointestinal upper and lower; minimally invasive surgery; laparoscopy and endoscopy.
PRIVATE: Foscote Private Hospital, Foscote Rise, Banbury, Oxfordshire OX16 9XP.
Tel: 01295 229 207 Fax: 01295 272 877

Staffordshire

Mr Terence J Duffy MA BM BCh FRCS
YEAR QUALIFIED: 1972
NHS POST: Consultant Surgeon (Lead), North Staffordshire Hospital Trust.
SPECIAL INTEREST: Breast surgery (benign and malignant), diagnosis and management breast disease, breast screening.
PRIVATE: North Staffordshire Nuffield Hospital, Clayton Road, Newcastle-under-Lyme, Staffordshire ST5 4DB. Tel: 01782 625431 Fax: 01782 712748

Mr Roderic Hutchinson MBBS FRCS
YEAR QUALIFIED: 1984
NHS POST: Consultant Surgeon and Coloproctologist, Staffordshire General Hospital.
SPECIAL INTEREST: General surgery with colorectal interest; special coloproctological interests in rapid diagnosis of rectal bleeding; colonoscopy; faecal incontinence and pelvic floor disorders; colorectal cancer and inflammatory bowel disease.
PRIVATE: The Stafford Clinic, Staffordshire General Hospital, Weston Road, Stafford, Staffs ST16 3SA. Tel: 01785 246025, 224796 Sct 4653 Fax: 01785 245211

Surrey

Mr Robert McFarland MChir FRCS
NHS POST: Consultant in Vascular & General Surgery, Epsom General Hospital.
SPECIAL INTEREST: Vascular surgery.
PRIVATE: Epsom General Hospital (Trust), Dorking Road, Epsom, Surrey, KT18 7EG.
Tel: 01372 735 735
Ashtead Hospital, The Warren, Ashtead, Surrey KT21 2SB.
Tel: 01372 276 161

Mr Eoghan R T C Owen FRCS Gen FRCSI FRCS Ed
YEAR QUALIFIED: 1978
NHS POST: Consultant in General and Colorectal Surgery Crawley Hospital
SPECIAL INTEREST: Colonoscopy; colorectal cancer; medical and surgical treatment of inflammatory bowel disease; anorectal surgical problems; laparoscopic and hernia surgery; surgical treatment of morbid obesity.
PRIVATE: Gatwick Park Hospital, Povey Cross Road, Horley, Surrey RH6 0BB.
Tel: 01293 785 511 Fax: 01403 242 904

Miss Asha Senapati PhD FRCS
YEAR QUALIFIED: 1974
NHS POST: Consultant, Queen Alexandra Hospital, Portsmouth.
SPECIAL INTEREST: General surgery; coloproctology.
PRIVATE: Bunchfield, Lynchmere Ridge, near Haslemere, Surrey GU27 3PP.
Tel: 01428 652000 Fax: 01428 645304

West Sussex

Mr Eoghan R T C Owen FRCS Gen FRCSI FRCS Ed
YEAR QUALIFIED: 1978
NHS POST: Consultant in General and Colorectal Surgery Crawley Hospital
SPECIAL INTEREST: Colonoscopy; colorectal cancer; medical and surgical treatment of inflammatory bowel disease; anorectal surgical problems; laparoscopic and hernia surgery; surgical treatment of morbid obesity.
PRIVATE: Ashdown Hospital, Burrell Road, Haywards Heath, West Sussex RH16 1UD.
Tel: 01403 242904

SURGERY - Hepatobiliary

Kent

Mrs Marie South MS FRCS
YEAR QUALIFIED: 1968
NHS POST: Consultant General Surgeon, Maidstone Hospital.
SPECIAL INTEREST: Vascular, laparoscopic, endocrine and paediatric surgery; minimally invasive procedures e.g. laparoscopic cholecystectomy, laparoscopic fundoplication, laparoscopic hernia repair and thoracoscopic cervical sympathectomy for hyperhydrosis.
PRIVATE: Somerfield Hospital, 63-77 London Road, Maidstone, Kent, ME16 0DU.
Tel: 01622 672829 Fax: 01622 672829

SURGERY - Neurology

Bristol

Professor Hugh Coakham BSc MB BS FRCP FRCS
- YEAR QUALIFIED: 1968
- NHS POST: Consultant Neurosurgeon, Frenchay Hospital, Bristol.
- SPECIAL INTEREST: Trigeminal neuralgias, cerebral tumours, especially acoustic neuromas and all skull based tumours; spinal surgery - cervical and lumbar.
- PRIVATE: Litfield House Medical Centre, 1 Litfield Place, Clifton Down, Bristol BS8 3LS. Tel: 0117 973 1323 Fax: 0117 973 3303

Cleveland

Mr Fred P Nath MBChB FRCS
- YEAR QUALIFIED: 1974
- NHS POST: Consultant Neurosurgeon, Middlesbrough General Hospital.
- SPECIAL INTEREST: Acoustic neuroma; cervical and lumbar surgery; trigeminal neuralgia.
- PRIVATE: Middlesbrough General Hospital, Ayresome Green Lane, Middlesbrough, Cleveland TS5 5AZ. Tel: 01642 854317, Home: 01642 786997 Fax: 01642 854118
E-mail: fred.nath@onyx.octacon.co.uk

Mr Roger Strachan MD FRCS(SN)
- YEAR QUALIFIED: 1979
- NHS POST: Consultant Neurosurgeon, Middlesbrough General Hospital.
- SPECIAL INTEREST: Routine spinal surgery including lumbar decompressive surgery, microdiscectomy and cervical decompressive surgery and fusion; functional neurosurgery including epilepsy surgery; intracranial tumour surgery.
- PRIVATE: Parkview Medical Clinic, 276 Marton Road, Middlesbrough, Cleveland TS4 2NS. Tel: 01642 242357 Fax: 01642 854118

Kent

Mr Michael M Sharr MBBS MRCP FRCS
- NHS POST: Consultant Neurosurgeon Kings College Hospital
- SPECIAL INTEREST: Cranial, neck and spinal surgery; neurovascular surgery; tumour surgery.
- PRIVATE: BMI Sloane Hospital, 125 Albermarle Road, Beckenham, Kent, BR3 2HS. Tel: 0181 313 0249 Fax: 0181 313 9547
Chelsfield Park Hospital, Bucks Cross Road, Chelsfield, Kent, BR6 7RG. Tel: 01689 877 855 Fax: 01689 837 439

London

Mr Farhad Afshar BSc(Hon) MBBS(Hon) MRCS LRCP MD FRCS
- NHS POST: Consultant Neuro-Surgeon, The Royal London Hospital and St. Bartholomew's Hospital.
- SPECIAL INTEREST: Neck and back pain; brain and spinal tumours; pituitary disorders and movement disorders.
- PRIVATE: The London Clinic, 149 Harley Street, London, W1N 2DE.
  Tel: 0171 935 7505 Fax: 0171 935 7245

Mr Robert Bradford BSc MD FRCS
- YEAR QUALIFIED: 1979
- NHS POST: Consultant Neurosurgeon The Royal Free NHS Trust
- SPECIAL INTEREST: All aspects of spinal surgery. Neuro-oncology particularly stereotactic techniques of diagnosis and treatment. Skull base surgery particularly the management of acoustic schwannomas.
- PRIVATE: Wellington Hospital,, Wellington Place, St John's Wood, London NW8 9LE.
  Tel: 0171 722 1224 Fax: 0171 722 3141

Mr Peter Bullock FRCS MRCP
- NHS POST: Consultant Neurosurgeon, King's College Hospital, Guy's and St Thomas' Hospital Trust.
- SPECIAL INTEREST: Adult and Paediatric Neurosurgery, Brain and Spinal tumours, Pituitary tumours, Aneurysms and AVMs, Cervical and Lumbar disc disease, Trigeminal neuralgia.
- PRIVATE: Private Consulting Rooms, 149 Harley Street, London W1N 2DE.
  Tel: Appointments Tel: 0171 616 7693 Fax: 0171 616 7633

Mr Michael M Sharr MBBS MRCP FRCS
- NHS POST: Consultant Neurosurgeon Kings College Hospital
- SPECIAL INTEREST: Cranial, neck and spinal surgery; neurovascular surgery; tumour surgery.
- PRIVATE: King's College Hospital, Denmark Hill, London, SE5 9RS.
  Tel: 0171 346 3287 / 737 4000 Fax: 0171 346 3280
  BMI Blackheath Hospital, 40-42 Lee Terrace, Blackheath, London SE3 9UD.
  Tel: 0181 318 7722 Fax: 0181 318 2542

Mr Anthony J Strong MA DM MB ChB FRCSEd
- YEAR QUALIFIED: 1966
- NHS POST: Consultant Surgeon, King's College Hospital.
- SPECIAL INTEREST: Neurology; surgery.
- PRIVATE: King's College Hospital, Denmark Hill, London, SE5 9RS.
  Tel: 0171 346 3282

Mr John Sutcliffe MBChB FRCS
- NHS POST: Consultant Neuro Surgeon Royal London Hospital
- SPECIAL INTEREST: Spinal surgery; neurostimulation; pain; trauma; paediatric neuro surgery.
- PRIVATE: The London Clinic, 147 Harley Street, London W1N 2DH.
  Tel: 0171 486 3760 Fax: 0171 486 4601

Nottinghamshire

Mr Terence Hope MB ChB FRCS ChM
YEAR QUALIFIED: 1970
NHS POST: Consultant Neurosurgeon, University Hospital Nottingham.
SPECIAL INTEREST: Cervical and lumbar disc; headache; medico-legal reports; vascular (carotid) disease; giant aneurysms.
PRIVATE: QMC, Nottingham NG7 2UH.
Tel: 0115 970 9102 Fax: 0115 970 9104

South Yorkshire

Mr Robert D E Battersby MB BS FRCS (Eng)
YEAR QUALIFIED: 1973
NHS POST: Consultant Neurosurgeon, Royal Hallamshire Hospital, Sheffield, Honorary Lecturer.
SPECIAL INTEREST: Pituitary tumours; meningiomas; trigeminal neuralgia; medico-legal practice.
PRIVATE: Claremont Hospital, 401 Sandygate Road, Sheffield, South Yorkshire S10 5UB.
Tel: 0114 263 2109 Fax: 0114 263 2119

Mr David M C Forster MA MB BChir FRCS
YEAR QUALIFIED: 1960
NHS POST: Consultant Neurosurgeon, Royal Hallamshire Hospital.
SPECIAL INTEREST: Stereotactic radiosurgery; director of National Centre Stereotactic Radiosurgery.
PRIVATE: Stereotactic Radiosurgery Department, Royal Hallamshire Hospital, Glossop Road, Sheffield, South Yorkshire S10 2JF. Tel: 0114 271 3572 Fax: 0114 275 4930

Tyne & Wear

Professor A David Mendelow FRCS PhD
YEAR QUALIFIED: 1969
NHS POST: Honorary Consultant Neurosurgeon, Newcastle General Hospital.
SPECIAL INTEREST: Carotid endarterectomy and vascular surgery for aneurysms and cerebral arteriovenous malformations.
PRIVATE: Newcastle General Hospital, Westgate Road, Newcastle-upon-Tyne NE4 6BE.
Tel: 0191 219 5000 ext 22269 Fax: 0191 256 3267

Warwickshire

Mr Peter A Stanworth TD MA BM MCh DCH FRCS
YEAR QUALIFIED: 1969
NHS POST: Consultant Neurosurgeon, Walsgrave Hospitals NHS Trust, Coventry.
SPECIAL INTEREST: Lumbar disc disease; rehabilitation of back/neck pain.
PRIVATE: Long Meadow Farm, Hob Lane, Burton Green, Kenilworth, Warwickshire CV8 1QB.
Tel: 01203 466524 Fax: 01203 466524

SURGERY - Oncology

East Sussex

Mr Andrew Yelland MB BS FRCS(Ed) MS
YEAR QUALIFIED: 1986
NHS POST: Lead Consultant in Breast Surgery, Royal Sussex County Hospital, Brighton.
SPECIAL INTEREST: Surgical oncology of the breast; breast reconstruction, reduction and augmentation.
PRIVATE: Hove Nuffield Hospital, 55 New Church Road, Hove, East Sussex BN3 4BG.
Tel: 01273 627044

Gwent

Mr Winsor Bowsher MA MChir FRCS FRCS(Ucol) FEBU
YEAR QUALIFIED: 1981
NHS POST: Consultant Urological Surgeon, Royal Gwent Hospital, Wales.
SPECIAL INTEREST: Lead clinician, Department of Urology, for urological cancer services. Special interests in prostate cancer, laser surgery and laparoscopy.
PRIVATE: St. Joseph's Private Hospital, Harding Avenue, Malpas, Newport, South Wales NP9 6ZE.
Tel: 01633 820300 Fax: 01633 858164

Kent

Mr David B Jackson BSc MB FRCS
NHS POST: Consultant Surgeon, Kent & Canterbury Hospital.
SPECIAL INTEREST: Surgical oncology specialising in breast reconstruction and major pelvic surgery; ileo-anal pouch surgery and laparoscopic procedures.
PRIVATE: Winters Farm, Nackington Road, Canterbury, Kent CT4 7AY.
Tel: 01227 472 581 Fax: 01227 472 581 E-mail: davidjackson@uk-consultants.co.uk

Liverpool

Mr Michael Hershman MSc MS FRCS(Eng, Ed, Glas and Irel) FICS
YEAR QUALIFIED: 1980
NHS POST: Consultant Surgeon, Royal Liverpool University Hospital.
SPECIAL INTEREST: General surgery with particular interests in colorectal and minimal access surgery.
PRIVATE: Lourdes Hospital, 57 Greenbank Road, Liverpool, L18 1HQ.
Tel: 0151 733 7123 Fax: 0151 735 0446

London

Dr Alastair Deery BSc MBBS FRCPath
- YEAR QUALIFIED: 1978
- NHS POST: Consultant Cytopathologist, Royal Free Hampstead NHS Trust.
- SPECIAL INTEREST: Aspiration Diagnosis of Tumours of Head and Neck, Thyroid, Breast, Lymph Nodes, Skin and Soft Tissue.
- PRIVATE: Clinic 7, Royal Free Hospital, Pond Street, Hampstead, London, NW3 2QG.
  Tel: 0171 830 2944 Fax: 0171 830 2944

Sir Arnold Elton MS(Lond) FRCS(Eng) FICS
- NHS POST: Honorary Consulting Surgeon, Northwick Park Hospital.
- SPECIAL INTEREST: Breast surgery. Founder Officer Of British Association Of Surgical Oncology. Member European Society Of Surgical Oncology. Member Council and International Advisor World Federation of Surgery Oncology Societies. Member, Government Committee on National Breast Screening.
- PRIVATE: The Consulting Rooms, Wellington Hospital,, Wellington Place, St John's Wood, London NW8 9LE. Tel: 0171 935 4101 Fax: 0171 483 0297
  Web site: www.medicalnet.co.uk/sir.arnold.elton

Mr David Skidmore OBE MA MD FRCS(Ed) (Eng)
- YEAR QUALIFIED: 1964
- NHS POST: Honorary Senior Lecturer, University College London Hospital.
- SPECIAL INTEREST: Surgical Oncology - Breast and Colo-rectal Surgery; Endocrine Surgery
- PRIVATE: London Bridge Hospital, 27 Tooley Street, London SE1 2PR.
  Tel: 0181 318 6923
  Woolavington Wing, Middlesex Hospital, Mortimer Street, London, W1N 8AA.
  Tel: 0181 318 6923 Fax: 0181 852 6919
  BMI Blackheath Hospital, 40-42 Lee Terrace, London, SE3 9UD.
  Tel: 0181 318 6923 Fax: 0181 852 6919

Professor Irving Taylor MB ChB MD ChM FRCS
- YEAR QUALIFIED: 1968
- NHS POST: University College London Hospital Trust
- SPECIAL INTEREST: Surgical oncology which includes breast disease. Colorectal cancer and liver malignancy.
- PRIVATE: Woolavington Wing, Middlesex Hospital, Mortimer Street, London, W1N 8AA.
  Tel: 0171 504 9312 Fax: 0171 636 5176 E-mail: j.stumcke@ucl.ac.uk

Surrey

Mr William Allum BSc MD FRCS
- YEAR QUALIFIED: 1977
- NHS POST: Consultant Surgeon, Epsom General Hospital.
- SPECIAL INTEREST: Gastrointestinal and breast disease.
- PRIVATE: Ashtead Hospital, The Warren, Ashtead, Surrey KT21 2SB.
  Tel: 01372 275 161 Fax: 01372 277 494

SURGERY - Oral & Maxillofacial

Bedfordshire

Mr Michael T. Simpson MB BS BDS MRCS FFDRCS
NHS POST: Consultant in Oral and Maxillo-facial surgery Bedford Hospital, Lister Hospital Stevenage and Milton Keynes Hospital
SPECIAL INTEREST: Salivary gland disease / surgery; orofacial malignancy; osteotomies facial skeleton e.g. genioplasty and osseointegrated implants.
PRIVATE: Manor Hospital, Church End, Biddenham, Bedfordshire MK40 4AW.
Tel: 01234 364252 Fax: 01234 325001 Appointments: 01234 214998 Fax: 01234 214998

Bristol

Mr Phillip G Guest MB ChB BDS FDSRCS FRCS
YEAR QUALIFIED: 1979
NHS POST: Consultant in Oral and Maxillofacial Surgery, Bristol Royal Infirmary.
SPECIAL INTEREST: Head and neck cancer; facial deformity; cosmetic facial surgery; facial injuries.
PRIVATE: Litfield House Medical Centre, 1 Litfield Place, Clifton Down, Bristol BS8 3LS.
Tel: 0117 928 4392 Fax: 0117 928 4222

Mr Peter J Revington MScD FDS FRCS
YEAR QUALIFIED: 1976
NHS POST: Consultant Oral and Maxillofacial Surgeon, Frenchay Hospital.
SPECIAL INTEREST: Facial deformity; salivary gland disease; dento alveolar surgery; trauma and TMJ dysfunction.
PRIVATE: BUPA Hospital Bristol, Durdham Down, Redland Hill, Bristol BS6 6UT.
Tel: 0117 975 3997 Fax: 0117 975 3750 E-mail: prevington@aol.com

Dr Ian Malcolm Vickery MB ChB MRCS LRCP BDS LDRRCS FDS RCSY
YEAR QUALIFIED: 1958
SPECIAL INTEREST: Oral and maxillofacial surgery; dental implantology.
PRIVATE: The Newman Oral Surgery Clinic, 35 Lower Redland Road, Redland, Bristol BS6 6TB.
Tel: 0117 946 6188 Fax: 0117 946 6177 E-mail: ivickery@aol.com

Buckinghamshire

Mr Martin Mace MBBS BDS FDS MRCS
YEAR QUALIFIED: 1972
NHS POST: Consultant Oral and Maxillo-Facial Surgeon, Stoke Mandeville Hospital, Buckinghamshire.
SPECIAL INTEREST: Oral surgery and facial deformity including cleft lip and palate.
PRIVATE: Chiltern Hospital, Great Missenden, Buckinghamshire HP16 0EN.
Tel: 01494 890 890 Fax: 01494 892 215

SURGERY - Oral & Maxillofacial. Buckinghamshire

Mr Michael T. Simpson MB BS BDS MRCS FFDRCS
NHS POST: Consultant in Oral and Maxillo-facial surgery Bedford Hospital, Lister Hospital Stevenage and Milton Keynes Hospital
SPECIAL INTEREST: Salivary gland disease / surgery; orofacial malignancy; osteotomies facial skeleton e.g. genioplasty and osseointegrated implants.
PRIVATE: Saxon Clinic, Saxon Street, Eaglestone, Milton Keynes, Buckinghamshire MK6 5LR.
Tel: 01908 665 533 Fax: 01908 608 112 Appointments: 01234 214998 Fax: 01234 214998

Cambridgeshire

Mr David Maxwell Adlam MBBS BDS FRCS FDSRCS
YEAR QUALIFIED: 1982
NHS POST: Consultant Maxillofacial Surgeon, Addenbrooke's Hospital, Cambridge.
SPECIAL INTEREST: Oral surgery and oral medicine; facial deformity; salivary gland disease; oral malignancy and facial pain.
PRIVATE: Cambridge Lea Hospital, 30 New Road, Impington, CB4 9EL.
Tel: 01223 892427 Fax: 01223 890022

Essex

Mr James Evans MB BCh BDS FDSRCS
NHS POST: Consultant in Oral and Maxillo-facial Surgery, Whipps Cross Hospital, King George Hospital Ilford, St. Margaret's Hospital Epping and Herts and Essex Hospital Bishop's Stortford.
SPECIAL INTEREST: Jaw and salivary gland problems; dental implants; oral malignancy.
PRIVATE: BUPA Roding Hospital, Roding Lane South, Redbridge, Ilford, Essex IG4 5PZ.
Tel: 0181 551 1100/01992 812 611 appts. sec.
Holly House Hospital, High Road, Buckhurst Hill, Essex, IG9 5HX.
Tel: 0181 505 3311/01992 812 611 appts. sec.

Hampshire

Mr Barrie (Thomas) Evans FRCS(Edin) FDSRCS(Eng) FFDRCS(Ire)
YEAR QUALIFIED: 1971
NHS POST: Consultant in Oral and Maxillotacial Surgery, Southampton University Hospitals NHS Trust.
SPECIAL INTEREST: Salivary gland surgery, oral pathology, head and neck malignancy, oral implantology.
PRIVATE: BUPA Chalybeate Hospital, Chalybeate Close, Tremona Road, Southampton, Hampshire SO16 6UY. Tel: 01703 764336 Fax: 01703 773735
Wessex Nuffield Hospital, Winchester Road, Chandler's Ford, Eastleigh, Hampshire SO53 2DW. Tel: 01703 764336 Fax: 01703 773735

SURGERY - Oral & Maxillofacial. Hampshire

Mr Hugh Ogus BDS FDS
YEAR QUALIFIED: 1966
NHS POST: Consultant in Oral and Maxillofacial Surgery, North Hampshire Hospital, Basingstoke; Royal Surrey County Hospital, Guildford.
SPECIAL INTEREST: Temporomandibular joint problems; salivary gland surgery; facial pain.
PRIVATE: The Hampshire Clinic, Basing Road, Basingstoke, Hampshire RG24 7AL.
Tel: 01256 328190 Fax: 01256 329986 E-mail: hughogus@msn.com

Hertfordshire

Mr James Evans MB BCh BDS FDSRCS
NHS POST: Consultant in Oral and Maxillo-facial Surgery, Whipps Cross Hospital, King George Hospital Ilford, St. Margaret's Hospital Epping and Herts and Essex Hospital Bishop's Stortford.
SPECIAL INTEREST: Jaw and salivary gland problems; dental implants; oral malignancy.
PRIVATE: The Rivers Hospital Thomas Rivers Medical Centre, High Wych Road, Sawbridgeworth, Hertfordshire, CM21 0HH. Tel: 01279 600282/01992 812 611 appts. sec.

Mr Michael T. Simpson MB BS BDS MRCS FFDRCS
NHS POST: Consultant in Oral and Maxillo-facial surgery Bedford Hospital, Lister Hospital Stevenage and Milton Keynes Hospital
SPECIAL INTEREST: Salivary gland disease / surgery; orofacial malignancy; osteotomies facial skeleton e.g. genioplasty and osseointegrated implants.
PRIVATE: Pinehill Hospital, Benslow Lane, Hitchin, Hertfordshire SG4 9QZ.
Tel: 01462 422 822 Fax: 01462 421 986 Appointments: 01234 214998
Fax: 01234 214998

London

Mr Peter T Blenkinsopp FRCS FDS RCS
NHS POST: Consultant Maxillofacial Surgeon, Roehampton, Kingston and St. Helier Hospitals.
PRIVATE: Parkside Hospital, 53 Parkside, Wimbledon, London, SW19 5NX.
Tel: 0181 971 8000 Fax: 0181 971 8002

Mr John Bowerman FRCS FDSRCS
NHS POST: Honorary Consulting Maxillofacial Surgeon, Queen Mary's Hospital and Chelsea & Westminster Hospital.
SPECIAL INTEREST: Salivary gland disease; temporo-mandibular joint disorders; medico-legal cases
PRIVATE: Princess Grace Hospital, 42-52 Nottingham Place, London, W1M 3FD.
Tel: 0171 486 1234 xt 4646 Fax: 0171 487 4676

Mr Martin Danford BDS LDS RCS MBBS FFDRCSI FRCS
YEAR QUALIFIED: 1975
NHS POST: Consultant Oral & Maxillofacial Surgeon, King's College Dental Institute.
SPECIAL INTEREST: Head and neck cancer and reconstruction; salivary gland disease; facial aesthetic/plastic surgery.
PRIVATE: The Lister Hospital, Chelsea Bridge Road, London, SW1W 8RH.
Tel: 0171 730 3417 Fax: 0171 824 8867

SURGERY - Oral & Maxillofacial. London

Mr David R James FRCS FDSRCS
- NHS POST: Consultant Oral and Maxillofacial Surgeon, Hospital for Sick Children, Great Ormond St
- SPECIAL INTEREST: Facial deformity; facial trauma; temporomandibular joint problems; salivary gland surgery; medico-legal cases.
- PRIVATE: 57 Portland Place, London W1N 3AH.
  Tel: 0171 436 0381/636 4781   Fax: 0171 580 8837   E-mail: drjmaxfac@aol.com

Mr Martin Mace MBBS BDS FDS MRCS
- YEAR QUALIFIED: 1972
- NHS POST: Consultant Oral and Maxillo-Facial Surgeon, Stoke Mandeville Hospital, Buckinghamshire.
- SPECIAL INTEREST: Oral surgery and facial deformity including cleft lip and palate.
- PRIVATE: 90 Harley Street, London W1N 1AF.
  Tel: 0171 935 2249   Fax: 0171 224 4158

Mr B Royston Sillers MB ChB BChD LDS
- SPECIAL INTEREST: Removal of wisdom teeth, cysts and tumour biopsy, bone augmentation with implantology, TMJ dysfunction.
- PRIVATE: Wellington Hospital North, Circus Road, St. John's Wood, London NW8 9JS.
  Tel: 0171 586 5959
  111 Harley Street, London W1N 1DG.
  Tel: 0171 935 3083   Fax: 0171 586 0673
  H R House, 447 High Road, Finchley, London N12 0AZ.
  Tel: 0181 346 8434   Fax: 0181 343 1869

Surrey

Mr John Bowerman FRCS FDSRCS
- NHS POST: Honorary Consulting Maxillofacial Surgeon, Queen Mary's Hospital and Chelsea & Westminster Hospital.
- SPECIAL INTEREST: Salivary gland disease; temporo-mandibular joint disorders; medico-legal cases
- PRIVATE: St. Anthony's Hospital, London Road, North Cheam, Surrey, SM3 9DW.
  Tel: 0181 337 6691 xt Out patients   Fax: 0181 330 1037

Mr Martin Danford BDS LDS RCS MBBS FFDRCSI FRCS
- YEAR QUALIFIED: 1975
- NHS POST: Consultant Oral & Maxillofacial Surgeon, King's College Dental Institute.
- SPECIAL INTEREST: Head and neck cancer and reconstruction; salivary gland disease; facial aesthetic/plastic surgery.
- PRIVATE: Frimley Park Hospital, Portsmouth Road, Frimley, Camberley, Surrey GU16 5UJ.
  Tel: 01276 604 604   Fax: 01276 604 148
  7 Woodlands Close, Claygate, Esher, Surrey KT10 OJF.
  Tel: 01372 462177   Fax: 01372 462170
  Shirley Oaks Hospital, Poppy Lane, Shirley Oaks Village, Surrey, CR9 8AB.
  Tel: 0181 655 2255   Fax: 0181 656 2868
  St. Anthony's Hospital, London Road, North Cheam, Surrey, SM3 9DW.
  Tel: 0181 337 6691   Fax: 0181 335 3325

Warwickshire

Mr John Fagan MA MB BChir FDSRCS
YEAR QUALIFIED: 1975
NHS POST: Consultant Oral and Maxillofacial Surgeon, George Eliot Hospital, Nuneaton and Coventry and Warwickshire Hospital Coventry.
SPECIAL INTEREST: Salivary gland surgery, oral medicine and all oral and dento-alveolar surgery, surgical correction of facial deformity, removal of facial lesions, mouth preparation and insertion of dental implants.
PRIVATE: Warwickshire Nuffield Hospital, The Chase, Old Milverton Lane, Leamington Spa, Warwickshire CV32 6RW. Tel: 01926 427971
Nuneaton Private Hospital, 132 Coventry Road, Nuneaton, Warwickshire CV10 7AD. Tel: 01203 353000

West Midlands

Mr John Fagan MA MB BChir FDSRCS
YEAR QUALIFIED: 1975
NHS POST: Consultant Oral and Maxillofacial Surgeon, George Eliot Hospital, Nuneaton and Coventry and Warwickshire Hospital Coventry.
SPECIAL INTEREST: Salivary gland surgery, oral medicine and all oral and dento-alveolar surgery, surgical correction of facial deformity, removal of facial lesions, mouth preparation and insertion of dental implants.
PRIVATE: Coventry Consulting Rooms, 11 Dalton Road, Earlesdon, Coventry, West Midlands CV5 6PD. Tel: 01203 677444 Fax: 01203 691436

SURGERY - Plastic

Avon

Mr Nigel S G Mercer MB ChB CLM FRCS FRCPCH
- YEAR QUALIFIED: 1980
- NHS POST: Consultant Plastic and Reconstructive Surgeon, Frenchay Hospital.
- SPECIAL INTEREST: Cleft and craniofacial disorders; paediatric plastic surgery; aesthetic surgery.
- PRIVATE: 2 Clifton Park, Clifton, Bristol, BS8 3BS.
  Tel: 0117 973 9998
  The Bath Clinic, Claverton Down Road, Combe Down, Bath BA2 7BR.
  Tel: 01225 835555

Bedfordshire

Mr Anthony I Attwood MBBS FRCS(Ed)
- YEAR QUALIFIED: 1972
- NHS POST: Consultant Advisor in Plastic Surgery to the Royal Air Force (Formerly).
- SPECIAL INTEREST: Cosmetic surgery and skin cancer.
- PRIVATE: Manor Hospital, Church End, Biddenham, Bedfordshire MK40 4AW.
  Tel: 01234 364 252 Fax: 01234 325 001

Professor Roy Sanders BSc MB BS FRCS
- YEAR QUALIFIED: 1962
- NHS POST: Consultant Plastic & Reconstructive Surgeon, Mount Vernon Hospital and Luton & Dunstable, RNOH Stanmore
- SPECIAL INTEREST: Aesthetic surgery; head and neck cancer; cleft lip & palate; orthopaedic complications.
- PRIVATE: BUPA Hospital Harpenden, Ambrose Lane, Harpenden, Herts, AL5 4BP.
  Tel: 01582 497433

Berkshire

Mr David M Evans MBBS FRCS
- YEAR QUALIFIED: 1965
- NHS POST: Consultant Hand Surgeon, Royal National Orthopaedic Hospital, & St. Thomas' Hospital, London.
- SPECIAL INTEREST: Hand surgery and rehabilitation. Surgery for congenital malformations of the hand, trauma and rheumatoid arthritis. Disorders of the wrist, Dupuytren's contracture, and peripheral nerve injury and compression.
- PRIVATE: The Hand Clinic, Oakley Green, Windsor, Berks SL4 4LH.
  Tel: 01753 831 333 Fax: 01753 832 109

Mr David L Martin FRCS
- NHS POST: Consultant Plastic & Reconstructive Surgeon, Chelsea & Westminster Hospital.
- SPECIAL INTEREST: General plastic surgery; cosmetic surgery; breast surgery; hand surgery.
- PRIVATE: The Hand Clinic, Oakley Green, Windsor, Berks SL4 4LH.
Tel: 01753 831 333 Fax: 01753 832 109

Bristol

Mr Phillip G Guest MB ChB BDS FDSRCS FRCS
- YEAR QUALIFIED: 1979
- NHS POST: Consultant in Oral and Maxillofacial Surgery, Bristol Royal Infirmary.
- SPECIAL INTEREST: Head and neck cancer; facial deformity; cosmetic facial surgery; facial injuries.
- PRIVATE: The Glen BUPA Hospital, Redland Hill, Durdham Down, Bristol BS6 6UT.
Tel: 0117 973 2562

Mr Donald Sammut FRCS FRCS(Plast)
- YEAR QUALIFIED: 1980
- NHS POST: Consultant Plastic and Hand Surgeon, Frenchay Hospital NHS Trust, Bristol.
- SPECIAL INTEREST: Hand surgery; plastic surgery.
- PRIVATE: The Chesterfield Hospital, 3 Clifton Hill, Bristol BS8 1BP.
Tel: 0117 973 5544 Fax: 0117 973 0323

Buckinghamshire

Mr Anthony I Attwood MBBS FRCS(Ed)
- YEAR QUALIFIED: 1972
- NHS POST: Consultant Advisor in Plastic Surgery to the Royal Air Force (Formerly).
- SPECIAL INTEREST: Cosmetic surgery and skin cancer.
- PRIVATE: The Chiltern Hospital, London Road, Great Missenden, Buckinghamshire HP16 0EN.
Tel: 01494 892288 (Appointments) Fax: 01494 890250
The Paddocks Hospital, Aylesbury Road, Princes Risborough, Buckinghamshire HP27 0JS. Tel: 01844 346 951 Fax: 01844 344 521
Saxon Clinic, Saxon Street, Eaglestone, Milton Keynes, Buckinghamshire MK6 5LR.
Tel: 01908 665533 Fax: 01908 608 112

Mr Alan Godfrey MB BCh FRCSEd
- YEAR QUALIFIED: 1968
- SPECIAL INTEREST: Breast and facial cosmetic surgery; laser surgery and reconstructive surgery.
- PRIVATE: The Paddocks Hospital, Aylesbury Road, Princes Risborough, Buckinghamshire HP27 0JS. Tel: 01865 244421 Fax: 01844 344521 E-mail: secretary@eslas.com

Cambridgeshire

Mr David Charles Herbert MB BS FRCSEd FRCSEng
- YEAR QUALIFIED: 1961
- SPECIAL INTEREST: Surgery of facial ageing and facial reconstruction; breast reduction and breast surgery; rhinoplasty.
- PRIVATE: Cromwell Clinic, Huntingdon, Cambridgeshire PE18 6DP. Tel: 01480 411411

Cornwall

Mr David J Hanley FRCS
- YEAR QUALIFIED: 1965
- NHS POST: Consultant Plastic Reconstructive and Hand Surgeon, Derriford Hospital, Plymouth.
- SPECIAL INTEREST: Hand surgery including congenital and rheumatoid hand conditions.
- PRIVATE: Duchy Hospital Truro Correspondence to Nuffield Hospital, Deniford Road, Plymouth, PL6 8BG. Tel: 01752 761835

Devon

Mr David J Hanley FRCS
- YEAR QUALIFIED: 1965
- NHS POST: Consultant Plastic Reconstructive and Hand Surgeon, Derriford Hospital, Plymouth.
- SPECIAL INTEREST: Hand surgery including congenital and rheumatoid hand conditions.
- PRIVATE: Nuffield Hospital, Derriford Road, Plymouth, Devon PL6 8BG. Tel: 01752 761835 Fax: 01752 768969

East Sussex

Mr N S Brent Tanner MA FRCS
- NHS POST: Honorary Consultant Plastic Surgeon Queen Victoria Hospital
- SPECIAL INTEREST: All forms of aesthetic surgery & Skin Care including laser and endoscopic surgery
- PRIVATE: The Sussex Nuffield Hospital, Warren Road, Woodingdean, Brighton, East Sussex BN2 6DX. Tel: 01273 624488 Fax: 01273 620101

East Yorkshire

Mr Nicholas Hart MBBS FRCS
- YEAR QUALIFIED: 1973
- NHS POST: Consultant Plastic Surgeon, Kingston General Hospital, Hull.
- SPECIAL INTEREST: Aesthetic and constructive plastic surgery; skin cancer, especially malignant melanoma; reconstructive microsurgery; endoscopic plastic surgery; lower limb reconstruction and hand surgery; head and neck surgery.
- PRIVATE: Hull Nuffield Hospital, 81 Westbourne Avenue, Hull, East Yorkshire HU5 3HP. Tel: 01482 342377 Fax: 01482 346364

Enfield Middlesex

Mr Nigel Carver MS FRCS FRCS(Plast)
- NHS POST: Consultant Plastic Surgeon, St. Bartholomew's Hospital And Royal London Hospital.
- SPECIAL INTEREST: Plastic reconstructive and aesthetic surgery; cosmetic facial surgery; rhinoplasty; breast reconstruction; skin cancer and hand surgery.
- PRIVATE: The King's Oak Hospital, Chase Farm Hospital (North Side), The Ridgeway, Enfield, Middlesex EN2 8SD. Tel: 0181 370 9500. Private secretary-0181 850 1020.

Essex

Mr Nigel Carver MS FRCS FRCS(Plast)
- NHS POST: Consultant Plastic Surgeon, St. Bartholomew's Hospital And Royal London Hospital.
- SPECIAL INTEREST: Plastic reconstructive and aesthetic surgery; cosmetic facial surgery; rhinoplasty; breast reconstruction; skin cancer and hand surgery.
- PRIVATE: Holly House Hospital, High Road, Buckhurst Hill, Essex, IG9 5HX.
Tel: 0181 505 3311. Private secretary-0181 850 1020.
BUPA Roding Hospital, Roding Lane South, Redbridge, Ilford, Essex IG4 5PZ.
Tel: 0181 551 1100. Private secretary-0181 850 1020.

Mr David Elliot MA FRCS
- YEAR QUALIFIED: 1975
- NHS POST: Consultant Hand & Reconstructive Surgeon, Southend General Hospital & St. Andrew's Hospital - Secretary 01245 516124
- SPECIAL INTEREST: Skin cancer and benign skin lesions; cosmetic surgery; hand surgery, especially Dupuytren's contracture; nerve injury and compression, and secondary upper limb trauma surgery.
- PRIVATE: BUPA Wellesley Hospital, Eastern Avenue, Southend on Sea SS2 4XH.
Tel: 01621 857362 Fax: 01621 841127 E-mail: info@david-elliot.co.uk
Springfield Hospital, Lawn Lane, Springfield, Chelmsford, Essex CM1 7GU.
Tel: 01621 857362 E-mail: info@david-elliot.co.uk

Mr James D Frame FRCS FRCS(Plast)
- YEAR QUALIFIED: 1977
- NHS POST: Consultant Plastic & Reconstructive Surgeon, St. Andrew's Centre For Plastic Surgery & Burns, Chelmsford, Essex.
- SPECIAL INTEREST: Lower limb trauma; burns; breast reconstruction; soft tissue sports injury; cosmetic surgery.
- PRIVATE: Springfield Hospital, Lawn Lane, Springfield, Chelmsford, Essex CM1 7GU.
Tel: 01245 460981-secretary Fax: 01245 460 981
Essex Nuffield Hospital, Shenfield Road, Brentwood, Essex, CM15 8EH.
Tel: 01245 460 981-secretary

SURGERY - Plastic. Essex

Mr Brian C Sommerlad MB BS FRCS
- NHS POST: Consultant Plastic Surgeon, Gt. Ormond St. Hospital; Royal London Hospital; St. Andrew's Centre for Plastic Surgery, Broomfield Hospital, Chelmsford.
- SPECIAL INTEREST: Congenital deformity; especially cleft lip and palate; hand deformities and hypospadias; skin cancer and benign skin lesions; head and neck surgery; especially parotid surgery; hand surgery especially Dupuytren's contracture.
- PRIVATE: Essex Nuffield Hospital, Shenfield Road, Brentwood, Essex, CM15 8EH. Tel: 01245 422 477
Springfield Hospital, Lawn Lane, Springfield, Chelmsford, Essex CM1 7GU. Tel: 01245 422 477
Oaks Hospital, Mile End Road, Colchester, Essex CO4 5XR. Tel: 01245 422 477

Gloucestershire

Mr Alan Godfrey MB BCh FRCSEd
- YEAR QUALIFIED: 1968
- SPECIAL INTEREST: Breast and facial cosmetic surgery; laser surgery and reconstructive surgery.
- PRIVATE: The Winfield Hospital, Tewkesbury Road, Longford, Gloucester, Gloucestershire GL2 9WH. Tel: 01452 331111 Fax: 01452 331200 E-mail: secretary@eslas.com

Hertfordshire

Mr Anthony I Attwood MBBS FRCS(Ed)
- YEAR QUALIFIED: 1972
- NHS POST: Consultant Advisor in Plastic Surgery to the Royal Air Force (Formerly).
- SPECIAL INTEREST: Cosmetic surgery and skin cancer.
- PRIVATE: BUPA Hospital Harpenden, Ambrose Lane, Harpenden, Herts, AL5 4BP. Tel: 01582 763191 Fax: 01582 712 312

Mr James D Frame FRCS FRCS(Plast)
- YEAR QUALIFIED: 1977
- NHS POST: Consultant Plastic & Reconstructive Surgeon, St. Andrew's Centre For Plastic Surgery & Burns, Chelmsford, Essex.
- SPECIAL INTEREST: Lower limb trauma; burns; breast reconstruction; soft tissue sports injury; cosmetic surgery.
- PRIVATE: The Rivers Hospital Thomas Rivers Medical Centre, High Wych Road, Sawbridgeworth, Hertfordshire, CM21 0HH. Tel: 01245 460 981-secretary Fax: 01245 460 981

Professor Roy Sanders BSc MB BS FRCS
- YEAR QUALIFIED: 1962
- NHS POST: Consultant Plastic & Reconstructive Surgeon, Mount Vernon Hospital and Luton & Dunstable, RNOH Stanmore
- SPECIAL INTEREST: Aesthetic surgery; head and neck cancer; cleft lip & palate; orthopaedic complications.
- PRIVATE: BUPA Hospital Harpenden, Ambrose Lane, Harpenden, Herts, AL5 4BP. Tel: 01582 763191 Fax: 01582 761358

Kent

Mr Roger W Smith MChir FRCS
- YEAR QUALIFIED: 1990
- NHS POST: Consultant Plastic Surgery, Queen Victoria Hospital, W. Sussex
- SPECIAL INTEREST: Head and neck surgery; breast cancer surgery; cosmetic surgery to the face, breast and trunk.
- PRIVATE: Fawkham Manor Hospital, Manor Lane, Fawkham, Longfield, Kent DA3 8ND. Tel: 01474 879900 Fax: 01474 879892
Somerfield Hospital, 63-77 London Road, Maidstone, Kent, ME16 0DU. Tel: 01622 686581 Fax: 01622 674706
The Tunbridge Wells Nuffield Hospital, Kingswood Road, Tunbridge Wells, Kent TN2 4UL. Tel: 01892 531 111 Fax: 01892 515 689
BUPA Hospital Tunbridge Wells, Fordcombe Road, Fordcombe, Tunbridge Wells, Kent TN3 0RD. Tel: 01892 740 047 Fax: 01892 740 046

Mr N S Brent Tanner MA FRCS
- NHS POST: Honorary Consultant Plastic Surgeon Queen Victoria Hospital
- SPECIAL INTEREST: All forms of aesthetic surgery & Skin Care including laser and endoscopic surgery
- PRIVATE: BUPA Hospital Tunbridge Wells, Fordcombe Road, Fordcombe, Tunbridge Wells, Kent TN3 0RD. Tel: 01892 740044 Fax: 01892 740085

Leicestershire

Mr Sanjay Varma MBBS MS FRCSED(Plastic Surgery)
- YEAR QUALIFIED: 1976
- NHS POST: Consultant Plastic Surgeon, Leicester Royal Infirmary NHS Trust.
- SPECIAL INTEREST: Breast plastic surgery; facial plastic surgery; aesthetic surgery; hand surgery; skin cancer; breast reconstruction.
- PRIVATE: Leicester Nuffield Hospital, Scraptoft Lane, Leicester, Leicestershire LE5 1HY.

London

Ms Lena Anderson MD Dr. med
- NHS POST: Consultant Plastic Surgeon, Royal London and St. Bartholomew's Hospitals until 1997. Present at St. Helier Hospital Jersey.
- SPECIAL INTEREST: Breast surgery; breast reconstruction; aesthetic plastic surgery; rhinoplasty; medico-legal work accepted.
- PRIVATE: Anelcia Clinic, 27 Devonshire Place, London W1N 1PD. Tel: 0171 224 4333 Fax: 0171 224 4606
E-mail: anelca@anelca.com; Internet: www.anelca.com

SURGERY - Plastic. London

Mr Anthony I Attwood MBBS FRCS(Ed)
- YEAR QUALIFIED: 1972
- NHS POST: Consultant Advisor in Plastic Surgery to the Royal Air Force (Formerly).
- SPECIAL INTEREST: Cosmetic surgery and skin cancer.
- PRIVATE: BMI Blackheath Hospital, 40-42 Lee Terrace, London, SE3 9UD.
  Tel: 0181 318 7722 Fax: 0181 318 2542 E-mail:tony.attwood@dial.pipex.com

Mr Awad M Awwad MB BCh MSc FRCS
- SPECIAL INTEREST: Cosmetic and reconstructive surgery; laser surgery; hand surgery and wound care management.
- PRIVATE: Cromwell Hospital, Cromwell Road, London SW5 0TU.
  Tel: 0171 460 5700 Fax: 0171 460 5555
  The Portland Hospital, 205-209 Great Portland Street, London W1N 6AH.
  Tel: 0171 460 5663

Mr Colin Bishop MB BS LRCP MRCS FRCS MAE
- YEAR QUALIFIED: 1971
- SPECIAL INTEREST: Facial cosmetic plastic surgery; rhinoplasty; blepharoplasty
- PRIVATE: Consulting Rooms, 79 Harley Street, London W1N 1DE.
  Tel: 0171 486 1104 Fax: 0171 935 9850

Mr Nigel Carver MS FRCS FRCS(Plast)
- NHS POST: Consultant Plastic Surgeon, St. Bartholomew's Hospital And Royal London Hospital.
- SPECIAL INTEREST: Plastic reconstructive and aesthetic surgery; cosmetic facial surgery; rhinoplasty; breast reconstruction; skin cancer and hand surgery.
- PRIVATE: 40 Harley Street, London W1N 1AB.
  Tel: Private secretary-0181 850 1020
  London Independent Hospital, 1 Beaumont Square, Stepney Green, London E1 4NL.
  Tel: 0171 790 0990

Mr John Clarke MB FRCS
- YEAR QUALIFIED: 1963
- NHS POST: Consultant Plastic Surgeon, I/C Burns Unit, Queen Mary's Hospital.
- SPECIAL INTEREST: Acute burn management; burns reconstruction; paediatric and adult reconstruction; plastic surgery.
- PRIVATE: Queen Mary's Hospital, Roehampton Lane, London, SW15 5PN.
  Tel: 0181 789 6611 Fax: 0181 788 8417
  Parkside Hospital, 53 Parkside, Wimbledon, London, SW19 5NX.
  Tel: 0181 944 5659 Fax: 0181 944 8461

Mr Dai Davies MB BS FRCS
- NHS POST: Consultant Plastic Surgeon Charing Cross Hospital
- SPECIAL INTEREST: Rhinoplasty, Carpal Tunnel Syndrome, Breast Reconstruction
- PRIVATE: 55 Harley Street, London W1N 1DD.
  Tel: 0181 631 3927 Fax: 0171 636 6573
  The Stanford Hospital, Ravenscourt Park, London W6 0TN.
  Tel: 0171 735 6060 Fax: 0171 735 6061

SURGERY - Plastic. London

Mr Peter Davis MS FRCS
- YEAR QUALIFIED: 1959
- SPECIAL INTEREST: Cosmetic surgery
- PRIVATE: Consulting Rooms, New Victoria Hospital, 184 Coombe Lane West, Kingston Upon Thames, Surrey, KT2 7EG. Tel: 0181 949 9000. Private Secretary: 0181 949 1111

Mr James D Frame FRCS FRCS(Plast)
- YEAR QUALIFIED: 1977
- NHS POST: Consultant Plastic & Reconstructive Surgeon, St. Andrew's Centre For Plastic Surgery & Burns, Chelmsford, Essex.
- SPECIAL INTEREST: Lower limb trauma; burns; breast reconstruction; soft tissue sports injury; cosmetic surgery.
- PRIVATE: The Princess Grace Hospital, 42-52 Nottingham Place, London W1M 3FD.
Tel: 01245 460 981-secretary. Fax: 01245 460 981
108 Harley Street, London W1N 2ET.
Tel: 01245 460 981-secretary Fax: 01245 460 981

Mr Philip Y Graham MBBS(Hons) FRCS
- YEAR QUALIFIED: 1979
- SPECIAL INTEREST: Cosmetic surgery; rhinoplasty; breast surgery; facial plastic surgery; medico-legal.
- PRIVATE: London Independent Hospital, 1 Beaumont Square, Stepney Green, London E1 4NL.
Tel: 0171 790 0990
Cromwell Hospital, Cromwell Road, London SW5 0TU.
Tel: 01784 469 017
10 Harley Street, London W1N 1AA.
Tel: 01784 469 017

Mr David Charles Herbert MB BS FRCSEd FRCSEng
- YEAR QUALIFIED: 1961
- SPECIAL INTEREST: Surgery of facial ageing and facial reconstruction; breast reduction and breast surgery; rhinoplasty.
- PRIVATE: 9A Winbraham Place, Sloane Square, London SW1X 9AE.
Tel: 0171 730 7928

Mr Saifuddin Khan MBBS FRCS
- YEAR QUALIFIED: 1983
- SPECIAL INTEREST: Cosmetic surgery; facelift; rhinoplasty; blepharoplasty; liposuction; otoplasty; cosmetic surgery of the breast and trunk.
- PRIVATE: Highgate Private Hospital, 17-19 View Road, Highgate, London N6 4DJ.
Tel: 07970 600317

Mr David L Martin FRCS
- NHS POST: Consultant Plastic & Reconstructive Surgeon, Chelsea & Westminster Hospital.
- SPECIAL INTEREST: General plastic surgery; cosmetic surgery; breast surgery; hand surgery.
- PRIVATE: Parkside Hospital, 53 Parkside, Wimbledon, London, SW19 5NX.
Tel: 0181 971 8000 Fax: 0181 971 8002

SURGERY - Plastic. London

Mr Basim A Matti MB ChB FRCS
- YEAR QUALIFIED: 1973
- NHS POST: Consultant Plastic Surgeon, Charing Cross Hospital.
- SPECIAL INTEREST: Cosmetic surgery; face lift; rhinoplasty; liposuction; breast.
- PRIVATE: Flat 2, 30 Harley Street, London W1N 7AB.
  Tel: 0171 637 9595 Fax: 0171 636 1639

Mr Bryan J Mayou MB ChB FRCS
- YEAR QUALIFIED: 1969
- NHS POST: Consultant Plastic Surgeon St Thomas' Hospital
- SPECIAL INTEREST: Aesthetic Surgery including Endoscopic Facelift, Liposuction, Laser Surgery, Hand Surgery, Birthmarks, Epidermolysis Bullosa.
- PRIVATE: Lister Hospital, Chelsea Bridge Road, London, SW1W 8RH.
  Tel: 0171 824 8080 Fax: 0171 259 9887

Mrs Dalia V Nield MB BCh FRCS(Ed) T(PS)
- NHS POST: Consultant Plastic Surgeon St. Bartholomew's Hospital (Formerly)
- SPECIAL INTEREST: General plastic surgery; cosmetic surgery; breast reconstruction; liposculpture; laser re-surfacing.
- PRIVATE: 149 Harley Street, London W1N 2DE.
  Tel: 0171 935 4444 xt 4160 Fax: 0171 935 5091

Mr Nicholas Parkhouse DM(Oxon) MCh FRCS
- NHS POST: Consultant Plastic Surgeon, Queen Victoria Hospital, East Grinstead
- SPECIAL INTEREST: Reconstructive surgery of disfigurement and scarring; post burn scarring. Cosmetic/aesthetic facial surgery, rhinoplasty and cosmetic surgery of the breasts and trunk; dermatological surgery.
- PRIVATE: The London Clinic, 149 Harley Street, London, W1N 2DE.
  Tel: 0171 224 0864 / 0171 935 4444 - appointments.

Assoc. Professor B Povlsen MD PhD
- YEAR QUALIFIED: 1984
- NHS POST: Consultant, Guy's and St Thomas' Hospital: St. Thomas' Hospital, Lambeth Palace Road, London SE1 7EH. Tel: 0171 928 9292. Guy's Hospital, St. Thomas Street, London SE1 9RT. Tel: 0171 955 5000.
- SPECIAL INTEREST: Hand and micro surgery.
- PRIVATE: Churchill Clinic, 80 Lambeth Road, London, SE1 7PW.
  Tel: 0171 620 1590 Fax: 0171 928 1702 E-mail: bo@povlsen.u-net.com

Mr Riad Roomi MB ChB FICS
- YEAR QUALIFIED: 1977
- SPECIAL INTEREST: Hair restoration surgery (hair transplantation/scalp lifting); fat transplantation (for breast enlargement, face & lip augmentation); liposuction / liposculpture; laser. Diplomat of the American Board of Hair Restoration Surgery.
- PRIVATE: The 'New You' Clinic for Laser and Cosmetic Surgery, 591 Fulham Road, London SW6 5UA. Tel: 0171 385 3922 Fax: 0171 381 8180

SURGERY - Plastic. London

Professor Roy Sanders BSc MB BS FRCS
- YEAR QUALIFIED: 1962
- NHS POST: Consultant Plastic & Reconstructive Surgeon, Mount Vernon Hospital and Luton & Dunstable, RNOH Stanmore
- SPECIAL INTEREST: Aesthetic surgery; head and neck cancer; cleft lip & palate; orthopaedic complications.
- PRIVATE: The Consulting Suite, 82 Portland Place, London W1N 3DH.
Tel: 0171 580 3541 Fax: 0171 436 2954

Mr Adam Searle BDS MB BS FRCS FRCS(Plast)
- NHS POST: Consultant Plastic Surgeon Charing Cross Hospital
- SPECIAL INTEREST: Breast surgery; head and neck surgery; microsurgery; oncology reconstruction; laser treatment; aesthetic surgery.
- PRIVATE: Charing Cross Hospital, Fulham Palace Road, London, W6 8RF.
Tel: 0181 846 1173 Fax: 0181 846 1719
Lister Hospital, Chelsea Bridge Road, London, SW1W 8RH.
Tel: 0171 730 0135 Fax: 0171 730 0137

Mr Brian C Sommerlad MB BS FRCS
- NHS POST: Consultant Plastic Surgeon, Gt. Ormond St. Hospital; Royal London Hospital; St. Andrew's Centre for Plastic Surgery, Broomfield Hospital, Chelmsford.
- SPECIAL INTEREST: Congenital deformity; especially cleft lip and palate; hand deformities and hypospadias; skin cancer and benign skin lesions; head and neck surgery; especially parotid surgery; hand surgery especially Dupuytren's contracture.
- PRIVATE: The London Independent Hospital, 1 Beaumont Square, Stepney Green, London E1 4NL. Tel: 01245 422477
Great Ormond Street Hospital for Children NHS Trust, Great Ormond Street, London WC1N 3JH. Tel: 01245 422 477

Mr Norman Waterhouse MBChB FRCS FRCS(Plastic Surgery)
- NHS POST: Consultant Plastic Surgeon Chelsea & Westminster Hospital
- SPECIAL INTEREST: Craniofacial surgery; congenital, traumatic and neoplastic disorders; all aesthetic surgery.
- PRIVATE: 55 Harley Street, London, W1N 1DD.
Tel: 0171 636 4073 Fax: 0171 636 6417 E-mail: wtrhouse@globelnet.co.uk

Nottinghamshire

Mr David Charles Herbert MB BS FRCSEd FRCSEng
- YEAR QUALIFIED: 1961
- SPECIAL INTEREST: Surgery of facial ageing and facial reconstruction; breast reduction and breast surgery; rhinoplasty.
- PRIVATE: 30A Regent Street, Nottingham, Nottinghamshire NG1 5BT.
Tel: 0115 950 4363

Oxfordshire

Mr Alan Godfrey MB BCh FRCSEd
YEAR QUALIFIED: 1968
SPECIAL INTEREST: Breast and facial cosmetic surgery; laser surgery and reconstructive surgery.
PRIVATE: The Acland Hospital, 25 Banbury Road, Oxford, Oxfordshire OX2 6NX.
Tel: 01865 244421 Fax: 01865 244421 E-mail: secretary@eslas.com

Surrey

Mr Peter Davis MS FRCS
YEAR QUALIFIED: 1959
SPECIAL INTEREST: Cosmetic surgery
PRIVATE: New Victoria Hospital, 184 Coombe Lane West, Kingston Upon Thames, Surrey, KT2 7EG. Tel: 0181 949 9000. Private Secretary: 0181 949 1111.
St. Anthony's Hospital, London Road, North Cheam, Surrey, SM3 9DW. Tel: 0181 337 6691. Private Secretary: 0181 949 1111

Mr David L Martin FRCS
NHS POST: Consultant Plastic & Reconstructive Surgeon, Chelsea & Westminster Hospital.
SPECIAL INTEREST: General plastic surgery; cosmetic surgery; breast surgery; hand surgery.
PRIVATE: Runnymede Hospital, Guildford Road, Ottershaw, Surrey, KT16 0RQ.
Tel: 01932 877 800 Fax: 01932 875 433

Mr N S Brent Tanner MA FRCS
NHS POST: Honorary Consultant Plastic Surgeon Queen Victoria Hospital
SPECIAL INTEREST: All forms of aesthetic surgery & Skin Care including laser and endoscopic surgery
PRIVATE: North Downs Hospital, 46 Tupwood Lane, Caterham, Surrey CR3 6DP.
Tel: 01883 348 981 Fax: 01883 341 163

Mr Christopher Ward BSc MA FRCS
YEAR QUALIFIED: 1965
SPECIAL INTEREST: Reconstructive and aesthetic breast surgery; surgery of the ageing face; rhinoplasty; abdominoplasty; 'See and Treat' approach to minor surgery.
PRIVATE: 15 Cumberland Road, Kew, Richmond, Surrey TW9 3HJ.
Tel: 0181 948 4990 Fax: 0181 332 7770

Warwickshire

Mr Richard N Matthews MB BS FRCS FRCS(Edin)
- YEAR QUALIFIED: 1972
- NHS POST: Consultant Plastic, Reconstructive and Hand Surgeon, Department of Plastic and Reconstructive Surgery.
- SPECIAL INTEREST: Cosmetic surgery; surgery for skin cancer and 'lumps and bumps'; vascular and pigmented birthmarks and other paediatric plastic surgery including hypospadias; breast reconstructions; hand surgery.
- PRIVATE: The Warwickshire Nuffield Hospital, Old Milverton Lane, Leamington Spa, Warwickshire CV32 6RW. Tel: 01926 427971 Fax: 01926 428791
  The Nuneaton Private Hospital, 132 Coventry Road, Hilltop, Nuneaton, Warwickshire CV10 7AD. Tel: 01203 353000 Fax: 01203 346645
  The Rooms, The Old Hall, Lilbourne Road, Clifton-upon-Dunsmore, Warwickshire CV23 0BD. Tel: 01788 561057

West Midlands

Mr Richard N Matthews MB BS FRCS FRCS(Edin)
- YEAR QUALIFIED: 1972
- NHS POST: Consultant Plastic, Reconstructive and Hand Surgeon, Department of Plastic and Reconstructive Surgery.
- SPECIAL INTEREST: Cosmetic surgery; surgery for skin cancer and 'lumps and bumps'; vascular and pigmented birthmarks and other paediatric plastic surgery including hypospadias; breast reconstructions; hand surgery.
- PRIVATE: Coventry Consulting Rooms, 11 Dalton Road, Earlesdon, Coventry, West Midlands CV5 6PD. Tel: 01203 677443

West Sussex

Mr Nicholas Parkhouse DM(Oxon) MCh FRCS
- NHS POST: Consultant Plastic Surgeon, Queen Victoria Hospital, East Grinstead
- SPECIAL INTEREST: Reconstructive surgery of disfigurement and scarring; post burn scarring. Cosmetic/aesthetic facial surgery, rhinoplasty and cosmetic surgery of the breasts and trunk; dermatological surgery.
- PRIVATE: Ashdown Nuffield Hospital, Burrell Road, Haywards Heath, West Sussex RH16 1UD. Tel: 01444 456999 Fax: 01444 454111
  King Edward VII Hospital, Midhurst, West Sussex, GU29 0BL. Tel: 01730 812341 Fax: 01730 817364
  Goring Hall Hospital, Bodiam Avenue, Goring-By-Sea, West Sussex BN12 4UX. Tel: 01903 506699 Fax: 01903 700782

Mr Roger W Smith MChir FRCS
- YEAR QUALIFIED: 1990
- NHS POST: Consultant Plastic Surgery, Queen Victoria Hospital, W. Sussex
- SPECIAL INTEREST: Head and neck surgery; breast cancer surgery; cosmetic surgery to the face, breast and trunk.
- PRIVATE: Queen Victoria Hospital, Holtye Road, East Grinstead, West Sussex RH19 2PU. Tel: 01342 300904 Fax: 01342 317959

Wiltshire

Mr Alan Godfrey MB BCh FRCSEd
- YEAR QUALIFIED: 1968
- SPECIAL INTEREST: Breast and facial cosmetic surgery; laser surgery and reconstructive surgery.
- PRIVATE: The Ridgeway Hospital, Moormead Road, Wroughton, Swindon, Wiltshire SN4 9DD. Tel: 01865 244421 Fax: 01793 814852 E-mail: secretary@eslas.com

SURGERY - Plastic - Hand Surgery

Bristol

Mr Donald Sammut FRCS FRCS(Plast)
- YEAR QUALIFIED: 1980
- NHS POST: Consultant Plastic and Hand Surgeon, Frenchay Hospital NHS Trust, Bristol.
- SPECIAL INTEREST: Hand surgery; plastic surgery.
- PRIVATE: The Chesterfield Hospital, 3 Clifton Hill, Bristol BS8 1BP.
  Tel: 0117 973 5544 Fax: 0117 973 0323

SURGERY - Spinal

Buckinghamshire

Mr Brian Gardner MA(oxon) BM BCh FRCS FRCP(Lon + Edin)
- YEAR QUALIFIED: 1973
- NHS POST: Consultant In Spinal Cord Injuries, Stoke Mandeville Hospital.
- SPECIAL INTEREST: Spinal cord paralysed - paraplegia and tetraplegia.
- PRIVATE: Stoke Mandeville Hospital, Mandeville Road, Aylesbury, Buckinghamshire HP21 8AL.
Tel: 01296 315 849 Fax: 01296 424627

London

Mr John P O'Brien PhD FRCS(Ed) FACS FRACS
- YEAR QUALIFIED: 1960
- SPECIAL INTEREST: Female back pain; back surgery.
- PRIVATE: The London Clinic, 149 Harley Street, London, W1N 2DE.
Tel: 0171 935 4444 Fax: 0171 486 5222 E-mail: obrien_spine@msn.com

SURGERY - Thoracic

London

Mr Peter Goldstraw FRCS
- NHS POST: Royal Brompton & National Heart Hospital
- SPECIAL INTEREST: Surgery/Thoracic
- PRIVATE: Private Consulting Rooms, Royal Brompton National Heart & Lung Hospital, Fulham Road, London, SW3 6HP.
  Tel: 0171 351 8558

SURGERY - Varicose Vein

Devon

Mr Denis Charles Wilkins MB ChB FRCS MD
- YEAR QUALIFIED: 1966
- NHS POST: Consultant General and Vascular Surgeon, Derriford Hospital, Plymouth.
- SPECIAL INTEREST: General surgery; hernia; endocrine; thyroid; hyperhydrosis; medico-legal; arterial surgery; carotid disease; peripheral vascular disease; aneurysms; varicose veins; aortic surgery; vibratory white finger; parathyroid; cholecystectomy.
- PRIVATE: Nuffield Hospital, Derriford Road, Plymouth, Devon PL6 8BG.
  Tel: 01752 778892 Fax: 01752 778421

East Sussex

Mr Brian J Stoodley MA MChir FRCS
- NHS POST: Consultant Surgeon Eastbourne District General & Uckfield Hospitals
- SPECIAL INTEREST: Colorectal and gastrointestinal/breast/varicose vein surgery.
- PRIVATE: Consulting Rooms, 21 Lushington Road, Eastbourne, East Sussex BN26 5UX.
  Tel: 01323 410 441 Fax: 01323 410 978

Hampshire

Mr Nicholas M Wilson MBBS BSc MS FRCS
- YEAR QUALIFIED: 1981
- NHS POST: Consultant Surgeon, Royal Hampshire County Hospital.
- SPECIAL INTEREST: General surgery, subspecialty vascular and varicose vein surgery.
- PRIVATE: Private Hospital, Sarum Road, Winchester, Hampshire SO22 5HA.
  Tel: 01962 826105

Kent

Mr David B Jackson BSc MB FRCS
- NHS POST: Consultant Surgeon, Kent & Canterbury Hospital.
- SPECIAL INTEREST: Surgical oncology specialising in breast reconstruction and major pelvic surgery; ileo-anal pouch surgery and laparoscopic procedures.
- PRIVATE: Winters Farm, Nackington Road, Canterbury, Kent CT4 7AY.
  Tel: 01227 472 581 Fax: 01227 472 581 E-mail: davidjackson@uk-consultants.co.uk

Mrs Marie South MS FRCS
- YEAR QUALIFIED: 1968
- NHS POST: Consultant General Surgeon, Maidstone Hospital.
- SPECIAL INTEREST: Vascular, laparoscopic, endocrine and paediatric surgery; minimally invasive procedures e.g. laparoscopic cholecystectomy, laparoscopic fundoplication, laparoscopic hernia repair and thoracoscopic cervical sympathectomy for hyperhydrosis.
- PRIVATE: Somerfield Hospital, 63-77 London Road, Maidstone, Kent, ME16 0DU.
Tel: 01622 672829 Fax: 01622 672829

Liverpool

Mr Michael Hershman MSc MS FRCS(Eng, Ed, Glas and Irel) FICS
- YEAR QUALIFIED: 1980
- NHS POST: Consultant Surgeon, Royal Liverpool University Hospital.
- SPECIAL INTEREST: General surgery with particular interests in colorectal and minimal access surgery.
- PRIVATE: Lourdes Hospital, 57 Greenbank Road, Liverpool, L18 1HQ.
Tel: 0151 733 7123 Fax: 0151 735 0446

London

Mr Mohan Adiseshiah MA MS FRCS MRCP
- NHS POST: Consultant Vascular Surgeon, University College & Middlesex Hospitals.
- SPECIAL INTEREST: Arterial and endovascular surgery.
- PRIVATE: The London Clinic, 149 Harley Street, London, W1N 2DE.
Tel: 0171 935 4444 E-mail: m.adis@lonclin.co.uk

Mr Christopher Bishop MChir FRCS
- NHS POST: Consultant Surgeon, Middlesex Hospital.
- SPECIAL INTEREST: Vascular and varicose vein surgery; carotid artery surgery; aneurysm surgery.
- PRIVATE: Lister Hospital, Chelsea Bridge Road, London, SW1W 8RH.
Tel: 0171 235 6086 Fax: 0171 730 2840
149 Harley Street, London W1N 2DE.
Tel: 0171 235 6086 Fax: 0171 730 2840
Cromwell Hospital, Cromwell Road, London SW5 0TU.
Tel: 0171 235 6086 Fax: 0171 730 2840
Humana Hospital Wellington, Wellington Place, St Johns Wood, London, NW8 9LE.
Tel: 0171 235 6086 Fax: 0171 730 2840

Professor Kevin Guiver Burnand MBBS FRCS MS
- NHS POST: Honorary Consultant Surgeon, St. Thomas' Hospital.
- SPECIAL INTEREST: Carotid, aortic and peripheral vascular disease; varicose veins, *** limb and lymphoedema.
- PRIVATE: St. Thomas' Hospital, Lambeth Palace Road, London, SE1 7EH.
Tel: 0171 928 9292 xt 2428 Fax: 0171 928 8742 E-mail: k.burnand@unds.ac.uk

Professor Josef J Pflug MD PhD FACS
- NHS POST: Consultant Surgeon Hammersmith Hospital
- SPECIAL INTEREST: Surgical treatment of non-healing venous ulcers and of chronic lymphoedema of the arm and leg.
- PRIVATE: Robert and Lisa Sainsbury Wing, Hammersmith Hospital, Du Cane Road, London, W12 OHS. Tel: 0181 740 3113 Fax: 0181 746 1127

South Glamorgan

Mr William Tudor Davies MD FRCS(Eng)
- YEAR QUALIFIED: 1963
- NHS POST: Consultant General and Vascular Surgeon, University Hospital of Wales.
- SPECIAL INTEREST: Varicose veins, all general surgery, arterial problems, vaseltomy, medico-legal work.
- PRIVATE: Glamorgan House, BUPA Hospital, Croescadarn Road, Pentwyn, Cardiff, South Glamorgan CF2 7XL. Tel: 01222 735825, 736011

Surrey

Mr Robert McFarland MChir FRCS
- NHS POST: Consultant in Vascular & General Surgery, Epsom General Hospital.
- SPECIAL INTEREST: Vascular surgery.
- PRIVATE: Epsom General Hospital (Trust), Dorking Road, Epsom, Surrey, KT18 7EG. Tel: 01372 735 735
  Ashtead Hospital, The Warren, Ashtead, Surrey KT21 2SB. Tel: 01372 276 161

West Midlands

Mr Mark Xavier Gannon MB ChB MD FRCS(Ed) FRCS(Eng)
- YEAR QUALIFIED: 1979
- NHS POST: Consultant surgeon, Birmingham Heartlands and Solihull NHS Trust (Teaching).
- SPECIAL INTEREST: Specialist vascular surgeon with interest in all aspects of arterial and venous disease including management of aneurysm, cerebro-vascular disease, peripheral vascular disease and venous problems.
- PRIVATE: BUPA Parkway Hospital, Damson parkway, Solihull, West Midlands B91 2PP. Tel: 0121 704 1451

SURGERY - Vascular

Cheshire

Professor David Charlesworth DSc MD FRCS MBCuB
- YEAR QUALIFIED: 1959
- NHS POST: Consultant Surgeon, South Manchester University Hospital Trust.
- SPECIAL INTEREST: Vascular surgery; aortic surgery; surgery for stroke (carotid); claudication and critical ischaemia of the legs.
- PRIVATE: Alexandra Hospital, Mill Lane, Cheadle, Cheshire SK8 2PX.
  Tel: 0161 291 4725 Fax: 01565 654813

County Durham

Mr Nigel Bruce Corner MB BS FRCS
- YEAR QUALIFIED: 1981
- NHS POST: Consultant General and Vascular Surgeon, Darlington Memorial Hospital.
- SPECIAL INTEREST: Venous and arterial surgery.
- PRIVATE: St. Cuthbert's Consulting Rooms, St. Cuthbert's Way, Darlington, County Durham DL1 1GB. Tel: 01325 364624 Fax: 01325 364624

Devon

Mr Denis Charles Wilkins MB ChB FRCS MD
- YEAR QUALIFIED: 1966
- NHS POST: Consultant General and Vascular Surgeon, Derriford Hospital, Plymouth.
- SPECIAL INTEREST: General surgery; hernia; endocrine; thyroid; hyperhydrosis; medico-legal; arterial surgery; carotid disease; peripheral vascular disease; aneurysms; varicose veins; aortic surgery; vibratory white finger; parathyroid; cholecystectomy.
- PRIVATE: Nuffield Hospital, Derriford Road, Plymouth, Devon PL6 8BG.
  Tel: 01752 778892 Fax: 01752 778421

Essex

Mr Alan Murray MB BS MS FRCS
- YEAR QUALIFIED: 1979
- NHS POST: Consultant Vascular and General Surgeon, Southend Hospital.
- SPECIAL INTEREST: Varicose veins; carotid surgery; aortic aneurysm surgery; distal grafting; endoscopic sympathectomy; thyroid and laparoscopic surgery.
- PRIVATE: BUPA Wellesley Hospital, Eastern Avenue, Southend on Sea SS2 4XH.

Glasgow

Mr Robert Paul Teenan MD FRCS
- YEAR QUALIFIED: 1981
- NHS POST: Consultant Surgeon, Stobhill NHS Trust, Glasgow.
- SPECIAL INTEREST: General surgery with a major interest in vascular disease, both arterial and venous.
- PRIVATE: Ross Hall Hospital, 221 Crookston Road, Glasgow G52 3NQ.
  Tel: 0141 810 3151 Fax: 0141 882 7439

Hampshire

Mr Nicholas M Wilson MBBS BSc MS FRCS
- YEAR QUALIFIED: 1981
- NHS POST: Consultant Surgeon, Royal Hampshire County Hospital.
- SPECIAL INTEREST: General surgery, subspecialty vascular and varicose vein surgery.
- PRIVATE: Private Hospital, Sarum Road, Winchester, Hampshire SO22 5HA.
  Tel: 01962 826105

Kent

Mrs Marie South MS FRCS
- YEAR QUALIFIED: 1968
- NHS POST: Consultant General Surgeon, Maidstone Hospital.
- SPECIAL INTEREST: Vascular, laparoscopic, endocrine and paediatric surgery; minimally invasive procedures e.g. laparoscopic cholecystectomy, laparoscopic fundoplication, laparoscopic hernia repair and thoracoscopic cervical sympathectomy for hyperhydrosis.
- PRIVATE: Somerfield Hospital, 63-77 London Road, Maidstone, Kent, ME16 0DU.
  Tel: 01622 672829 Fax: 01622 672829

Lincolnshire

Mr Andrew Lamerton FRCS MRCP
- YEAR QUALIFIED: 1970
- NHS POST: Consultant General and Vascular Surgeon, Lincoln and Louth NHS Hospitals Trust.
- SPECIAL INTEREST: General and vascular surgery; surgery of thoracic outlet compression syndrome.
- PRIVATE: The Manor House, Church Lane, Cherry Willingham, Lincolnshire LN3 4DB.
  Tel: 01522 751377 Fax: 01522 595536

London

Mr Daryll Baker PhD FRCS
- YEAR QUALIFIED: 1986
- NHS POST: Consultant Vascular and General Surgeon, Royal Free Hospital, London.
- SPECIAL INTEREST: All complex vascular surgery, venous surgery including varicose veins.
- PRIVATE: The Wellington Hospital, Wellington Place, London, NW8 9LE.
  Tel: 0171 722 7370 Fax: 0171 722 7406

Mr Christopher Bishop MChir FRCS
- NHS POST: Consultant Surgeon, Middlesex Hospital.
- SPECIAL INTEREST: Vascular and varicose vein surgery; carotid artery surgery; aneurysm surgery.
- PRIVATE: 149 Harley Street, London W1N 2DE.
  Tel: 0171 235 6086 Fax: 0171 730 2840

Professor Kevin Guiver Burnand MBBS FRCS MS
- NHS POST: Honorary Consultant Surgeon, St. Thomas' Hospital.
- SPECIAL INTEREST: Carotid, aortic and peripheral vascular disease; varicose veins, limb and lymphoedema.
- PRIVATE: St. Thomas' Hospital, Lambeth Palace Road, London, SE1 7EH.
  Tel: 0171 928 9292 xt 2428 Fax: 0171 928 8742 E-mail: k.burnand@unds.ac.uk

Mr Frank W Cross MB MS FRCS
- YEAR QUALIFIED: 1975
- NHS POST: Consultant Surgeon Royal London Hospital
- SPECIAL INTEREST: Vascular surgery and varicose vein. Laser surgery of veins.
- PRIVATE: The London Clinic, 149 Harley Street, London W1N 2HG.
  Tel: 0171 935 4444 / 0171 486 4688 - direct line. Fax: 0171 487 5479
  E-mail: f.cross@dial.pipex.com

Professor Roger M Greenhalgh MA MD MChir(Cantab) FRCS(Eng)
- YEAR QUALIFIED: 1966
- NHS POST: Chief of Vascular Surgery, Charing Cross Hospital (Hammersmith Hospitals Trust).
- SPECIAL INTEREST: Vascular surgery; aortic aneurysms; surgery for minor stroke; limb salvage; intermittent claudication; varicose veins; venous ulcers.
- PRIVATE: Regional Vascular Service, Charing Cross Hospital, Fulham Palace Road, London, W6 8RF. Tel: 0181 846 1555/7313 Fax: 0181 846 7330 E-mail: r.greenhalgh@ic.ac.uk

Mr David Nott BSc MD FRCS
- YEAR QUALIFIED: 1981
- NHS POST: Consultant Surgeon Chelsea & Westminster Hospital
- SPECIAL INTEREST: All aspects of arterial and venous surgery.
- PRIVATE: Seretary at, Chelsea & Westminster Hospital, 396 Fulham Road, London SW10 9TH.
  Tel: 0181 746 8464
  Lister Hospital, Chelsea Bridge Road, London, SW1W 8RH.
  Tel: 0171 730 3417
  Cromwell Hospital, Cromwell Road, London SW5 0TU.
  Tel: 0171 370 4233
  King Edward VII Hospital, Beaumont Street, London, W1N 2AA.
  Tel: 0171 486 4411

SURGERY - Vascular. London

Professor Josef J Pflug MD PhD FACS
- NHS POST: Consultant Surgeon Hammersmith Hospital
- SPECIAL INTEREST: Surgical treatment of non-healing venous ulcers and of chronic lymphoedema of the arm and leg.
- PRIVATE: Robert and Lisa Sainsbury Wing, Hammersmith Hospital, Du Cane Road, London, W12 OHS. Tel: 0181 740 3113 Fax: 0181 746 1127

Mr John H N Wolfe MBBS FRCS MS
- NHS POST: Vascular Surgeon St. Mary's Hospital, Imperial College Medical School
- SPECIAL INTEREST: Arterial disease; venous disease; lymphatic disease.
- PRIVATE: 66 Harley Street, London W1N 1AE.
  Tel: 0171 580 5030 Fax: 0171 631 5341

Merseyside

Mr Peter Lyon Harris MD FRCS
- YEAR QUALIFIED: 1967
- NHS POST: Consultant Vascular Surgeon, Royal Liverpool University Hospital.
- SPECIAL INTEREST: Aortic aneurysms; carotid artery disease; lower limb ischaemia and varicose veins.
- PRIVATE: 88 Rodney Street, Liverpool, Merseyside L1 9AR.
  Tel: 0151 709 0669 Fax: 0151 709 7279

Surrey

Mr Robert McFarland MChir FRCS
- NHS POST: Consultant in Vascular & General Surgery, Epsom General Hospital.
- SPECIAL INTEREST: Vascular surgery.
- PRIVATE: Epsom General Hospital (Trust), Dorking Road, Epsom, Surrey, KT18 7EG.
  Tel: 01372 735 735
  Ashtead Hospital, The Warren, Ashtead, Surrey KT21 2SB.
  Tel: 01372 276 161

West Midlands

Mr Mark Xavier Gannon MB ChB MD FRCS(Ed) FRCS(Eng)
- YEAR QUALIFIED: 1979
- NHS POST: Consultant surgeon, Birmingham Heartlands and Solihull NHS Trust (Teaching).
- SPECIAL INTEREST: Specialist vascular surgeon with interest in all aspects of arterial and venous disease including management of aneurysm, cerebro-vascular disease, peripheral vascular disease and venous problems.
- PRIVATE: BUPA Parkway Hospital, Damson parkway, Solihull, West Midlands B91 2PP.
  Tel: 0121 704 1451

Sexual Medicine

London

Professor Tom Robin Caine Boyde MB BS MD FRCPath
- YEAR QUALIFIED: 1955
- SPECIAL INTEREST: Chemical pathology.
- PRIVATE: 21D Devonshire Place, London W1N 1PD.
  Tel: 0171 487 4884 Fax: 0171 487 2926

Dr John Kellett MB BChir FRCP FRCPsych
- NHS POST: Consultant Psychiatrist, Pathfinder Trust.
- SPECIAL INTEREST: Psychiatry of old age - especially dementia and sexual dysfunction.
- PRIVATE: Priory Hospital, Priory Lane, Roehampton, London, SW15 5JJ.
  Tel: 0181 876 8261 ext 347

Suffolk

Dr Fran Reader MB BS FRCOG MFFP
- YEAR QUALIFIED: 1973
- NHS POST: Consultant in Family Planning and Reproductive Health Care, Ipswich Hospital.
- SPECIAL INTEREST: Sexual and relationship problems; contraception; unplanned pregnancy; menopause; pre-menstrual syndrome.
- PRIVATE: Christchurch Park Hospital, 57-61 Fonnereau Road, Ipswich, Suffolk IP1 3JN.
  Tel: 01473 256071 Fax: 01473 288053

Sports Medicine & Surgery

Essex

Dr Thomas Crisp TD BSc MB BS Dip Sports Medicine
- YEAR QUALIFIED: 1973
- NHS POST: Sports Physician, Royal London Hospital.
- SPECIAL INTEREST: Sports and orthopaedic medicine; overuse and running injuries; shoulder and knee injuries.
- PRIVATE: Springfield Hospital, Lawn Lane, Springfield, Chelmsford, Essex CM1 7GU.
  Tel: 01245 461777 Fax: 01245 460169 E-mail: tomcrisp@aol.com

Miss Janet Porter MB BChir FRCS FFAEM
- YEAR QUALIFIED: 1971
- NHS POST: Accident & Emergency Consultant, Southend Hospital.
- SPECIAL INTEREST: Soft tissue injuries; shoulder and hand problems.
- PRIVATE: 114 Woodside, Leigh-on-sea, Essex SS9 4RB.
  Tel: 01702 421661 Fax: 01702 421661

London

Dr Thomas Crisp TD BSc MB BS Dip Sports Medicine
- YEAR QUALIFIED: 1973
- NHS POST: Sports Physician, Royal London Hospital.
- SPECIAL INTEREST: Sports and orthopaedic medicine; overuse and running injuries; shoulder and knee injuries.
- PRIVATE: London Independent Hospital, 1 Beaumont Square, Stepney Green, London E1 4NL.
  Tel: 0171 790 0990 (Direct Line) Fax: 0171 791 2594 E-mail: tomcrisp@aol.com

Dr Colin Peter Crosby MA (Oxon) MB,BS(Lond) LRCP MRCP
- YEAR QUALIFIED: 1979
- SPECIAL INTEREST: Sports and exercise medicine; general sports injuries; health related fitness; exercise prescription.
- PRIVATE: The Garden Hospital, 46-50 Sunny Gardens Road, Hendon, London, NW4 1RX.
  Tel: 0181 203 0111 Fax: 0181 203 4343
  29-31 Devonshire Street, London W1N 1RF.
  Tel: 0171 486 7131 Fax: 0171 486 0090

Dr Susan Daniel BSc MBBS MD FRCPath
- YEAR QUALIFIED: 1979
- NHS POST: Honorary Consultant, National Hospital for Neurology and Neurosurgery, Senior Lecturer.
- SPECIAL INTEREST: Research into diseases of ageing, instructor of BUPA approved Shaw method of swimming with special interest in disorders of movement, fitness and health.
- PRIVATE: Laboratory Spa and Health Club, The Avenue, Muswell Hill, London N10 2QJ.
  Tel: 0181 482 3000

Sports Medicine & Surgery. London

Professor John Elfed Davies MRCS D.Phys.Med Dip.SportsMed PM Rehab (EU)
- NHS POST: Consultant Physician In Sports Medicine, Physical Medicine And Rehabilitation Guy's Hospital, London
- SPECIAL INTEREST: Rehabilitation of low back pain and diagnosis of musculo-skeletal sports injuries; treatment of fibro myalgia and chronic fatigue syndrome; foot problems; bio-mechanics and surgery.
- PRIVATE: The Harley Street Sports Clinic, Devonshire Hospital, Devonshire Street, London, W1. Tel: 0171 486 2494 Fax: 0171 486 0090

Mr Graham M N Holloway MB ChB FRCS
- YEAR QUALIFIED: 1969
- SPECIAL INTEREST:
- PRIVATE: Sports Injury Clinic, London Bridge Hospital, 27 Tooley Street, London SE1 2PR. Tel: 0171 407 3100 Fax: 0171 407 3162

Dr Stephen Motto BM, Dip Med Ac, D M-S Med, Dip Sports Med.
- NHS POST: British Olympic Medical Centre, Northwick Park Hospital and Royal London Homoeopathic Hospital.
- SPECIAL INTEREST: All exertional muscle and tendon injuries, particularly Achilles tendon disorders. The treatment of back pain using spinal manipulation, injections and acupuncture; anterior knee pain.
- PRIVATE: London Bridge Hospital, Emblem House, 27 Tooley Street, London SE1 2PR. Tel: 0171 815 3660 Fax: 0171 815 3654 Mobile-0958 274 984. E-mail: info@smsportmed.co.uk

Mr Simon Moyes MB FRCS FRCS.Orth D.Sports Med
- YEAR QUALIFIED: 1982
- SPECIAL INTEREST: Minimally invasive surgery of the knee, shoulder, foot and ankle.
- PRIVATE: 86 Harley Street, London W1N 1AE. Tel: 0171 323 0040 Fax: 0171 323 0080 E-mail:simonmoyes@aol.com

Dr John Price MBBS MRCS LRCP DRCOB DPhMed
- YEAR QUALIFIED: 1958
- SPECIAL INTEREST: Cervical and lumbo-sacral disc lesions and spondylosis; joint injuries and sports injuries; rehabilitation for degenerative joint disease.
- PRIVATE: 12 Fitzjames Avenue, East Croydon, Surrey CR0 5DH. Tel: 0181 654 3862 Fax: 0171 935 5972

Wiltshire

Mr Graham M N Holloway MB ChB FRCS
- YEAR QUALIFIED: 1969
- SPECIAL INTEREST:
- PRIVATE: Sports Injury Clinic, Ridgeway Hospital, Moormead Road, Wroughton, Swindon, Wilts SN4 9DD. Tel: 01793 814848 Fax: 01793 814852

Thoracic Medicine

Berkshire

Dr James Lyall MD FRCP
- YEAR QUALIFIED: 1969
- NHS POST: Consultant Physician, Battle Hospital.
- SPECIAL INTEREST: Sleep related breathing disorders.
- PRIVATE: Berkshire Independent Hospital, Wensley Road, Coley Park, Reading, Berkshire RG1 6UZ. Tel: 0118 956 0056 Fax: 0118 956 6333

London

Professor K Fan Chung MD FRCP
- NHS POST: Consultant Physician, Royal Brompton Hospital, London.
- SPECIAL INTEREST: Respiratory medicine including asthma and bronchitis.
- PRIVATE: Private Consulting Rooms, Royal Brompton Hospital, Sydney Street, London SW3 6NP. Tel: 0171 351 8995 - apointments Fax: 0171 351 8085

Dr Duncan Empey FRCP
- NHS POST: Consultant Physician, The Royal London Hospital and London Chest Hospital.
- SPECIAL INTEREST: Bronchoscopy, Asthma, Chronic Bronchitis, Sleep-disordered breathing, Chronic cough.
- PRIVATE: 18 Upper Wimpole Street, London W1M 7TB. Tel: 0171 935 2977 Fax: 0171 935 2740

Professor Timothy W Evans BSc MD FRCP PhD
- NHS POST: Consultant, Royal Brompton Hospital.
- SPECIAL INTEREST: Asthma; intensive care.
- PRIVATE: Royal Brompton Hospital, Sydney Street, London SW3 6NP. Tel: 0171 351 8523 Fax: 0171 351 8524

Dr Philip Jeremy M George MA MSc MD FRCP
- YEAR QUALIFIED: 1979
- NHS POST: Consultant Physician in General and Thoracic Medicine, The Middlesex Hospital and University College Hospitals.
- SPECIAL INTEREST: All aspects of thoracic medicine particularly lung cancer, diagnostic and therapeutic bronchoscopy; laser treatment; airway stenting and endobronchial radiotherapy.
- PRIVATE: Private Patients Wing, University College Hospital, 25 Grafton Way, London, WC1E 6DB. Tel: 0171 380 9851

Dr Geoffrey K Knowles MD FRCP
- YEAR QUALIFIED: 1970
- NHS POST: Consultant Physician, Kingston Hospital.
- SPECIAL INTEREST: All aspects of respiratory medicine including asthma, allergy, infections and cancer.
- PRIVATE: Parkside Hospital, 53 Parkside, Wimbledon, London, SW19 5NX. Tel: 0181 946 4202 Fax: 0181 946 7775

Thoracic Medicine. London

Dr David Mitchell MA MD FRCP
NHS POST: Consultant Physician, General & Respiratory Medicine, St. Mary's Hospital.
SPECIAL INTEREST: Allergy; asthma; sarcoidosis; TB.
PRIVATE: 55 Harley Street, London W1N 1DD.
Tel: 0171 886 1082 Fax: 0171 886 1613

Professor Stephen J G Semple MD FRCP
SPECIAL INTEREST: General medicine; respiratory (thoracic) medicine.
PRIVATE: The Middlesex Hospital Woolavington Wing, Mortimer Street, London W1N 8AA.
Tel: 0171 504 9443 Fax: 0171 380 9117
Cromwell Hospital, Cromwell Road, London SW5 0TU.
Tel: 0171 460 5700 Fax: 0171 460 5555

Surrey

Dr Geoffrey K Knowles MD FRCP
YEAR QUALIFIED: 1970
NHS POST: Consultant Physician, Kingston Hospital.
SPECIAL INTEREST: All aspects of respiratory medicine including asthma, allergy, infections and cancer.
PRIVATE: New Victoria Hospital, 184 Coombe Lane West, Kingston Upon Thames, Surrey, KT2 7EG. Tel: 0181 949 9000 Fax: 0181 949 9099
Coombe Wing, Kingston Hospital, Galsworthy Road, Kingston Upon Thames, Surrey, KT2 7QB. Tel: 0181 546 6677 Fax: 0181 541 5613

West Sussex

Dr John Evans FRCP MBBS MRCS LRCP BSc
NHS POST: Consultant Physician, Worthing & Southlands Hospital Medical Trust.
SPECIAL INTEREST: Bronchial asthma; chronic obstructive pulmonary disease; lung cancer; allergic conditions of the respiratory system.
PRIVATE: Chilton, 93 Warren Road, Worthing, Sussex BN14 9QU.
Tel: 01903 260 086 Fax: 01903 260 086
Goring Hall Hospital, Bodiam Avenue, Goring-By-Sea, West Sussex BN12 4UX.
Tel: 01903 506 699

Worcestershire

Dr Arumugam Santi Vathenen BM(Soton) MRCP(UK) DM(Soton)
YEAR QUALIFIED: 1980
NHS POST: Consultant Physician, Alexandra Hospital, Worcs.
SPECIAL INTEREST: General internal medicine with a special interest in respiratory medicine.
PRIVATE: Droitwich Spa Hospital, St. Andrew's Road, Droitwich, Worcestershire WR9 8DN.
Tel: 01789 763994 Fax: 01527 512000

Urology

Antrim

Mr Richard Donaldson MSSc BSc MB BCh FRCSEd
YEAR QUALIFIED: 1969
NHS POST: Consultant Urologist, Belfast City Hospital.
SPECIAL INTEREST: Cystitis and interstitial cystitis, renal calculous disease.
PRIVATE: 4 The Cairns, Belfast, Antrim BT4 2JQ.
Tel: 01232 654866 Fax: 01232 655857

Berkshire

Mr Ravi Kulkarni MS FRCS
YEAR QUALIFIED: 1976
NHS POST: Consultant Urological Surgeon, Ashford Hospital.
SPECIAL INTEREST: Radical prostectomy; stone disease; female incontinence; andrology; BPH; ureteric disease.
PRIVATE: The Princess Margaret Hospital, Osborne Road, Windsor, Berkshire SL4 3SJ.
Tel: 01784 884 059 Fax: 01784 884 393

Buckinghamshire

Mr Manoah Pancharatnam MBBS FRCS
YEAR QUALIFIED: 1974
NHS POST: Consultant Urologist St Albans & Hemel Hempstead Trust Hospitals
SPECIAL INTEREST: Reconstructive surgery; hypospadias repair; prostatic disease; andrology and sup bladder carcinoma.
PRIVATE: The Chiltern Hospital, London Road, Great Missenden, Buckinghamshire HP16 0EN.
Tel: 01494 890 890 Fax: 01494 890 250

Mr Jonathan Ramsay MS FRCS FRCS Urol
YEAR QUALIFIED: 1977
NHS POST: Consultant Urologist and Director of Lithotripsy Unit Charing Cross and Chelsea Westminster Hospitals
SPECIAL INTEREST: Male infertility including vasectomy reversal and storage of sperm for IVF/ICSI. Treatment of stones including all forms of lithotripsy.
PRIVATE: The Thames Valley Nuffield Hospital, Wexham Street, Slough, Buckinghamshire SL3 6NH. Tel: 0181 846 7669/1146 Fax: 0181 846 7696

Enfield Middlesex

Miss Jean McDonald MBBS FRCS(Ed) DipUrol(Lon)
- YEAR QUALIFIED: 1973
- NHS POST: Consultant Urologist North Middlesex Hospital
- SPECIAL INTEREST: Benign prostate disease, stones, infertility, impotence.
- PRIVATE: Kings Oak Hospital, Chase Farm (North side), The Ridgeway, Enfield, Middlesex EN2 8SD. Tel: 0181 370 9505 (appts) Fax: 0181 370 9501 Email: JMcdon2395@aol.com

Essex

Mr Henry Lewi FRCS
- YEAR QUALIFIED: 1974
- NHS POST: Consultant Urological Surgeon, Broomfield Hospital.
- SPECIAL INTEREST: Andrology and penile reconstructive surgery.
- PRIVATE: Springfield Hospital, Lawn Lane, Springfield, Chelmsford, Essex CM1 7GU. Tel: 01245 461 777 xt 341 Fax: 0245 462 151 Tel/Fax

Mr Jaspal Virdi MCh MS FRCS FRCS(Urol) FEBU
- NHS POST: Consultant Urological Surgeon Princess Alexandra Hospital NHS Trust
- SPECIAL INTEREST: Prostatic hyperplasia - laser; minimally invasive technique; urinary incontinence. stone disease; andrology.
- PRIVATE: Holly House Hospital, High Road, Buckhurst Hill, Essex, IG9 5HX. Tel: 0181 505 3311

Gwent

Mr Winsor Bowsher MA MChir FRCS FRCS(Ucol) FEBU
- YEAR QUALIFIED: 1981
- NHS POST: Consultant Urological Surgeon, Royal Gwent Hospital, Wales.
- SPECIAL INTEREST: Lead clinician, Department of Urology, for urological cancer services. Special interests in prostate cancer, laser surgery and laparoscopy.
- PRIVATE: St. Joseph's Private Hospital, Harding Avenue, Malpas, Newport, South Wales NP9 6ZE. Tel: 01633 820300 Fax: 01633 858164

Hertfordshire

Mr John Charles Crisp MBBS FRCS
- YEAR QUALIFIED: 1966
- NHS POST: Consultant Urologist Mount Vernon & Watford General Hospital Trust
- SPECIAL INTEREST: Benign and malignant prostatic disease.
- PRIVATE: BUPA Hospital Bushey, Heathbourne Rd, Bushey, Watford, Hertfordshire WD2 1RD. Tel: 0181 901 5555 Fax: 0181 421 8514 Phone/Fax: 01923 225514.
  E-mail: crispyjc@aol.com

Urology. Hertfordshire

Mr Manoah Pancharatnam MBBS FRCS
- YEAR QUALIFIED: 1974
- NHS POST: Consultant Urologist St Albans & Hemel Hempstead Trust Hospitals
- SPECIAL INTEREST: Reconstructive surgery; hypospadias repair; prostatic disease; andrology and sup bladder carcinoma.
- PRIVATE: BUPA Hospital Harpenden, Ambrose Lane, Harpenden, Herts, AL5 4BP. Tel: 01582 763 191/0800 585 112 - free phone
Hemel Hempstead General Hospital Hillfield Road, Hemel Hempstead, Herts, HP2 4AD. Tel: 01442 213 141 xt 2713

Mr Jaspal Virdi MCh MS FRCS FRCS(Urol) FEBU
- NHS POST: Consultant Urological Surgeon Princess Alexandra Hospital NHS Trust
- SPECIAL INTEREST: Prostatic hyperplasia - laser; minimally invasive technique; urinary incontinence. stone disease; andrology.
- PRIVATE: Thomas Rivers Medical Centre, High Wych Road, Sawbridgeworth, Hertfordshire CM21 0HH. Tel: 01279 600282 ext 2237 Fax: 01279 600212

Kent

Mr James L Lewis MS MRCP(UK) FRCS (Eng)
- NHS POST: Consultant Urologist & General Surgeon, Kent & Sussex Hospital.
- SPECIAL INTEREST: General urology; prostate and bladder cancer; minimal access surgery.
- PRIVATE: BUPA Hospital Tunbridge Wells, Fordcombe Road, Fordcombe, Tunbridge Wells, Kent TN3 0RD. Tel: 01892 740037 Fax: 01892 740037

London

Mr David Badenoch DM MCh FEBU FRCS (Urol)
- NHS POST: Consultant Urologist, St. Bartholomew's Hospital, London and Royal London Hospital.
- SPECIAL INTEREST: Stone disease; prostatic disease; male fertility and potency.
- PRIVATE: 123 Harley Street, London W1N 1HE. Tel: 0171 935 3881 Fax: 0171 224 6481

Mr Simon Carter MBBS FRCS
- YEAR QUALIFIED: 1976
- NHS POST: Consultant Urologist, Charing Cross Hospital.
- SPECIAL INTEREST: Minimally invasive urology; benign prostatic disease.
- PRIVATE: 147 Harley Street, London, W1N 1DL. Tel: 0171 487 4426 Fax: 0171 935 5608 E-mail:100753.21@compuserve.com
The London Clinic, 20 Devonshire Place, London, W1N 2DH. Tel: 0171 935 4444 Fax: 0171 935 5608

Mr Francis Chinegwundoh MS FRCS(Urol) FRCSEd FEBU
- YEAR QUALIFIED: 1984
- NHS POST: Consultant Urologist, The Royal Hospitals NHS Trust and Newham Healthcare Trust.
- SPECIAL INTEREST: Urological oncology, especially prostate cancer; sexual dysfunction; incontinence.
- PRIVATE: 144 Harley Street, London, W1N 1AH. Tel: 0171 935 0023 Fax: 0171 935 5792 / 0181 926 9618

Urology. London

Mr Patrick G Duffy MB BCh BAO FRCS(I)
- YEAR QUALIFIED: 1973
- NHS POST: Consultant Paediatric Urologist, Great Ormond Street Hospital for Children NHS Trust.
- SPECIAL INTEREST: Paediatric urology; reconstruction urinary tract; undescended testicles; hypospadias.
- PRIVATE: Private Consulting Rooms, 234 Great Portland Street, London W1N 5PH.
  Tel: 0171 390 8322 Fax: 0171 390 8324

Mr William Hendry MD ChM FRCS
- YEAR QUALIFIED: 1961
- NHS POST: Consultant Urologist, St. Bartholomew's and Royal Marsden Hospitals
- SPECIAL INTEREST: Cancer and infertility.
- PRIVATE: The London Clinic, 149 Harley Street, London, W1N 2DE.
  Tel: 0171 636 7426 Fax: 0171 935 5765

Mr Roger S Kirby MA MD FRCS(Urol) FEBU
- YEAR QUALIFIED: 1975
- NHS POST: Consultant Urologist, St. George's Hospital, London SW17.
- SPECIAL INTEREST: Prostate cancer/prostate disease; male erectile dysfunction; urethral strictures.
- PRIVATE: 149 Harley Street, London W1N 2DE.
  Tel: 0171 935 9720. 0171 487 3738 Fax: 0171 224 5706
  E-mail:rogerkirby@compuserve.com

Mr Ravi Kulkarni MS FRCS
- YEAR QUALIFIED: 1976
- NHS POST: Consultant Urological Surgeon, Ashford Hospital.
- SPECIAL INTEREST: Radical prostatectomy; stone disease; female incontinence; andrology; BPH; ureteric disease.
- PRIVATE: London Medical Centre, 144 Harley Street, London, W1N 1AH.
  Tel: 0171 935 0023 Fax: 0171 935 5972

Miss Jean McDonald MBBS FRCS(Ed) DipUrol(Lon)
- YEAR QUALIFIED: 1973
- NHS POST: Consultant Urologist North Middlesex Hospital
- SPECIAL INTEREST: Benign prostate disease, stones, infertility, impotence.
- PRIVATE: North Middlesex Hospital, Sterling Way, Edmonton, London, N18 1QX.
  Tel: 0181 887 2431 Fax: 0181 887 4661 Email: JMcdon2395@aol.com
  Cromwell Hospital, Cromwell Road, London SW5 OTU.
  Tel: 0171 460 5700 (appts) Fax: 0171 460 5555 Email: JMcdon2395@aol.com

Mr A David Mee MB ChB FRCS
- YEAR QUALIFIED: 1964
- NHS POST: Consultant Urologist, Northwick Park & St Mark's NHS Trust.
- SPECIAL INTEREST: General urology; oncology; incontinence.
- PRIVATE: Clementine Churchill Hospital, Sudbury Hill, Harrow, Middlesex, HA1 3RX.
  Tel: 0181 872 3872, 01895 232 275 Fax: 01895 810 120
  Northwick Park Hospital, Watford Road, Harrow, Middlesex, HA1 3UJ.
  Tel: 0181 869 2616 Fax: 0181 869 2577

Urology. London

Mr Ronald A Miller MB BS MS FRCS FRGS
YEAR QUALIFIED: 1974
NHS POST: Consultant Urologist, Whittington Hospital and Honorary Senior Lecturer, Institute Urology, Middlesex Hospital.
SPECIAL INTEREST: Minimally invasive surgery; prostate disease; stones; urological cancer.
PRIVATE: The Garden Hospital, 46-50 Sunny Gardens Road, Hendon, London, NW4 1RX.
Tel: 0181 341 3422 Fax: 0181 340 1376
Hospital of St. John & St. Elizabeth, 60 Grove End Road, St Johns Wood, London, NW8 9NH. Tel: 0181 341 3422 Fax: 0181 340 1376
Highgate Private Hospital, 17 View Road, Highgate, London N6 4DJ.
Tel: 0181 341 3422 Fax: 0181 340 1376
Hospital of St. John & St. Elizabeth, 60 Grove End Road, St Johns Wood, London, NW8 9NH. Tel: 0181 341 3422 Fax: 0181 340 1376
Wellington Hospital South, Wellington Place, London NW8 9LE.
Tel: 0181 341 3422 Fax: 0181 340 1376

Mr Robert J Morgan MA BM BCh(Oxon) FRCS(Eng)
NHS POST: Consultant Urological Surgeon, Royal Free Hospital Trust.
SPECIAL INTEREST: Prostatic and bladder surgery; urinary stone disease; paediatric urology; endoscopic surgery.
PRIVATE: 147 Harley Street, London W1N 1DL.
Tel: 0171 486 3345 Fax: 0171 486 3782

Mrs Helen Parkhouse FRCS FRCS(Urol) FEBU
YEAR QUALIFIED: 1978
NHS POST: Honorary Consultant Urologist, King Edward VII Hospital, Midhurst.
SPECIAL INTEREST: Female, Paediatric & Reconstructive Urology
PRIVATE: 149 Harley Street, London W1N 2DE.
Tel: 0171 935 8391 Fax: 0171 486 3782 E-mail: h.parkhouse@thelondonclinic.co.uk

Mr Jonathan Ramsay MS FRCS FRCS Urol
YEAR QUALIFIED: 1977
NHS POST: Consultant Urologist and Director of Lithotripsy Unit Charing Cross and Chelsea Westminster Hospitals
SPECIAL INTEREST: Male infertility including vasectomy reversal and storage of sperm for IVF/ICSI. Treatment of stones including all forms of lithotripsy.
PRIVATE: The London Clinic, 149 Harley Street, London, W1N 2DE.
Tel: 0181 846 7669/1146 Fax: 0181 846 7696
15th Floor, Charing Cross Hospital, Fulham Palace Road, London, W6 8RF.
Tel: 0181 846 7669/1146 Fax: 0181 846 7696
Cromwell Hospital, Cromwell Road, London SW5 OTU.
Tel: 0171 370 4233

Mr Justin Vale MS FRCSurol
- NHS POST: Consultant Urological Surgeon St. Mary's Hospital Paddington W2
- SPECIAL INTEREST: Urological cancer; prostate disease; impotence.
- PRIVATE: Hospital of St. John & St. Elizabeth, 60 Grove End Road, St Johns Wood, London, NW8 9NH. Tel: 0171 286 3040 Fax: 0171 286 6961
  The Lindo Wing, St. Mary's Hospital, South Wharf Road, Paddington, London W2 1NY. Tel: 0171 286 3040 Fax: 0171 286 6961

Mr Hugh Whitfield MA MCHIR FRCS
- YEAR QUALIFIED: 1968
- NHS POST: Consultant Urologist, Institute of Urology & Nephrology, and Central Middlesex Hospital
- SPECIAL INTEREST: Stone disease, minimally invasive alternatives to TURP.
- PRIVATE: 43 Wimpole Street, London W1M 7AF. Tel: 0171 935 3095 Fax: 0171 935 3147
  Stone Clinic, Institute of Urology and Nephrology, 48 Riding House Street, London W1P 7PN. Tel: 0171 380 9179 Fax: 0171 637 7076

Mr Christopher R J Woodhouse MB FRCS FEBU
- YEAR QUALIFIED: 1970
- NHS POST: Reader in Urology, Middlesex Hospital. Consultant Urologist, Royal Marsden Hospital.
- SPECIAL INTEREST: Urological cancer and reconstruction; adolescent urology.
- PRIVATE: The Lister Hospital, Chelsea Bridge Road, London, SW1W 8RH. Tel: 0171 730 6204 Fax: 0171 730 6204
  The Royal Marsden Hospital, Fulham Road, London, SW3 6JJ. Tel: 0171 352 8171 xt 2789 Fax: 0171 376 5425
  Royal Free & UCL Medical School The Middlesex Hospital, Mortimer Street, London, W1N 8AA. Tel: 0171 380 9210 Fax: 0171 637 7076

Middlesex

Mr Brian W Ellis MB FRCS
- YEAR QUALIFIED: 1970
- NHS POST: Consultant Urologist, Ashford & St. Peter's Hospitals NHS Trust.
- SPECIAL INTEREST: Bladder and prostate.
- PRIVATE: The Shakespeare Suite, Ashford Hospital, London Road, Ashford, TW15 3AA. Tel: 01932 873 254 Fax: 01932 873 254 E-mail: brian.ellis@dial.pipex.com

Norfolk

Mr Gokarakonda Suresh MBBS
- YEAR QUALIFIED: 1979
- NHS POST: Consultant Urologist, James Paget Hospital, Gt. Yarmouth.
- SPECIAL INTEREST: Urological cancer and female urinary incontinence.
- PRIVATE: Coastal Clinic, 4 Park Road, Gorleston, Great Yarmouth, Norfolk Tel: 01493 601770
  BUPA Hospital Norwich, Old Watton Road, Colney, Norwhich, Norfolk NR4 7TD. Tel: 01603 456181 Fax: 01603 250968

North Wales

Miss Christine Mary Evans MD FRCS FRCSEd
- YEAR QUALIFIED: 1966
- NHS POST: Consultant Urologist, Glan Clwyd Hospital.
- SPECIAL INTEREST: Erectile Dysfunction and penile deformity / implants; male to female gender reassignment; bladder reconstruction and surgery for stress incontinence.
- PRIVATE: Glan Clwyd Hospital, Bodelwydden, Rhyl, North Wales LL18 5WJ.
  Tel: 01745 534091 Fax: 01745 583910

Surrey

Mr Michael J Bailey MBBS MS FRCS
- NHS POST: Consultant Urologist, St. George's Hospital Tooting and Epsom General Hospital.
- SPECIAL INTEREST: Uro-oncology and prostatic diseases including treatment with new technology (lasers; thermotherapy).
- PRIVATE: Ashtead Hospital, The Warren, Ashtead, Surrey KT21 2SB.
  Tel: 01372 275161 Fax: 01372 277494

Mr John Davies BSc MB BS FRCS(Urol)
- YEAR QUALIFIED: 1979
- NHS POST: Consultant Urological Surgeon, Royal Surrey County Hospital, Egerton Road, Guildford GU2 5XX. Tel: 01483 563122 ext 4878; Fax: 01483 454871.
- SPECIAL INTEREST: Urological Oncology. Prostatic disease Uro-andrology and bladder dysfunction.
- PRIVATE: Guildford Nuffield Hospital, Stirling Road, Guildford, Surrey GU2 6RF.
  Tel: 01483 567517 Fax: 01483 455488
  Woking Nuffield Hospital, Shores Road, Woking, Surrey, GU21 4BY.
  Tel: 01483 567517 Fax: 01483 455488
  Private Consulting Rooms, Mount Alvernia Hospital, Harvey Road, Guildford, Surrey GU1 3LX. Tel: 01483 567517 Fax: 01483 455488

Mr Brian W Ellis MB FRCS
- YEAR QUALIFIED: 1970
- NHS POST: Consultant Urologist, Ashford & St. Peter's Hospitals NHS Trust.
- SPECIAL INTEREST: Bladder and prostate.
- PRIVATE: Runnymede Hospital, Guildford Road, Ottershaw, Surrey, KT16 0RQ.
  Tel: 01932 873254 Fax: 01932 873254 E-mail: brian.ellis@dial.pipex.com

West Sussex

Mr John Davies BSc MB BS FRCS(Urol)
- YEAR QUALIFIED: 1979
- NHS POST: Consultant Urological Surgeon, Royal Surrey County Hospital, Egerton Road, Guildford GU2 5XX. Tel: 01483 563122 ext 4878; Fax: 01483 454871.
- SPECIAL INTEREST: Urological Oncology. Prostatic disease Uro-andrology and bladder dysfunction.
- PRIVATE: King Edward VII Hospital, Midhurst, West Sussex, GU29 0BL.
  Tel: 01483 567517 Fax: 01483 455488

West Yorkshire

Mr Michael Flannigan MB ChB ChM FRCS
- YEAR QUALIFIED: 1975
- NHS POST: Consultant Urologist, Bradford Royal Infirmary.
- SPECIAL INTEREST: General urology and paediatric urology.
- PRIVATE: The Yorkshire Clinic, Bradford Road, Bingley, West Yorkshire BD16 1TW. Tel: 01274 511973

Mr Karol Marian Rogawski FRCS FCS(SA)
- YEAR QUALIFIED: 1980
- NHS POST: Consultant Urologist, Royal Halifax Infirmary.
- PRIVATE: BUPA Hospital Elland, Elland Lane, Elland, Halifax, West Yorkshire HX5 9EB. Tel: 01422 324000 Fax: 01422 377501

Wrexham

Mr Alan Robert De Bolla MD FRCSEd FRCSEng FEBU
- YEAR QUALIFIED: 1975
- NHS POST: Consultant Urologist, Wrexham Maelor Hospital.
- SPECIAL INTEREST: URO oncology, incontinence andrology.
- PRIVATE: The Gables, Ruthin Road, Minera, Wrexham LL11 3UT. Tel: 01978 291306 Fax: 01978 291397

Consultant Index

A

Abdalla, Mr Hossam 89
Abraham, Dr Ralph 38,49,65
Abramovich, Mr Solomon 28,33
Abrams, Mr David 104
Acheson, Mr James 104
Ackroyd, Mr Christopher E 115
Adams, Dr Alistair 110
Adams, Dr Bernard 153
Adiseshiah, Mr Mohan 232
Adlam, Mr David Maxwell 211
Afshar, Mr Farhad 206
Albert, Mr David M 28
Al-Haddad, Mr Hassan B 120
Ali, Mr S 34,69
Allan, Dr Laurie 144
Allard, Dr Simon 171
Allen, Mr Paul R 118
Allen-Mersh, Professor Timothy G 185
Allum, Mr William 179,189,209
Almeyda, Dr John James Ryan 17,19
Amies, Dr Peter 160
Anderson, Ms Lena 220
Ang, Miss Swee 120
Annan, Mr Henry 85
Ardeman, Dr Simon 59
Ashraf, Dr Waseem 42
Ashton, Dr Richard Eric 18
Attwood, Mr Anthony I 215,216,219,221
Auchincloss, Dr Jeremy M 131
August, Dr Paul J 17,22
Austin, Mr Michael William 114
Awwad, Mr Awad M 221
Axon, Professor Anthony 47
Aylward, Mr G William 104

B

Badenoch, Mr David 245
Badrawy, Dr Galal A 148,153
Bailey, Mr C Martin 28,135
Bailey, Mr Michael J 249
Baird, Mr Peter 120
Baker, Dr Anthony 160
Baker, Dr Harvey 19
Baker, Dr Laurence R I 49,72,168
Baker, Mr Daryll 236

Balen, Mr Adam H 88
Barkley, Dr Alastair 19
Barnes, Dr Colin G 172
Barr, Mr Lester 178,200
Barrie, Dr Margaret 74,75
Barton, Dr Simon 55
Bataille, Dr Veronique 20
Bates, Mr Grant James 34
Battersby, Mr Robert D E 207
Baynes, Dr Christopher 40
Bean, Dr Brenda E 87
Beaney, Dr Ronald 96
Beare, Dr John D L 105,113
Behr, Dr Harold 153
Bentovim, Dr Arnon 153
Berry, Dr Hedley 172,174
Berth-Jones, Dr John 19,23
Bevan, Mr Kemal 35,36
Bicknell, Mr Philip G 24
Bingham, Dr John B 166
Bird, Dr Julian 152
Bishop, Mr Christopher 197,232,236
Bishop, Mr Colin 221
Black, Dr Martin M 20
Blackie, Dr Stuart 69,147
Blake, Dr Peter 96
Blenkinsopp, Mr Peter T 212
Booker, Mr Michael 94
Bose-Haider, Dr Bratati 137
Boston, Mr Derek A 117
Bowdler, Mr David Anthony 26,28
Bowen, Mr David Ivor 112
Bowerman, Mr John 212,213
Bowsher, Mr Winsor 208,244
Boyde, Professor Tom Robin Caine 147,238
Bradford, Mr Robert 206
Brecker, Dr Stephen J D 12,15
Brewer, Dr Colin 150,153
Bridges, Dr Paul 153
Bridle, Mr Simon 120,127
Brook, Professor Charles G D 38,138
Brostoff, Professor Jonathan 4
Browett, Mr John Peter 120
Brown, Dr Edwina A 72
Brown, Mr Peter M 24
Bryan, Dr Elizabeth 138
Buchanan, Dr Charles R 138
Bucknall, Dr Cliff 11,12

Consultant Index

Bucknall, Mr Timothy Eric 179
Bulgen, Dr Dianne 170
Bullock, Mr Peter 206
Bunker, Dr Christopher 20
Burke, Dr Michael J 171
Burnand, Professor Kevin Guiver 197,232,236
Burroughs, Dr Andrew K 43

C

Campbell, Dr Alastair 137
Campbell, Dr Lachlan 154
Cannon, Dr Paul 166
Cannon, Mr Stephen R 118,120,126
Cantopher, Dr Tim G A 161
Carlstedt, Mr Thomas P 131
Carnwath, Dr Thomas 149
Carruthers, Dr Malcolm 6
Carter, Mr Simon 245
Carver, Mr Nigel 218,221
Catte, Mr Anthony 121
Catterall, Mr Anthony 121
Chakravarty, Dr Kuntal 170
Chambers, Dr John 11,12
Chapman, Mr Patrick 35
Chapman, Mrs Roxana 89
Charlesworth, Professor David 234
Chesterton, Mr James 105
Chevretton, Miss Elfy B 28
Chinegwundoh, Mr Francis 245
Choa, Mr Dennis I 25,29
Chowdhury, Mr Chitta Ranjan 25
Christie-Brown, Dr Jeremy 154
Christie-Brown, Dr Margaret 162
Chung, Professor K Fan 241
Ciclitira, Professor Paul J 43,49
Claoué, Mr Charles 101,105
Clarke, Mr John 221
Clearkin, Mr Louis 111
Clein, Dr Lewis J 154
Clements, Dr Michael R .37,40,48,53,65,66,70,71
Coakes, Mr Roger 105,113
Coakham, Professor Hugh 205
Cobb, Dr Carol Anne 42
Cobb, Mr Justin 121
Coburn, Dr Peter R 23
Cochrane, Mr Geoffrey W 86
Cohen, Dr Simon L 50
Cohen, Mr Brian 121,132

Collier, Mr David St. John 194
Collis, Dr Christopher H 96
Condon, Mr Richard W 113
Coombs, Mr Richard R H 121
Coote, Dr Nadia 144
Corner, Mr Nigel Bruce 234
Cory, Mr Charles 113
Costa, Dr Durval 82
Cowan, Mr Dickinson B 89
Cox, Mr Simon J 176
Cripps, Dr Timothy 9
Crisp, Dr Thomas 239
Crisp, Mr John Charles 244
Crock, Mr Henry V 134
Croft, Dr Desmond N 38,50
Croft, Mr Charles B 29
Croker, Dr John 43,57
Crosby, Dr Colin Peter 239
Cross, Mr Frank W 197,236
Crouchman, Dr Marion 76,138
Crumplin, Mr Michael K H 190
Curran, Mr Frank 190
Curry, Dr Paul V L 11,12

D

Dalton, Miss Maureen 95
Danford, Mr Martin 212,213
Daniel, Dr Susan 239
Daniel, Mr Reginald 102,105
Daniel, Mr Rhodri D 101,106
Dann, Dr Thomas Charles 54
Darby, Dr David 106
Dart, Mr John K G 106
Darzi, Professor A 185,188,197,201
Davey, Miss Clare 106
Davidson, Dr Robert N 63
Davidson, Mr Tim 177,197
Davies, Dr David Denison 144
Davies, Dr Wyn 12
Davies, Mr Dai 221
Davies, Mr John 249
Davies, Mr William Tudor 233
Davies, Professor John Elfed 172,240
Davis, Mr Peter 222,225
Daya, Mr Sheraz M 106,114
Daymond, Professor Terence John 175
de Belder, Dr Mark Andrew 15,16
De Bolla, Mr Alan Robert 250

Consultant Index

de Zulueta, Dr Felicity I S 158,163
Deanfield, Professor John 13,138
Deeble, Dr Terence John 60
Deery, Dr Alastair..209
Deighton, Dr Chris 174
Deutsch, Dr George P..96
Dilke, Dr Timothy F W 172
Dodd, Mr Christopher 110
Donaldson, Mr Richard 243
Dorrell, Mr David 101
Drake, Mr David Paul.......................................135
Drew, Mr Nicholas C..87
Duffy, Mr Patrick G 135,246
Duffy, Mr Terence J 179,202
Dymond, Dr Duncan S.......................................13

E

East, Mr Charles A 29
Eben, Ms Friedericke 89
Edgar, Mr M A 134
Edwards, Dr Christopher 147
Elliot, Mr David 218
Elliott, Mr Martin 135,180
Ellis, Mr Brian W 248,249
Elrington, Dr Giles 74,76
Elton, Sir Arnold 177,209
Emens, Mr J Michael 83
Emery, Mr Roger J H 121
Empey, Dr Duncan 241
Espir, Dr Michael..76
Evans, Dr John..242
Evans, Miss Christine Mary 6,7,249
Evans, Mr Barrie (Thomas) 211
Evans, Mr D Andrew 185
Evans, Mr David M.....................................131,215
Evans, Mr James 211,212
Evans, Mr Michael John 122
Evans, Professor Timothy W 241
Ewins, Dr David..37

F

Fabri, Mr Brian M...181
Fagan, Mr John 214
Fahy, Mr Gerald T 104
Fairbank, Mr Adrian C................................122,127
Falcon, Mr Michael 106
Falkowski, Dr Jan..154
Fallon, Mr Timothy 107

Farewell, Dr Joan 162
Farmer, Dr Simon Francis 76
Farthing, Mr Alan 90
Fawcett, Mr Ivan 102,103
Fearn, Mr Barry...116
Featherstone, Dr Terence 165
Fell, Dr Richard 143
Fenton, Dr David A...20
Ferguson, Mrs Veronica M G 107
Ficker, Miss Linda Anne 107
Field, Mr Ellis S...198
Field, Mr Richard..127
Finch, Dr Peter 46
Findley, Professor Leslie 75
Fisher, Mr ffolliott Francis 99
Fisk, Professor Nicholas 90
Flanagan, Mr Jamie...117
Flannigan, Mr Michael 250
Flower, Dr Paul 154
Foale, Dr Rodney A 9,13
Fogarty, Dr Paul..85
Foley, Mr Roberts J E 193
Ford, Dr Michael 150
Fordyce, Mr Michael...118
Forster, Mr David M C 207
Foster, Mr George 183,193
Fowler, Dr P Bruce S 50
Fozard, Dr John...145
Frame, Mr James D 218,219,222
Frank, Dr Stephen 154
Franklin, Dr Alan 137
Franklin, Dr Rodney 141
Fraser, Dr Alan A 151
Fraser, Mr Ian 29,35
Fry, Dr Anthony H 155
Furniss, Dr Stephen 16

G

Gallannaugh, Mr Charles 116
Gannon, Mr Mark Xavier 233,237
Gardner, Mr Brian 229
Garfield Davies, Mr David..................................29
Garvie, Dr Neil Wardlaw..................................166
Gauci, Dr Charles A 143,144
Gawler, Dr Jeffrey 76
George, Dr Philip Jeremy M 241
Gibb, Dr William 75
Gillard, Mr Malcolm G 90

Consultant Index

Gilmore, Mr Jerry 177,198
Glazer, Mr Geoffrey 198
Gledhill, Dr Maureen 163
Gleeson, Dr Catherine 53,54
Gleeson, Professor Michael 29
Glynn, Dr Christopher J 145
Glynn, Dr Michael J 44
Glynne-Jones, Dr Robert 98
Godfrey, Mr Alan 216,219,225,227
Golding, Dr Douglas 170
Golding-Wood, Mr David 27
Goldstraw, Mr Peter 230
Goodwin, Dr Stewart 50,63
Gopalji, Mr Bipin 118
Gordon, Mr Yehudi 90
Goswamy, Mr Rajat K 83,88,90
Graham, Dr Robert 22
Graham, Mr Philip Y 222
Grahame, Professor Rodney 172
Grant, Mr Henry R 30
Gravett, Dr Peter J 59
Green, Dr Malcolm 169
Greenberg, Dr Maurice 155,163
Greenhalgh, Professor Roger M 236
Gregor, Mr Zdenek J 107
Gregory, Dr Ralph Peter 74,79
Griffiths, Mr Carl Lindsay 201
Guest, Mr Phillip G 210,216
Guiloff, Dr Roberto J 76

H
Hackett, Dr David 10
Hacking, Dr Nigel 165
Hakin, Mr Kim Neal 112
Hall, Dr Michael J 43
Hall, Mr Anthony John 122
Hallan, Mr Rodney 184,195
Hanham, Dr Iain W F 97
Hanley, Mr David J 217
Hann, Dr Ian 60,97,139
Hariri, Dr Mohamed 8,30
Harrington, Dr Christine I 22,69
Harris, Dr David 20
Harris, Mr Peter Lyon 237
Harris, Mr Thomas Martin 30
Hart, Dr Jerome 152,155,159
Hart, Mr Nicholas 217
Hashmi, Mr Manzoor S 102

Hatton, Miss Marion 90
Hawk, Professor John L M 17
Hawkins, Dr David A 56
Hawley, Mr Peter R 186
Hay, Mr David John 183
Heath, Dr Peter Desmond 81
Heckmatt, Dr John Zia 137
Hems, Mr Timothy E J 131
Hendry, Mr William 246
Henry, Mr Richard 85
Herbert, Mr David Charles 217,222,224
Hershman, Mr Michael 185,196,208,232
Herst, Dr Edward Richard 163
Higton, Mr Ian 195
Hill, Mr John 33
Hill, Mr Robert A 122
Hine, Dr Keith R 54
Hingorani, Dr Kishin 175
Hirons, Dr Ruth Margaret 162
Hislop, Dr William Stuart 42
Hobbiss, Mr John Holland 185
Hodges, Dr Neville 53
Hoffbrand, Dr Barry I 50
Hoffbrand, Professor A Victor 60
Hoile, Mr Ronald 195
Hollingworth, Mr Antony 86
Holloway, Mr Graham M N 240
Holmes, Mr Keith 136
Hope, Mr Terence 207
Hosking, Dr Gwilym 77,139
Houlton, Dr Peter 145
Howard, Dr Robin 77
Howells, Dr Roger B 155
Hubbard, Dr William N 9
Hughes, Dr Louis 6
Hughes, Dr Rodney 175
Hughes, Professor Sean 122
Hull, Professor Michael G R 83
Hutchinson, Mr Roderic 189,202
Hykin, Mr Philip G 107

I
Ibrahim, Mr Zaky H Z 95
Iffland, Miss Claire 87
Igboaka, Dr Gilbert 147
Ikkos, Dr George 68,155
Innes, Mr Anthony J 33
Irvine, Dr Allan 166

Consultant Index

J

Jackson, Dr Rodwin 37,38,48,50,57
Jackson, Mr Andrew 123
Jackson, Mr David B 176,184,196,208,231
Jacobs, Professor Howard S 38
Jagger, Mr Jonathan 107
James, Dr Martin 17
James, Mr David R 213
Jameson Evans, Mr David 116
Jenkins, Mr Howard 84
Jepson, Mr Keith 69,129
Jewitt, Dr David E 13
John, Mr Anthony C 30,35
Johns, Mr Andrew N 27
Johnson, Mr Jonathan R 123
Johnson, Professor Gordon J 112
Johnston, Dr Colin 37,48
Johnston, Mr David 24,26
Jones, Dr Lydia 61
Jones, Mr Jonathan R 115
Jones, Mr Nicholas P 100
Jones, Mr Philip Hodgson 24

K

Kamlana, Dr Sikandar Hayat 149,162
Katz, Dr Maurice 38,91
Kaufmann, Dr Peter 77
Kaye, Mr Jeremy 130
Keet, Dr John P D 51,57,58
Keir, Dr Peter 10
Kellett, Dr John 238
Khan, Mr Jamsheed 30
Khan, Mr Omar 196
Khan, Mr Saifuddin 222
Kiely, Mr Edward M 136
King, Mr Richard 117,123
Kingswood, Dr John C 48,62,72
Kinnear, Mr Paul 108
Kirby, Mr Roger S 246
Kirkham, Mr John Squire 186
Knight, Dr Ronald K 54
Knight, Mr Jeffrey R 35
Knight, Mr Michael James 198
Knowles, Dr Geoffrey K 51,54,241,242
Kobza Black, Dr Anne 20
Konotey-Ahulu, Dr Felix I D 51,63
Kotecha, Mr Bhik 26,30
Kulkarni, Mr Ravi 243,246

L

Lam, Mr Soli 119,123
Lamb, Mr Martin Piers 89
Lamerton, Mr Andrew 235
Lancer, Mr Jack Michael 34
Lane, Dr Russell J M 74,77,79
Lang-Stevenson, Mr Andrew 117
Lask, Dr Bryan 148,156
Latham, Dr John Bannerman 82,167
Leatherbarrow, Mr Brian 100,110
Ledermann, Dr Eric 163
Lee, Mr Cheng-Lian 86
Lee, Mr Nicholas 100,108,111
Lee, Mr Robin John 33
Lee, Professor Tak 4
Legg, Dr Nigel John 77
Leigh, Professor Irene M 21
Leighton, Mrs Susanna 31
Leonard, Mr Timothy J K 108
Levantine, Dr Ashley V 23
Lewi, Mr Henry 6,244
Lewis, Mr James L 196,245
Lewis, Mr Terence 181
Libby, Dr Gerald 156
Lim, Dr Frederick 56
Lipkin, Dr Bron 156
Lipkin, Dr David P 11,13
Little, Mr James Timothy 34
Littlewood, Dr T J 60
Lloyd, Dr Geoffrey J 39,44
Lloyd, Dr Helen 164
Lock, Mr M Russell 186,198
Lolin, Dr Yvette I 70,147
Lourie, Mr John 116
Lower, Mr Adrian 91
Luck, Mr Jonathan 99
Ludman, Mr Harold 31
Luzzi, Dr Graz 55
Lyall, Dr James 241
Lynn, Mr John 177,191

M

Maberly, Dr Jonathan 4
MacDonald, Dr Lesley 167
MacDonald, Mr David A 130
Mace, Mr Martin 210,213
Mackie, Dr Peter H 59
Mackworth-Young, Dr Charles 172

Page 255

Consultant Index

Maddocks, Dr John Leyshon 53,69
Maddocks, Dr Peter D 148
Mahady, Mr Ian William 88
Mahendran, Dr Bhanu 5
Malone-Lee, Professor James 51,58
Maltz, Dr Milton B 51
Manning, Dr Eileen 70
Manning, Mr E A Dermot 94
Markey, Dr Andrew C 21
Marsh, Dr Frank 51,72
Martin, Dr Vivian M 173
Martin, Mr David L 216,222,225
Martin, Mr Michael 86
Marwood, Mr Roger P 91
Mathew, Dr George 152,156
Matthews, Mr Richard N 226
Matti, Mr Basim A 223
Maurice, Dr Paul 18
Maw, Dr D S Jonathan 49
Maynard, Mr John D 186,198
Mayou, Mr Bryan J 223
McAuliffe, Mr Tom 117
McDonald, Miss Jean 244,246
McDonald, Mr Peter 201
McDonnell, Mr Peter 99
McFarland, Mr Robert 202,233,237
McHugh, Mr Dominic 108
McLeod, Mr Fraser Neil 83
McNeil, Dr Neil Ian 44
Mee, Mr A David 246
Meeran, Dr Karim 39
Mellett, Dr Peter George 156,161
Melville, Mr David 183,186,194
Mendelow, Professor A David 207
Mercer, Mr Nigel S G 215
Migdal, Mr Clive 108
Miller, Mr John 128
Miller, Mr Ronald A 247
Mills, Dr Peter R 43
Mills, Miss Angela M 91
Milton, Miss Catherine 27
Minasian, Mr Harvey 178,186,198
Mintowt-Czyz, Mr Witer 127
Misiewicz, Dr J J 44,46
Mitchell, Dr David 242
Monteiro, Dr Brendan Thomas 149,152,159
Montgomery, Dr Donald H 157,163
Morgan, Mr Robert J 247

Moriarty, Mr Anthony Peter 100
Morrison, Mr Gavin A J 31
Morsman, Mr John M 85
Mortensen, Mr Neil James M 189
Motto, Dr Stephen 240
Mowbray, Mr Michael A S 128
Moyes, Mr Simon 123,240
Mugliston, Mr Terence 31
Muir, Dr John R 13
Munton, Mr Charles G.F. 103
Murphy, Mr Karl 91
Murray T D, Dr Dermot 55
Murray, Mr Alan 234
Murray-Lyon, Dr Iain M 44
Murugananthan, Dr Nagalingam 159

N
Nairne, Mr James 103
Nancekievill, Dr David 5
Nashef, Mr Samer A M 180
Nath, Mr Fred P 205
Negus, Mr David 199
Nethisinghe, Dr Shelton 146
Nevelos, Mr Akos Bela 130
Newman, Dr Claus G H 139,141
Newman, Mr John Howard 115
Nicholls, Professor R John 186
Nield, Mrs Dalia V 223
Niven, Mr Peter Ashley R 84
Nixon, Mr John E 119,123
Noble, Mr Jonathan 125
Noble, Mrs Joan L 111
Nockler, Dr Ingeborg 167
Northover, Mr John 187
Nott, Mr David 199,236
Novelli, Dr Vas 64,139

O
O'Brien, Mr John P 229
O'Callaghan, Dr Abina C 144,145
O'Connell, Dr Morgan Ross 151,157
O'Flynn, Dr Richard 149,150,160
O'Flynn, Mr Paul 31
Oakley, Dr Nigel 39
Odemuyiwa, Dr Olusola 16
Ogus, Mr Hugh 212
Oldham, Dr Roger 171
Ornstein, Mr Markus 199

Consultant Index

Osborne, Mr Jonathan 25
Outhwaite, Dr John Martin 173
Owen, Mr Eoghan R T C 202,203
Owens, Mr Owen 87,91
Oxbury, Dr John Michael 78,79

P
Palmer, Dr Andrew B D 72,73
Panayi, Professor Gabriel 173
Pancharatnam, Mr Manoah 243,245
Pappin, Dr John C 5
Parker, Mr Barrie 128
Parker, Mr Michael 177,184,196
Parkhouse, Mr Nicholas 223,226
Parkhouse, Mrs Helen 247
Parkinson, Mr Richard W 125
Patel, Mr Kalpesh S 26,32
Paterson, Mr J Mark H 124
Patterson, Mr Marc 128,129
Pattison, Mr Charles William 180
Patton, Professor Michael 67
Pearson, Mr Russell 102
Peatfield, Dr Richard 78,79
Percy, Mr Anthony J L 124
Perkin, Dr G D 78
Perks, Mr Nigel 92
Perry, Dr J David 173
Perry, Dr Raphael Adam 11
Persaud, Dr Raj 157
Pfeffer, Dr Jeremy M 157
Pflug, Professor Josef J 233,237
Phillips, Mr David Esmond 36
Phillips, Mr Robin 188
Pickering, Dr David 96
Pitt, Professor Brice 150
Plant, Dr Gordon 78,108
Pokorny, Dr Michael R. 163
Pool, Mr Rowan 128
Porter, Miss Janet 68,239
Potts, Mr Michael 99
Povlsen, Assoc. Professor B 68,132,223
Prentice, Professor H Grant 60
Price, Dr John 124,240
Price, Dr Len 97
Price, Dr Pat 97
Price, Dr Thomas Richard 171,173
Priddy, Mr Alvan 92
Pyper, Mr Richard J D 95

Q
Quiney, Mr Robert E 32
Qureshi, Dr Shakeel Ahmed 139

R
Raimundo, Dr Ana H. 45
Ramsay, Dr Ian 37,39
Ramsay, Mr Jonathan 243,247
Rao, Mr Sudhir 119,124
Ratnesar, Mr Padman 27
Reader, Dr Fran 238
Rees, Dr Richard G 173,174
Reilly, Mr David Tempest 201
Revington, Mr Peter J 210
Richardson, Dr Ricky 140
Rickards, Dr Anthony 14
Rigby, Dr Michael 14,140
Robb, Mr Peter J 36
Roberts, Mr David 32
Robinson, Dr Trevor W E 21
Robinson, Miss Patricia 27
Robinson, Mr David Derek 130
Rogawski, Mr Karol Marian 250
Rogers, Mr John 187
Roomi, Mr Riad 223
Roques, Dr Antoine 61
Rosen, Mr Paul 108,112
Rosenthal, Dr Mark 140,142
Rosin, Mr R David 199
Rostron, Mr Chad K 109,113
Rouholamin, Mr Ebrahim 130
Rowland Payne, Dr Christopher 21
Rowlands, Dr Michael 161
Rudolf, Dr Noel 81
Russell Jones, Dr Robin 21,22
Russell, Mr R Christopher G 187
Rustin, Dr Malcolm 21

S
Sa' adu, Dr Alfa 48,52,57
Sacks, Mr Nigel P M 178,191,200
Sagor, Mr Geoffrey R 195
Saha, Mr Arabinda 89
Sammut, Mr Donald 216,228
Sanders, Professor Roy 215,219,224
Sanderson, Dr Jeremy 45
Sarner, Dr Martin 45
Sathanandan, Mr Satha-M 86

Page 257

Consultant Index

Saunders, Dr Brian Paul 45,46
Savage, Mr Adrian 190
Sayer, Mr Richard 180,182
Schapira, Professor Anthony 78
Schulenburg, Mr Edmund 109
Scott, Mr Gareth 124
Searle, Mr Adam 224
Seed, Dr Mary 65,66
Segal, Professor Anthony W 52
Semple, Professor Stephen J G 52,242
Senapati, Miss Asha 202
Seymour, Professor Carol 71
Shanahan, Mr Donal 187
Shanmugaraju, Mr Palaniappa 7
Sharp, Mr David John 134
Sharr, Mr Michael M 205,206
Shaw, Mr Laurence M A 88
Shawaf, Mr Talha 92
Shephard, Dr Edmund Peter 39,52
Shepherd, Mr John 92
Shinebourne, Dr Elliot 14,140
Sigwart, Dr Ulrich 14
Sillers, Mr B Royston 213
Sillince, Dr Claire 149
Silverman, Dr Maurice 151
Simcock, Mr Peter Reginald 101
Simpson, Mr Hamish 127
Simpson, Mr Michael T 210,211,212
Simson, Mr Jay N L 190
Singer, Professor Albert 92
Singh, Mr Chandra B 26
Sireling, Dr Lester 157
Sirimanna, Dr Kusum S 8,32
Skidmore, Mr David 178,187,209
Skinner, Mr Paul W 119
Slaney, Dr Mark 152
Slater, Mr Neil 119
Slevin, Dr Maurice L 97
Smith, Dr Alastair Gordon 59
Smith, Mr J Richard 92
Smith, Mr Peter 181
Smith, Mr Roger W 220,227
Sommerlad, Mr Brian C 219,224
Soucek, Dr Sava O F 8
South, Mrs Marie 191,196,204,232,235
Soutter, Mr William P 93
Spector, Dr Tim 173
Spence-Jones, Mr Clive 93

Spencer, Mr John D 124
Spittle, Dr Margaret F 97
Springall, Mr Roger G 188
Stanhope, Dr Richard 39,140
Stanworth, Mr Peter A 207
Steele, Mr Stuart 93
Steffen, Dr Hartmut 150
Stephens, Dr John 10,14
Stern, Dr Richard 161
Stewart, Mr Michael Peter M 126
Stoker, Mr David L 184,194
Stoodley, Mr Brian J 176,183,193,231
Strachan, Mr Roger 205
Strickland, Dr Ian 47
Strong, Mr Anthony J 206
Stroobant, Dr John 140
Strover, Mr Angus E 133
Studd, Mr John W W 93
Suresh, Mr Gokarakonda 248
Sutcliffe, Mr John 206
Sutton, Dr Vera E 52,158
Swan, Dr Jonathan 9,15
Swanson, Mr Alexander J G 129
Swanton, Dr Robert Howard 14

T

Tait, Dr Graeme W 10
Tang, Dr Alan 55
Tanner, Mr N S Brent 217,220,225
Tapp, Mr Andrew John S 94
Tattersall, Dr Mark 148
Taylor, Dr Alan 70
Taylor, Dr Christopher M 161
Taylor, Dr Jason 151
Taylor, Mr David S I 109
Taylor, Mr Philip 84
Taylor, Mr Robert 112
Taylor, Professor Irving 178,188,209
Tebbutt, Miss Isabel Helen 86
Teenan, Mr Robert Paul 194,235
Teoh, Mr T G 93
Terry, Mr Roland Mark 28
Thakkar, Dr Chandra 167
Thomas, Professor P K 78
Thompson, Mr Jeremy 200
Thompson, Professor Gilbert 65
Thomson, Dr Allan D 45
Thomson, Dr John 18

Consultant Index

Thorogood, Dr Alan 143
Toms, Dr David Anthony 160
Tonge, Dr Keith 167
Toplis, Mr Philip 95
Towler, Mr Hamish 102,109
Townsend, Mr Calver 109,111
Travis, Dr Simon 42
Treleaven, Dr Jennifer 61
Trend, Dr Patrick 80
Trew, Mr David 103
Trew, Mr Geoffrey 93
Tucker, Dr Sam Michael 141
Tucker, Mr John Keith 126
Tulloh, Dr Robert M R 14,141
Turner, Mr Peter J 133
Turnock, Mr Richard 136

U
Uppal, Mr Rakesh 181
Usherwood, Mr Martin 84

V
Vale, Mr Justin 248
Valentine, Dr Jonathan M J 145
Vallance-Owen, Professor John 39,52
Vanniasegaram, Mr Iynga 8,32,68
Vardi, Mr Glen 133
Varma, Mr Sanjay 220
Vathenen, Dr Arumugam Santi 242
Veale, Dr David 158,159
Vellacott, Mr Keith D 189
Venn, Dr Peter John 5
Venn, Mr Graham 181
Vicary, Dr Robin 46
Vickers, Mr Roger 125
Vickery, Dr Ian Malcolm 210
Vijayasingam-Henderson, Dr Sarah 18
Vijaykumar, Mr Annaswami 104,114
Villar, Mr Richard 116
Virdi, Mr Jaspal 244,245

W
Waldron, Dr Gillian 151,158
Walker, Dr John Malcolm 15
Walker, Dr Peter Elton 141,142,158
Walker, Mr Patrick 94
Wallace, Mr Colin E 33
Walsh, Dr William 148,159

Ward, Mr Christopher 225
Ward, Mr David A 125,129
Warren, Dr Martin John 165,166
Waterhouse, Mr Norman 224
Watson, Mr David M 109
Watson, Professor Anthony 188,200
Watts, Dr Richard W E 40,52,168
Wear, Dr Alan Nicholas 152
Webb-Peploe, Dr Michael Murray 15
Webster, Dr Jonathan 41
Wells, Mr Francis Charles 180
Wellwood, Mr James 176,184,200
Wenger, Mr R Julien J 118
Wharton, Dr Christopher F P 49
Wheeler, Professor Malcolm H 192
White, Dr Anthony 174
Whitelocke, Mr Rodger 110
Whitfield, Mr Hugh 248
Whittaker, Dr Sean 22
Whyte, Dr Robert 164
Wierzbicki, Dr Anthony 65
Wilkins, Mr Denis Charles .. 135,191,193,231,234
Wilkinson, Dr Mark L 46
Williams, Dr Wyn 170
Williams, Mr Hugh 110
Williams, Mr Keith 110
Williams, Mr Robert 114
Williamson, Mr John G 84
Wilson, Mr Nicholas M 195,231,235
Windle-Taylor, Mr Paul C 25
Winson, Mr Ian Geoffrey 115
Wiselka, Dr Martin 63
Witt, Mr Johan 125
Wolfe, Mr John H N 237
Woo, Professor Patricia 174
Wood, Dr David 158
Wood, Mr Peter 119
Woodhouse, Mr Christopher R J 248
Wright, Dr Michael 171,174
Wright, Dr Stephen G 64
Wright, Mr Charles 94
Wu, Dr Frederick C W 40

Y
Yelland, Mr Andrew 176,194,208
Younis, Mr Farouk 188

Buckinhgamshire

Dr Hamish Mason
Weylands
Beaconsfield Road
Farnham Royal
Buckinhgamshire, SL2 3BS
Tel: 01753 644465   Fax: 01753 644465

East Sussex

Dr Lal B Mandal
Telscombe Surgery
365 South Coast Road
Telscombe-Cliffs
East Sussex, BN10 7HA
Tel: 01273 583238   Fax: 01273 580586

Essex

Mr David Gibbins
Sutherland Lodge Surgery
115 Baddon Road
Chelmsford
Essex, CM2 7PY
Tel: 01245 351351   Fax: 01245 494192

Dr Q A Gillet-Waller
140 Station Lane
Hornchurch
Essex, RM12 6LU
Tel: 01708 440780   Fax: 01708 455489

Dr N K Gupta MBBS MS DCH
206 Mawney Road
Romford
Essex, RM7 8BU
Tel: 01708 739 379   Fax: 01708 780457

Mrs J Smith
The Surgery
Kings Road
Halstead
Essex, CO9 1HX
Tel: 01787 475944   Fax: 01787 474506

Hampshire

Dr Natverlal Shah
332 North Avenue
Southend-On-Sea
Hampshire, SS2 4EQ
Tel: 01702 467215   Fax: 01702 603160

Hertfordshire

Dr G M Cooray MBBS FFOM DIH DPH
C Av. Med.
Special Interest: Occupational Health; medical reports; surveys; aviation medicals; diving medicals.
8 Letchmore Road
Radlett, Hertfordshire, WD7 8HT
Tel: 01923 856017 Fax: 01923 856017

Dr Krishna M Mishra
Highfield Surgery
Jupiter Drive
Hemel Hempstead
Hertfordshire, HP1 5NU
Tel: 01442 65322   Fax: 01442 256641

Dr S I A Zaidi
Health Centre
Canterbury Way
Stevenage, Hertfordshire, SG1 4LH
Tel: 01438 357 411   Fax: 01438 720 523

Kent

Dr Toqeer Aslam MB ChB
Special Interest: Visectomy Clinic.
Princess Park Medical Centre
Dove Close
Walderslade, Chatham, Kent, ME5 7TD
Tel: 01634 201272   Fax: 01634 868156

Dr D Diggens
Northdown Surgery
St. Anthony's Way
Margate, Kent, CT9 2TR
Tel: 01843 296413

Kent *continued*

Dr K Jeganmohan
Southlands Surgery
46 Southlands Road
Bromley, Kent, BR2 9QP
Tel: 0181 289 3981   Fax: 0181 289 3245

Dr Anthony Stellon
The Abbey Practice
107 London Road
Temple Ewell, Nr Dover
Kent, CT16 3BY
Tel: 01304 821182   Fax: 01304 827 673

London

Dr Kamaruddin Afghan
104 Wades Hill
Winchmore Hill
London, N21 1AJ
Tel: 0181 360 4003   Fax: 0181 809 2640

Dr Barry Carruthers
55 Wimpole Street
London, W1M

Dr Maxwell Carter
Consulting Room
79 Harley Street
London, W1N 1DE
Tel: 0171 935 7403   Fax: 0181 992 0394

Dr Anil Kumar Chanda
266 Forest Road
London, E17 5JN
Tel: 0181 520 3556   Fax: 0181 520 3556

Dr Dhulipalli Choudary
43/51 Beechwood Road
London, E8 3DY
Tel: 0860 435566   Fax: 0181 809 6071

Dr Ann Cobbe
1 Avenue Crescent
Acton, London, W3 8ES
Tel: 0181 992 1963   Fax: 0181 896 2791

London *continued*

Dr Sean Cummings
Freedom Health
16-17 The Links
Shepherds Bush Centre
London, W12 8PP

Dr Ronald D'Silva
130 Harley Street
London, W1N 1AH
Tel: 0171 580 1736   Fax: 0171 935 2385

Dr Roshan R Dalal MBBS MRCOG
Special Interest: Gynaecology; paediatrics; general practice.
3 Carlton Gardens
London, W5 2AN
Tel: 0181 997 2076   Fax: 0181 989 4362

Dr Sohrab R Dalal MBBS DCH DRCOG MRCGP
Special Interest: Paediatrics; general practice; diploma in occupational medicine & sports medicine.
3 Carlton Gardens
London, W5 2AN
Tel: 0181 997 2076   Fax: 0181 989 4362

Dr Anil V Dalsania
Crest Medical Centre
157 Crest Road
London, NW2 7NA
Tel: 0181 452 5155   Fax: 0181 452 4570

Dr Rimah El-Borai MB BCh LMSSA(Lond) MRCS(Eng) MFFP
32 Eardley Crescent
London, SW5 9JZ
Tel: 0171 373 0140   Fax: 0171 244 6617

Dr Christine Elliot
Sterndale Clinic
74A Sterndale Road
London, W14 0HX
Tel: 0171 610 4560   Fax: 0171 371 3347

Private General Practitioners

London *continued*

Dr B Geffin
270 Chase Side
Southgate
London, N14 4PR
Tel: 0181 440 9301   Fax: 0181 449 9349

Dr Peter Simon Gugenheim
Willow Court Surgery
2 Willow Court
Stonegrove, Edgware
London, HA8 8AG

Ms Jean Hagberg
1st Floor
49 Emperor's Gate
London, SW7 4HJ
Tel: 0181 237 5333

Dr S A Hashmi
226 Mitcham Road
London, SW17 9NN
Tel: 0181 672 7868   Fax: 0181 672 6830

Dr Muhammed Jamil
50 Downton Avenue
London, SW2 3TR
Tel: 0181 671 1194

Dr Julius Kimerling MB MRCP
14 Horton Street
London, W8
Tel: 0171 9379520   Fax: 0171 937 9520

Dr Lionel Kopelowitz
10 Cumberland House
Clifton Gardens
London, W9 1DX
Tel: 0171 289 6375

Dr D K Kundu
The Surgery
18 St. John's Road
Tottenham, London, N15 6QP

London *continued*

Dr Thangarajah Maheswaran
276 Criclewood Lane
London, NW2 2PU
Tel: 0181 452 8822   Fax: 0181 208 0509
60 Cricklewood Broadway
London, NW2 3ET
Tel: 0181 452 9904

Dr Simon Moore MBS DRCOG MRCGP
Special Interest: Paediatrics; Obsterics & gynaecology.
10 Pennant Mews
Kensington
London, W8 5JN
Tel: 0171 460 5980   Fax: 0171 460 5981

Dr Simon Moore MRCGP DRCOG
1 Park Close
Knightsbridge
London, SW1X 7PQ
Tel: 0171 589 2006   Fax: 0171 225 1645

Dr Jonathan Munday MA(Oxon) MB BChir(Cantab) MRCGP
Special Interest: Andrology.
15 Denbigh Street
London, SW1V 2HF
Tel: 0171 834 6969   Fax: 0171 931 7747

Dr Adrian Naftalin MA MB BChir FRCS
79 Grays Inn Road
London, WC1X 8TP
Tel: 0171 405 9360   Fax: 0171 831 1964

Dr M B O Pieris
75 Pellatt Road
East Dulwich
London, SE22 9JG
Tel: 0181 693 5588

Mr Bo Povlsen
Churchill Clinic
80 Lambeth Road
London, SE1 7PW
Tel: 0171 620 1590   Fax: 0171 928 1702

London *continued*

Dr Athar Mushtaq Rana
Esme House Surgery
3 Esme House
1 Ludovick Walk
London, SW15 5LS

Dr Stuart Sanders
22 Harmont House
20 Harley Street
London, W1N 1AL
Tel: 0171 935 5687   Fax: 0171 436 4387

Dr Stuart Saunders MB ChB FRCGP
Special Interest: Private family practice and executive corporate healthcare.
22 Harmont House
20 Harley Street
London, W1N 1AL
Tel: 0171 935 5687   Fax: 0171 436 4387

Dr Dilip Shah
Jaina House Surgery
66 Arnos Grove
London, N14 7AR
Tel: 0181 886 4035   Fax: 0181 882 7024

Dr M M Shah
60 Market Square
Edmonton Green
London, N9 0TZ

Dr Rajinder Singh
15 High Road
Tottenham
London, N13 6LT
Tel: 0181 800 6507

Dr Upender Sobti
Brampton Health Centre
5 Brampton Road
London, NW9 9BY
Tel: 0181 204 6219
Dr David Suppree
91 Heath Street
London, NW3 6SS
Tel: 0171 435 0922   Fax: 0171 794 4101

London *continued*

Dr A M Vincent
11 Sloane Court West
Chelsea
London, SW3 4TD
Tel: 0171 730 1142   Fax: 0171 824 8905

Dr John Lewis Winkler
4 Kensington Mansions
Trebovir Road
London, SW5 9TF
Tel: 0171 373 2029

Middlesex

Dr A Gomes
193 High Street
Ponders End
Enfield, Middlesex, EN3 4DZ
Tel: 0181 804 1060

Dr K Lahon MBBS MRCOG
Special Interest: Obstetrics & gynaecology.
Languages: Hindi, Urdu, Punjabi, Bengali, some Arabic.
243 Western Road
Southall, Middlesex, UB2 5HS
Tel: 0181 571 5094   Fax: 0181 813 0335

Dr Nizar Merali
7 Welbeck Road
Harrow, Middlesex, HA2 0RQ
Tel: 0181 422 3021   Fax: 0181 422 6949

Dr Nigel O'Sullivan
Elm Park Clinic
69 Elm Park
Stanmore, Middlesex, HA7 4AU
Tel: 0181 954 8181/1333   Fax: 0181 420 7027

Dr Rajinder Saluja
81 Trinity Road
Southall, Middlesex, UB1 1ER
Tel: 0181 574 8136   Fax: 0181 574 0880

Middlesex *continued*

Dr Mansukh Unadkat MBBS
Special Interest: Hypertension.
Oak Lane Medical Centre
6 Oak Lane
Twickenham, Middlesex, TW1 3PA
Tel: 0181 774 0094/0067 Fax: 0181 892 1332

Southampton

Mrs Carolyn Hill
233a Brook Lane
Sarisbury Green
Southampton, SO31 7DQ
Tel: 01489 570022   Fax: 01489 570033

Surrey

Dr Apelles Econs MRCS LRCP
Special Interest: Investigation and treatment of all types of allergy & intolerence; desensitisation.
29 Hersham Road
Walton-On-Thames, Surrey, KT12 1LF
Tel: 01932 820578

Mr Terence Field
Merrow Park Surgery
Kingfisher Drive
Merrow, Guildford
Surrey, GU4 7EP

Dr W E Griffiths
37 Paradise Road
Richmond
Surrey, TW9 1SA
Tel: 0181 940 2423   Fax: 0181 332 6363

Dr Thomas F Guilder MB ChB MRCGP DRCOG
Special Interest: General practice.
Riverbank Surgery
Westcott Street
Westcott, Surrey, RH4 3PA
Tel: 01306 875 577   Fax: 01306 883 230

Dr M S Norton
Park Gates
The Green
Richmond
Surrey, TW9 1QG
Tel: 0181 940 4742

Dr Diana Samways MBBS (Lond)
Special Interest: Food and inhalant allergy; candida; overgrowth; environmental and nutritional illness; ME; chronic fatigue; alcoholism and addictions; overwieght and obesity.
PO Box 52, Haslemere
Surrey, GU27 1JA
Tel: 01428 643021, Fax: 01428 654850

Private Hospitals

Aberdeenshire

ALBYN HOSPITAL
21-24 Albyn Place, Aberdeen, Aberdeenshire, AB9 1RJ. Tel:(01224) 595993, Fax:(01224) 589869

Ayrshire

CHG CARRICK GLEN HOSPITAL
Dalmellington Rd., Ayr, Ayrshire, KA6 6PG. Tel:(01292) 288882, Fax:(01292) 283315

Bath

BATH CLINIC
Claverton Down Road, Combe Down, Bath, BA2 7BR. Tel:(01225) 835555, Fax:(01225) 835900

Bedforshire

MANOR HOSPITAL
Church End, Biddenham, Bedford, Bedforshire, MK40 4AW. Tel:(01234) 364252, Fax:(01234) 325001

Belfast

ULSTER INDEPENDENT CLINIC
245 Stranmillis Road, Belfast, BT9 5JH. Tel:(01232) 661 212

Berkshire

BMI THE PRINCESS MARGARET HOSPITAL
Osborne Road, Windsor, Berkshire, SL4 3SJ. Tel:(01753) 868292, Fax:(01753) 851749

BUPA DUNEDIN HOSPITAL
16 Bath Road, Reading, Berkshire, RG1 6NB. Tel:(01734) 587676, Fax:(01734) 503847

CARDINAL CLINIC
Bishops Lodge, Oakley Green, Windsor, Berkshire, SL4 5UL. Tel:(01753) 869755, Fax:(01753) 869755

Berkshire *continued*

CHG BERKSHIRE INDEPENDENT HOSPITAL
Wensley Road, Reading, Berkshire, RG1 6UZ. Tel:(01189) 560056, Fax:(01189) 566333

HRH PRINCESS CHRISTIAN'S HOSPITAL
12 Clarence Road, Windsor, Berkshire, SL4 5AG. Tel:(01753) 853121, Fax:(01753) 831185

HUNTERCOMBE MANOR HOSPITAL
Huntercombe Lane South, Taplow, Maidenhead, Berkshire, SL6 0PQ. Tel:(01628) 667881, Fax:(01628) 666989

LYNDEN HILL CLINIC
Linden Hill Lane, Kiln Green, near Twyford, Reading, Berkshire, RG10 9XP. Tel:(0118) 940 1234, Fax:(0118) 940 1424

THAMES VALLEY NUFFIELD HOSPITAL
Wexham Street, Wexham, Slough, Berkshire, SL3 6NH. Tel:(01753) 662241, Fax:(01753) 662129

Birmingham

BIRMINGHAM NUFFIELD HOSPITAL
22 Somerset Road, Edgbaston, Birmingham, B15 2QQ. Tel:(0121) 456 2000, Fax:(0121) 454 5293

BMI THE PRIORY HOSPITAL
Priory Road, Edgbaston, Birmingham, B5 7UG. Tel:(0121) 440 2323, Fax:(0121) 440 0804

MANOR CLINIC
23 Woodbourne Road, Edgbaston, Birmingham, B17 8BY. Tel:(0121) 434 4343,

ROBERT CLINIC
162 Station Road, Kings Norton, Birmingham, B30 1DB. Tel:(0121) 458 1483, Fax:(0121) 458 4320

THE CALTHORPE CLINIC
4 Arthur Road, Edgbaston, Birmingham, B15 2UL. Tel:(0121) 455 7585, Fax:(0121) 455 7684

Birmingham *continued*

WARWICKSHIRE ORTHOPAEDIC HOSPITAL
St Gerard's, Coventry Road, Coleshill, Birmingham, B46 3EB.
Tel:(01675) 463242, Fax:(01675) 467191

WOODBOURNE CLINIC
21 Woodbourne Road, Edgbaston, Birmingham, B17 8BY. Tel:(0121) 434 4343,

Bristol

CHESTERFIELD NUFFIELD HOSPITAL
3 Clifton Hill, Clifton, Bristol, BS8 1BP.
Tel:(0117) 9730391, Fax:(0117) 9467424

Buckinghamshire

BMI THE CHILTERN HOSPITAL
London Road, Great Missenden, Buckinghamshire, HP16 0EN.
Tel:(01494) 890890, Fax:(01494) 890250

BON SECOURS HOSPITAL
Candlemas Lane, Beaconsfield, Buckinghamshire, HP9 1AG.
Tel:(01494) 680111, Fax:(01494) 680166

PADDOCKS HOSPITAL
Aylesbury Road, Princes Risborough, Buckinghamshire, HP27 0JS.
Tel:(01844) 346951, Fax:(01844) 344521

SAXON CLINIC
Saxon Street, Eaglestone, Milton Keynes, Buckinghamshire, MK6 5LR.
Tel:(01908) 665533, Fax:(01908) 608112

Cambridgeshire

CROMWELL CLINIC
Cromwell House, 82 High Street, Huntingdon, Cambridgeshire, PE18 6DP.
Tel:(01480) 411 411, Fax:(01480) 411 411

Cambridgeshire *continued*

FITZWILLIAM HOSPITAL
Milton Way, South Bretton, Peterborough, Cambridgeshire, PE3 9AQ.
Tel:(01733) 261717, Fax:(01733) 332561

BOURN HALL CLINIC
Bourn, Cambridge, Cambridgeshire, CB3 7TR.
Tel:(01954) 719111, Fax:(01954) 718826

BUPA CAMBRIDGE LEA HOSPITAL
30 New Road, Impington, Cambridge, Cambridgeshire, CB4 4EL. Tel:(01223) 237474, Fax:(01223) 233421

EVELYN HOSPITAL, THE
4 Trumpington Road, Cambridge, Cambridgeshire, CB2 2AF. Tel:(01223) 303336, Fax:(01223) 316068

Cardiff

BUPA HOSPITAL CARDIFF
Croescadarn Road, Pentwyn, Cardiff, CF2 7XL.
Tel:(01222) 735515, Fax:(01222) 735821

Cheshire

ALTRINCHAM PRIORY HOSPITAL
Rappax Road, Hale, Altrincham, Cheshire, WA15 0NX. Tel:(0161) 904 0050, Fax:(0161) 980 4322

BMI THE ALEXANDRA HOSPITAL
Mill Lane, Cheadle, Cheshire, SK8 2PX.
Tel:(0161) 428 3656, Fax:(0161) 491 3867

BMI THE SOUTH CHESHIRE PRIVATE HOSPITAL
Leighton, Cheshire, CW1 4QP.
Tel:(01270) 500411, Fax:(01270) 583297

BUPA NORTH CHESHIRE HOSPITAL
Fir Tree Close, Stretton, Warrington, Cheshire, WA4 4LU. Tel:(01925) 265000, Fax:(01925) 604469

CHEADLE ROYAL HOSPITAL
100 Wilmslow Road, Cheadle, Cheshire, SK8 3DG. Tel:(0161) 428 9511, Fax:(0161) 428 1870

Cheshire *continued*

GROSVENOR NUFFIELD HOSPITAL
Wrexham Road, Chester, Cheshire, CH4 7QP.
Tel:(01244) 680444, Fax:(01244) 680812

REGENCY HOSPITAL, THE
West Street, Macclesfield, Cheshire, SK11 8DW.
Tel:(01625) 501150, Fax:(01625) 501800

Cleveland

CLEVELAND NUFFIELD HOSPITAL
Junction Road, Norton, Stockton-on-Tees,
Cleveland, TS20 1PX. Tel:(01642) 360100,
Fax:(01642) 556535

Clwyd

YALE HOSPITAL
Wrexham Technology Park, Groesnewydd Road,
Wrexham, Clwyd, LL13 7YP. Tel:(01978) 291306,
Fax:(01978) 291397

Cornwall

DUCHY HOSPITAL
Penventinnie Lane, Trelishe, Truro, Cornwall,
TR1 3UP. Tel:(01872) 226100, Fax:(01872)
74590

ST MICHAEL'S HOSPITAL
4 Trelissick Road, Hayle, Cornwall, TR27 4JA.
Tel:(01736) 753234, Fax:(01736) 753344

County Down

ST. JOHN OF GOD HOSPITAL
Courtney Hill, Newry, County Down, BT34 2EB.
Tel:(01693) 67711, Fax:(01693) 68492

County Dublin

BLACKROCK CLINIC
Rock Road, Blackrock, County Dublin.
Tel:(00 353) (1) 283 2222

Cumbria

CHG ABBEY PARK HOSPITAL
Dalton Lane, Barrow-in-Furness, Cumbria, LA14
4TP. Tel:(01229) 813388, Fax:(01229) 813366

CHG CALDEW HOSPITAL
64 Dalston Road, Carlisle, Cumbria, CA2 5NW.
Tel:(01228) 531713, Fax:(01228) 590158

CHG CUMBRIAN HOSPITAL
Branthwaite Road, Workington, Cumbria, CA14
4SS. Tel:(01900) 67111, Fax:(01900) 68339

Derbyshire

BMI CHATSWORTH SUITE
Chesterfield North Derbyshire Royal Hospital,
Calow, Chesterfield, Derbyshire, S44 5BL.
Tel:(01246) 550638, Fax:(01246) 205703

EAST MIDLANDS NUFFIELD HOSPITAL
Rykneld Road, Littleover, Derby, Derbyshire,
DE23 7SN. Tel:(01332) 517891, Fax:(01332)
512481

Devon

BROADREACH
465 Tavistock Road, Plymouth, Devon, PL6
7HE. Tel:(01752) 790000, Fax:(01752) 785750

EXETER NUFFIELD HOSPITAL
Wonford Road, Exeter, Devon, EX2 4UG.
Tel:(01392) 276591, Fax:(01392) 425147

MOUNT STUART HOSPITAL
St Vincents Road, Torquay, Devon, TQ1 4UP.
Tel:(01803) 313881, Fax:(01803) 314051

PLYMOUTH NUFFIELD HOSPITAL
Derriford Road, Plymouth, Devon, PL6 8BG.
Tel:(01752) 775861, Fax:(01752) 768969

THE HYPERBARIC MEDICAL CENTRE
(DDRC-Plymouth), Tamar Science Park,
Derriford Road, Plymouth, Devon, PL6 8BQ.
Tel:(01752) 209999, Fax:(01752) 209115

Private Hospitals

Dorset

BMI THE HARBOUR HOSPITAL
St Mary's Road, Poole, Dorset, BH15 2BH.
Tel:(01202) 244200, Fax:(01202) 244201

BOURNEMOUTH NUFFIELD HOSPITAL
67 Lansdowne Road, Bournemouth, Dorset, BH1 1RW. Tel:(01202) 291866, Fax:(01202) 294612

DEAN PARK CLINIC
23-25 Ophir Road, Bournemouth, Dorset, BH8 8LS. Tel:(01202) 556174, Fax:(01202) 554956

WINTERBOURNE HOSPITAL
Herringston Road, Dorchester, Dorset, DT1 2DR. Tel:(01305) 263252, Fax:(01305) 265424

Dundee

FERNBRAE HOSPITAL
329 Perth Road, Dundee, DD2 1LJ.
Tel:(01382) 667 203, Fax:(01382) 660 155

Dyfed

WERNDALE PRIVATE HOSPITAL
Bancyfelin, Carmarthen, Dyfed, SA33 5NE.
Tel:(01267) 211500, Fax:(01267) 211511

Edinburgh

BUPA MURRAYFIELD HOSPITAL
122 Corstorphine Road, Edinburgh, EH12 6UD.
Tel:(0131) 334 0363, Fax:(0131) 334 7338

Essex

BUPA HARTSWOOD HOSPITAL
Eagle Way, Brentwood, Essex, CM13 3LE.
Tel:(01277) 232525, Fax:(01277) 200128

BUPA RODING HOSPITAL
Roding Lane South, Ilford, Essex, IG4 5PZ.
Tel:(0181) 551 1100, Fax:(0181) 551 6415

Essex *continued*

BUPA WELLESLEY HOSPITAL
Eastern Avenue, Southend-on-Sea, Essex, SS2 4XH. Tel:(01702) 462944, Fax:(01702) 600160

DUKES PRIORY HOSPITAL
Stump Lane, Springfield Green, Springfield, Chelmsford, Essex, CM1 5SJ. Tel:(01245) 345345,

ELM PARK
Station Road, Ardleigh, Colchester, Essex, CO7 7RT. Tel:(01206) 231055, Fax:(01206) 231596

ESSEX NUFFIELD HOSPITAL
Shenfield Road, Brentwood, Essex, CM15 8EH.
Tel:(01277) 263263, Fax:(01277) 201158

HOLLY HOUSE HOSPITAL
High Road, Buckhurst Hill, Essex, IG9 5HX.
Tel:(0181) 505 3311, Fax:(0181) 506 1013

MARIE STOPES FAIRFIELD CLINIC
88 Russell Road, Buckhurst Hill, Essex, IG9 5QB.
Tel:(0181) 505 4641,

SPRINGFIELD MEDICAL CENTRE
Lawn Lane, Springfield, Chelmsford, Essex, CM1 5GU. Tel:(01245) 461777, Fax:(01245) 450317

SUTTON'S MANOR CLINIC
London Road, Stapleford Tawney, Essex, RM4 1SB. Tel:(01992) 814661, Fax:(01708) 688583

THE OAKS HOSPITAL
Oaks Place, Mile End Road, Colchester, Essex, CO4 5XR. Tel:(01206) 752121, Fax:(01206) 852701

Glamorgan (West)

SANCTA MARIA HOSPITAL
Ffynone Road, Swansea, Glamorgan (West), SA1 6DF. Tel:(01792) 479040, Fax:(01792) 641452

Glasgow

BMI ROSS HALL HOSPITAL
221 Crookston Road, Glasgow, G52 3NQ.
Tel:(0141) 810 3151, Fax:(0141) 882 7439

Glasgow *continued*

BON SECOURS HOSPITAL (GLASGOW)
36 Mansionhouse Road, Langside, Glasgow, G41 3DW. Tel:(0141) 632 9231, Fax:(0141) 636 5066

GLASGOW NUFFIELD HOSPITAL
25 Beaconsfield Road, Glasgow, G12 0PJ.
Tel:(0141) 334 9441, Fax:(0141) 339 1352

ST FRANCIS' NURSING HOME
42 Merryland St, Glasgow, G51 2QD.
Tel:(0141) 445 1118,

Gloucestershire

COTSWOLD NUFFIELD HOSPITAL
Talbot Road, Cheltenham, Gloucestershire, GL51 6QA. Tel:(01242) 232351, Fax:(01242) 251735

WINFIELD HOSPITAL
Tewkesbury Road, Longford, Gloucester, Gloucestershire, GL2 9EE. Tel:(01452) 331111, Fax:(01452) 331200

Gloucestershire (South)

BUPA HOSPITAL BRISTOL
The Glen, Redland Hill, Durdham Down, Bristol, Gloucestershire (South), BS6 6UT.
Tel:(0117_) 9732562, Fax:(0117) 9743203

HEATH HOUSE PRIORY HOSPITAL
Heath House Lane, off Bell Hill, Purdown, Bristol, Gloucestershire (South), BS16 1EQ.
Tel:(0117) 952 5255,

ST MARY'S HOSPITAL
Upper Byron Place, Clifton, Bristol, Gloucestershire (South), BS8 1JU.
Tel:(0117) 987 2727, Fax:(0117) 925 4909

Gwent

LLANARTH COURT HOSPITAL
Llanarth, Raglan, Gwent, NP5 2YD.
Tel:(01873) 840555,

ST JOSEPH'S PRIVATE HOSPITAL
Harding Avenue, Malpas, Newport, Gwent, NP9 6ZE. Tel:(01633) 858203, Fax:(01633) 858164

Gwynedd

NORTH WALES MEDICAL CENTRE
Queen's Road, Craig-y-Don, Llandudno, Gwynedd, LL30 1UD. Tel:(01492) 879031, Fax:(01492) 876754

Hampshire

BMI SARUM ROAD HOSPITAL
Sarum Road, Winchester, Hampshire, SO22 5HA. Tel:(01962) 844555, Fax:(01962) 842620

BUPA CHALYBEATE HOSPITAL
Chalybeate Close, Tremona Road, Southampton, Hampshire, SO16 6UY.
Tel:(01703) 775544, Fax:(01703) 701160

BUPA HOSPITAL PORTSMOUTH
Bartons Rd., Havant, Hampshire, PO9 5NP.
Tel:(01705) 454511, Fax:(01705) 452630

HAMPSHIRE CLINIC
Basing Rd., Old Basing, Basingstoke, Hampshire, RG24 7AL. Tel:(01256) 57111, Fax:(01256) 29986

MARCHWOOD PRIORY HOSPITAL
Hythe Road, Marchwood, Southampton, Hampshire, SO40 4WU. Tel:(01703) 840044, Fax:(01703) 207554

WESSEX NUFFIELD HOSPITAL
Winchester Road, Chandler's Ford, Eastleigh, Hampshire, SO53 2DW. Tel:(01703) 266377, Fax:(01703) 251525

Herefordshire

WYE VALLEY NUFFIELD HOSPITAL
Venns Lane, Hereford, Herefordshire, HR1 1DF.
Tel:(01432) 355131, Fax:(01432) 274979

Hertfordshire

BUPA HOSPITAL BUSHEY
Heathbourne Road, Bushey, Watford, Hertfordshire, WD2 1RD. Tel:(0181) 950 9090, Fax:(0181) 950 7556

Private Hospitals

Hertfordshire *continued*

BUPA HOSPITAL HARPENDEN
Ambrose La., Harpenden, Hertfordshire, AL5 4BP. Tel: (01582) 763191, Fax: (01582) 712312

CHATSWORTH CLINIC
76-78 Park Rd., New Barnet, Barnet, Hertfordshire, EN4 9QD.
Tel: (0181) 440 4217,

KNEESWORTH HOUSE HOSPITAL
Bassingbourn-cum-Kneesworth, Royston, Hertfordshire, SG8 5JP. Tel: (01763) 242911, Fax: (01763) 242011

PINEHILL HOSPITAL
Benslow Lane, Hitchin, Hertfordshire, SG4 9QZ. Tel: (01462) 422822, Fax: (01462) 421968

THE RIVERS HOSPITAL
Thomas Rivers Medical Centre, High Wych Road, Sawbridgeworth, Hertfordshire, CM21 0HH. Tel: (01279) 600282, Fax: (01279) 600212

Isle of Wight

ORCHARD HOSPITAL, THE
189 Fairlee Road, Newport, Isle of Wight, PO30 2EP. Tel: (01983) 520022, Fax: (01983) 528788

Kent

BENENDEN HOSPITAL
Goddards Green Road, Benenden, Cranbrook, Kent, TN17 4AX. Tel: (01580) 240333, Fax: (01580) 241877

BMI CHELSFIELD PARK HOSPITAL
Bucks Cross Road, Chelsfield, Orpington, Kent, BR6 7RG. Tel: (01689) 877855, Fax: (01689) 837439

BMI FAWKHAM MANOR HOSPITAL
Manor Lane, Fawkham, Longfield, Kent, DA3 8ND. Tel: (01474) 879900,

BMI SOMERFIELD HOSPITAL
63-77 London Road, Maidstone, Kent, ME16 0DU. Tel: (01622) 686581, Fax: (01622) 674706

Kent *continued*

BMI THE CHAUCER HOSPITAL
Nackington Road, Canterbury, Kent, CT4 7AR. Tel: (01227) 825100, Fax: (01227) 762733

BMI THE SLOANE HOSPITAL
125 Albemarle Road, Beckenham, Kent, BR3 5HS. Tel: (0181) 466 6911, Fax: (0181) 464 1443

BUPA ALEXANDRA HOSPITAL
Impton Lane, Walderslade, Chatham, Kent, ME5 9PG. Tel: (01634) 687166, Fax: (01634) 686162

BUPA ST SAVIOUR'S HOSPITAL
73 Seabrook Road, Hythe, Kent, CT21 5QW. Tel: (01303) 265581, Fax: (01303) 261441

GODDEN GREEN CLINIC
Godden Green, Sevenoaks, Kent, TN15 0JR. Tel: (01732) 763491, Fax: (01732) 763160

HAYES GROVE PRIORY HOSPITAL
Prestons Road, Hayes, Bromley, Kent, BR2 7AS. Tel: (0181) 462 7722,

TUNBRIDGE WELLS INDEPENDENT HOSPITAL
Fordcombe Road, Fordcombe, Tunbridge Wells, Kent, TN3 0RD. Tel: (01892) 740047, Fax: (01892) 740046

TUNBRIDGE WELLS NUFFIELD HOSPITAL
Kingswood Road, Tunbridge Wells, Kent, TN2 4UL. Tel: (01892) 531111, Fax: (01892) 515689

Lancashire

BMI THE BEARDWOOD HOSPITAL
Preston New Road, Blackburn, Lancashire, BB2 3AE. Tel: (01254) 564219, Fax: (01254) 695032

BMI THE BEAUMONT HOSPITAL
Old Hall Clough, Chorley New Road, Lostock, Bolton, Lancashire, BL6 4LA.
Tel: (01204) 404404, Fax: (01204) 848878

BMI THE HIGHFIELD HOSPITAL
Manchester Road, Rochdale, Lancashire, OL11 4LZ. Tel: (01706) 55121, Fax: (01706) 860719

Lancashire *continued*

CHG EUXTON HALL HOSPITAL
Wigan Road, Euxton, Chorley, Lancashire, PR7 6DY. Tel:(01257) 276261, Fax:(01257) 261882

CHG FULWOOD HALL HOSPITAL
Midgery Lane, Fulwood, Preston, Lancashire, PR2 9SZ. Tel:(01772) 704111, Fax:(01772) 795131

CHG RENACRES HALL HOSPITAL
Renacres Lane, Halsall, Ormskirk, Lancashire, L39 8SE. Tel:(01704) 841133, Fax:(01704) 841277

GISBURNE PARK PRIVATE HOSPITAL
Gisburne, Clitheroe, Lancashire, BB7 4HX. Tel:(01200) 445 693, Fax:(01200) 445 688

KEMPLE VIEW
Longsight Rd, Langho, Blackburn, Lancashire, BB6 8AD. Tel:(01254) 248 021,

LANCASTER & LAKELAND NUFFIELD HOSPITAL
Meadowside, Lancaster, Lancashire, LA1 3RH. Tel:(01524) 62345, Fax:(01524) 844725

Lankashire

BUPA FYLDE COAST HOSPITAL
St Walburgas Road, Blackpool, Lankashire, FY3 8BP. Tel:(01253) 394188, Fax:(01253) 397946

Leicestershire

LEICESTER NUFFIELD HOSPITAL, THE
Scraptoft Lane, Leicester, Leicestershire, LE5 1HY. Tel:(0116) 2769401, Fax:(0116) 2461076

SKETCHLEY HALL REHABILITATION CENTRE
Manor Way, Burbage, Hinckley, Leicestershire, LE10 3HT. Tel:(01455) 890023,

Leicestrshire

BUPA HOSPITAL LEICESTER
Gartree Rd., Oadby, Leicester, Leicestrshire, LE2 2FF. Tel:(0116) 2720888, Fax:(0116) 2720666

Lincolnshire

BROMHEAD HOSPITAL
Nettleham Road, Lincoln, Lincolnshire, LN2 1QU. Tel:(01522) 578000, Fax:(01522) 514021

London

BMI THE BLACKHEATH HOSPITAL
40-42 Lee Terrace, Blackheath, London, SE3 9UD. Tel:(0181) 318 7722, Fax:(0181) 318 2542

CHARTER CLINIC CHELSEA
1-5 Radnor Walk, London, SW3 4PB. Tel:(0171) 351 1272,

CHARTER NIGHTINGALE HOSPITAL
11-19 Lisson Grove, London, NW1 6SH. Tel:(0171) 258 3828, Fax:(0171) 724 8294

CHURCHILL PRIVATE CLINIC
80 Lambeth Road, London, SE1 7PW. Tel:(0171) 928 5633, Fax:(0171) 928 1702

CROMWELL HOSPITAL
Cromwell Road, London, SW5 0TU. Tel:(0171) 460 2000, Fax:(0171) 460 5555

DEVONSHIRE HOSPITAL
29-31 Devonshire Street, London, W1N 1RF. Tel:(0171) 486 7131, Fax:(0171) 486 7131

FITZROY NUFFIELD HOSPITAL
10-12 Bryanston Square, London, W1H 8BB. Tel:(0171) 723 1288, Fax:(0171) 262 6357

GARDEN HOSPITAL
46-50 Sunny Gardens Road, Hendon, London, NW4 1RX. Tel:(0181) 203 0111, Fax:(0181) 203 4343

GROVELANDS PRIORY HOSPITAL
The Bourne, Southgate, London, N14 6RA. Tel:(0181) 882 8191, Fax:(0181) 447 8138

HARLEY STREET CLINIC, THE
35 Weymouth Street., London, W1N 4BJ. Tel:(0171) 935 7700, Fax:(0171) 487 4415

London *continued*

HEATH CLINIC, THE
58 West Heath Drive, London, NW11 7QH.
Tel:(0181) 458 4416, Fax:(0181) 905 5274

HIGHGATE PRIVATE HOSPITAL LTD
17-19 View Road, Highgate, London, N6 4DJ.
Tel:(0181) 341 4182, Fax:(0181) 342 8347

HOSPITAL OF ST. JOHN & ST. ELIZABETH
60 Grove End Road, St Johns Wood, London, NW8 9NH. Tel:(0171) 286 5126, Fax:(0171) 266 4813

KING EDWARD VII'S HOSPITAL FOR OFFICERS
Beaumont Street, London, W1N 2AA.
Tel:(0171) 486 4411, Fax:(0171) 467 4303

LEIGHAM PRIVATE CLINIC
76 Leigham Court Road, Streatham, London, SW16 2QA. Tel:(0181) 677 5522,

LISTER HOSPITAL
Chelsea Bridge Road, London, SW1W 8RH.
Tel:(0171) 730 3417, Fax:(0171) 824 8867

LONDON BRIDGE HOSPITAL
27 Tooley Street, London, SE1 2PR.
Tel:(0171) 407 3100, Fax:(0171) 407 3162

LONDON INDEPENDENT HOSPITAL
1 Beaumont Square, Stepney Green, London, E1 4NL. Tel:(0171) 790 0990, Fax:(0171) 265 9032

MANOR HOUSE HOSPITAL LTD
North End Road, Golders Green, London, NW11 7HX. Tel:(0181) 455 6601, Fax:(0181) 458 4991

MARIE STOPES PARKVIEW CLINIC
87 Mattock Lane, Ealing, London, W5 5BJ.
Tel:(0181) 567 0102,

MARIE STOPES RALEIGH CLINIC
1A Raleigh Gardens, Briston Hill, Arodne Road, London, SW2 1AB.
Tel:(0181) 671 1541,

OLD COURT HOSPITAL
19 Montpelier Road, London, W5 2QT.
Tel:(0181) 998 2848, Fax:(0181) 997 5561

London *continued*

PARKSIDE HOSPITAL
53 Parkside, Wimbledon, London, SW19 5NX.
Tel:(0181) 946 4202, Fax:(0181) 946 7775

PORTLAND HOSPITAL FOR WOMEN AND CHILDREN, THE
205-209 Great Portland Street, London, W1N 6AH. Tel:(0171) 580 4400, Fax:(0171) 390 8012

PRINCESS GRACE HOSPITAL, THE
42-52 Nottingham Place, London, W1M 3FD.
Tel:(0171) 486 1234, Fax:(0171) 935 2198

PRIORY HOSPITAL
Priory Lane, Roehampton, London, SW15 5JJ.
Tel:(0181) 876 8261,

REDFORD LODGE
15 Church Street, Edmonton, London, N9 9DY.
Tel:(0181) 956 1234, Fax:(0181) 956 1230

ST LUKE'S HOSPITAL FOR THE CLERGY
14 Fitzroy Square, London, W1P 6AH.
Tel:(0171) 388 4954, Fax:(0171) 383 4812

THE LONDON CLINIC
20 Devonshire Place, London, W1N 2DH.
Tel:(0171) 935 4444, Fax:(0171) 486 3782

WELLINGTON HOSPITAL, THE
(Wellington South), 8a Wellington Place, London, NW8 9LE. Tel:(0171) 586 5959, Fax:(0171) 586 1960

WEST HAMPSTEAD CLINIC
9 Hilltop Road, London, NW6 2QA.
Tel:(0171) 624 7366,

Londonderry

NORTH WEST INDEPENDENT HOSPITAL
Church Hill House, Ballykelly, Londonderry, BT49 9HS. Tel:(01504) 763090, Fax:(01504) 768306

Manchester

BUPA HOSPITAL MANCHESTER
Russell Road, Whalley Range, Manchester, M16 8AJ. Tel:(0161) 226 0112, Fax:(0161) 227 9405

Manchester *continued*

CHG VICTORIA PARK HOSPITAL
Daisy Bank Road, Victoria Park, Manchester, M14 6QH. Tel: (0161) 257 2233, Fax: (0161) 256 3128

MARIE STOPES CENTRE
St John Street Mansions, 2 St John Street, Manchester, M3 4DB. Tel: (0161) 832 4260, Fax: (0161) 834 4872

Manchester (Greater)

CHG OAKLANDS HOSPITAL
19 Lancaster Road, Salford, Manchester (Greater), M6 8AQ. Tel: (0161) 787 7700, Fax: (0161) 787 8097

OAKLANDS HOSPITAL
11a-19 Lancaster Road, Salford, Manchester (Greater), M6 8AQ. Tel: (0161) 787 7700,

Merseyside

BUPA MURRAYFIELD HOSPITAL
Holmwood Drive, Thingwall, Wirral, Merseyside, L61 1AU. Tel: (0151) 648 7000, Fax: (0151) 648 0195

FAIRFIELD HOSPITAL
Crank, St Helens, Merseyside, WA11 7RS. Tel: (01744) 39311,

LOURDES HOSPITAL
57 Greenbank Road, Liverpool, Merseyside, L18 1HQ. Tel: (0151) 733 7123, Fax: (0151) 735 0446

MERSEYSIDE CLINIC
32 Parkfield Road, Liverpool, Merseyside, L17 8UJ. Tel: (0151) 727 1851, Fax: (0151) 726 950

PARK HOUSE NURSING HOME
Haigh Road, Waterloo, Liverpool, Merseyside, L22 3XS. Tel: (0151) 928 4343,

Middlesex

BMI BISHOPS WOOD HOSPITAL
Rickmansworth Road, Northwood, Middlesex, HA6 2JW. Tel: (01923) 835 814, Fax: (01923) 835 181

BMI THE CLEMENTINE CHURCHILL HOSPITAL
Sudbury Hill, Harrow, Middlesex, HA1 3RX. Tel: (0181) 422 3464, Fax: (0181) 864 1747

BMI THE KING'S OAK HOSPITAL
Chase Farm (North Side), The Ridgeway, Enfield, Middlesex, EN2 8SD. Tel: (0181) 364 5520, Fax: (0181) 364 6779

NORTH LONDON NUFFIELD HOSPITAL
Cavell Drive, Uplands Park Road, Enfield, Middlesex, EN2 7PR. Tel: (0181) 366 2122, Fax: (0181) 367 8032

ROSSLYN CLINIC
15 Rosslyn Road, East Twickenham, Middlesex, TW1 2AR. Tel: (0181) 891 3173,

ST ANDREW'S AT HARROW (BOWDEN HOUSE)
London Road, Harrow-on-the-Hill, Harrow, Middlesex, HA1 3JL. Tel: (0181) 966 7000, Fax: (0181) 864 6092

ST VINCENT'S ORTHOPAEDIC HOSPITAL
Eastcote, Pinner, Middlesex, HA5 2NB. Tel: (0181) 429 6200, Fax: (0181) 866 6512

Newcastle upon Tyne

NEWCASTLE NUFFIELD HOSPITAL
Clayton Road, Jesmond, Newcastle upon Tyne, NE2 1JP. Tel: (0191) 281 6131, Fax: (0191) 212 0113

Norfolk

BMI THE SANDRINGHAM HOSPITAL
Gayton Road, King's Lynn, Norfolk, PE30 4HJ. Tel: (01553) 769770, Fax: (01553) 767573

Norfolk *continued*

BUPA HOSPITAL NORWICH
Old Watton Rd., Colney, Norwich, Norfolk, NR4 7TD. Tel:(01603) 456181, Fax:(01603) 250968

BURSTON HOUSE
Rectory Road, Burston, Diss, Norfolk, IP22 3TU. Tel:(01379) 741562, Fax:(01379) 740558

ST JOHN'S HOUSE
Lion Road, Palgrave, Diss, Norfolk, IP22 1BA. Tel:(01379) 643334, Fax:(01379) 641455

North Lincolnshire

BARROW HALL NURSING HOME
Wold Road, Barrow-upon-Humber, North Lincolnshire, DN19 7DQ. Tel:(01469) 531281, Fax:(01469) 532544

North Yorkshire

DUCHY NUFFIELD HOSPITAL
Queens Road, Harrogate, North Yorkshire, HG2 0HF. Tel:(01423) 567136, Fax:(01423) 524381

Northamptonshire

CHG WOODLAND HOSPITAL
Rothwell Road, Kettering, Northamptonshire, NN16 8XF. Tel:(01536) 414515, Fax:(01536) 412155

GRAFTON MANOR
Grafton Regis, Towcester, Northamptonshire, NN12 7SS. Tel:(01908) 543131, Fax:(01908) 542644

ST ANDREW'S HOSPITAL
Billing Road, Northampton, Northamptonshire, NN1 5DG. Tel:(01604) 29696, Fax:(01604) 232325

ST MATTHEW'S PRIVATE HOSPITAL
St Matthew's Parade, Northampton, Northamptonshire, NN2 7EZ.
Tel:(01604) 711222, Fax:(01604) 711222

Northamptonshire *contd.*

THREE SHIRES HOSPITAL
The Avenue, Cliftonville, Northampton, Northamptonshire, NN1 5DR.
Tel:(01604) 20311, Fax:(01604) 29066

Nottinghamshire

BMI THE PARK HOSPITAL
Sherwood Lodge Drive, Burntstump Country Park, Arnold, Nottingham, Nottinghamshire, NG5 8RX. Tel:(0115) 967 0670, Fax:(0115) 967 0381

CONVENT HOSPITAL
748 Mansfield Road, Woodthorpe, Nottingham, Nottinghamshire, NG5 3FZ. Tel:(0115) 920 9209, Fax:(0115) 967 3005

Oxfordshire

ACLAND NUFFIELD HOSPITAL
Banbury Road, Oxford, Oxfordshire, OX2 6PD.
Tel:(01865) 404142, Fax:(01865) 556303

FOSCOTE PRIVATE HOSPITAL
2 Foscote Rise, Banbury, Oxfordshire, OX16 9XP. Tel:(01295) 252281, Fax:(01295) 272877

Peeblesshire

CASTLE CRAIG CLINIC
Blyth Bridge, West Linton, Peeblesshire, EH46 7DH. Tel:(01721) 752 625,

Shropshire

SHROPSHIRE NUFFIELD HOSPITAL
Longden Road, Shrewsbury, Shropshire, SY3 9DP.
Tel:(01743) 353441, Fax:(01743) 247575

Somerset

SOMERSET NUFFIELD HOSPITAL
Staplegrove Elm, Taunton, Somerset, TA2 6AN.
Tel:(01823) 286991, Fax:(01823) 338951

Somerset (North)

BROADWAY LODGE
Oldmixon Road, Weston Super Mare, Somerset (North), BS24 9NN. Tel: (01934) 812319, Fax: (01934) 815381

South Humberside

ST HUGH'S HOSPITAL
Prince's Road, Cleethorpes, South Humberside, DN35 8AP. Tel: (01472) 692834, Fax: (01472) 696630

ST HUGH'S HOSPITAL
Peaks Lane, Grimsby, South Humberside, DN32 9RP. Tel: (01472) 251100, Fax: (01472) 251130

Staffordshire

CHG ROWLEY HALL HOSPITAL
Rowley Park, Stafford, Staffordshire, ST17 9AQ. Tel: (01785) 223203, Fax: (01785) 249532

NORTH STAFFORDSHIRE NUFFIELD HOSPITAL
Clayton Road, Newcastle, Staffordshire, ST5 4DB. Tel: (01782) 625431, Fax: (01782) 712748

Stirling

CHG KING'S PARK HOSPITAL
Polmaise Road, Stirling, FK7 9PU. Tel: (01786) 451669, Fax: (01786) 465296

Suffolk

ALL HALLOWS HOSPITAL
Station Road, Ditchingham, Bungay, Suffolk, NR35 2QL. Tel: (01986) 892 728, Fax: (01986) 895 063

CHRISTCHURCH PARK HOSPITAL
57 Fonnereau Road, Ipswich, Suffolk, IP1 3JN. Tel: (01473) 256 071, Fax: (01473) 288 053

Suffolk *continued*

ST EDMUND HOSPITAL
St Mary's Square, Bury St. Edmunds, Suffolk, IP33 2AA. Tel: (01284) 701371, Fax: (01284) 769998

Surrey

ASHTEAD HOSPITAL
The Warren, Ashtead, Surrey, KT21 2SB. Tel: (01372) 276161, Fax: (01372) 278704

BMI THE RUNNYMEDE HOSPITAL
Guildford Road, Ottershaw, Chertsey, Surrey, KT16 0RQ. Tel: (01932) 872007, Fax: (01932) 875433

BUPA GATWICK PARK HOSPITAL
Povey Cross Road, Horley, Surrey, RH6 0BB. Tel: (01293) 785511, Fax: (01293) 774883

BUPA HOSPITAL CLARE PARK
Clare Park, Crondall Lane, Crondall, Farnham, Surrey, GU10 5XX. Tel: (01252) 850216, Fax: (01252) 850228

CHG NORTH DOWNS HOSPITAL
46 Tupwood Lane, Caterham, Surrey, CR3 6DP. Tel: (01883) 348981, Fax: (01883) 341163

CHILDREN'S TRUST, THE
Tadworth St, Tadworth, Surrey, KT20 5RU. Tel: (01737) 357 171, Fax: (01737) 373 848

FARM PLACE
Ockley, Dorking, Surrey, RH5 5NG. Tel: (01306) 627 742,

HOLY CROSS HOSPITAL
Hindhead Road, Haslemere, Surrey, GU27 1NQ. Tel: (01428) 643311, Fax: (01428) 644007

LYNBROOK PRIORY HOSPITAL
Chobham Road, Knaphill, Woking, Surrey, GU21 2QF. Tel: (01483) 489211, Fax: (01483) 797053

MOUNT ALVERNIA HOSPITAL
Harvey Road, Guildford, Surrey, GU1 3LX. Tel: (01483) 570 122, Fax: (01483) 325 54

Surrey *continued*

NEW VICTORIA HOSPITAL
184 Coombe Lane West, Kingston upon Thames, Surrey, KT2 7EG. Tel:(0181) 949 9000, Fax:(0181) 949 9099

SHIRLEY OAKS HOSPITAL
Poppy Lane, Shirley Oaks Village, Croydon, Surrey, CR9 8AB. Tel:(0181) 655 2255, Fax:(0181) 656 2868

ST ANTHONY'S HOSPITAL
London Road, North Cheam, Sutton, Surrey, SM3 9DW. Tel:(0181) 337 6691, Fax:(0181) 335 3325

STURT PRIORY HOSPITAL
Sturts Lane, Walton-on-the-Hill, Tadworth, Surrey, KT20 7RQ. Tel:(01737) 814488, Fax:(01737) 813926

WOKING NUFFIELD HOSPITAL
Shores Road, Woking, Surrey, GU21 4BY. Tel:(01483) 763511, Fax:(01483) 722966

Sussex

SUSSEX NUFFIELD HOSPITAL
Warren Road, Woodingdean, Brighton, Sussex, BN2 6DX. Tel:(01273) 624488, Fax:(01273) 620101

WISTONS CLINIC
138 Dyke Road, Brighton, Sussex, BN1 5PA. Tel:(01273) 506263, Fax:(01273) 562337

Sussex (East)

ESPERANCE PRIVATE HOSPITAL
Hartington Place, Eastbourne, Sussex (East), BN21 3BG. Tel:(01323) 411188, Fax:(01323) 410626

HOVE NUFFIELD HOSPITAL
55 New Church Road, Hove, Sussex (East), BN3 4BG. Tel:(01273) 779471, Fax:(01273) 220919

Sussex (East) *continued*

SUSSEX PRIVATE CLINIC, THE
The Green, St Leonards-on-Sea, Sussex (East), TN38 0SY. Tel:(01424) 439 439, Fax:(01424) 718 806

TICEHURST HOUSE HOSPITAL
Ticehurst, Wadhurst, Sussex (East), TN5 7HU. Tel:(01580) 200391, Fax:(01580) 201006

Sussex (West)

GORING HALL HOSPITAL
Bodiam Avenue, Goring-by-Sea, Worthing, Sussex (West), BN12 4AT. Tel:(01903) 506699, Fax:(01903) 242348

KING EDWARD VII HOSPITAL
Midhurst, Sussex (West), GU29 0BL. Tel:(01730) 811 178, Fax:(01730) 817 364

ST FRANCIS NURSING HOME
47 Church Street, Littlehampton, Sussex (West), BN17 5PY. Tel:(01903) 714 351,

Tyne and Wear

WASHINGTON HOSPITAL, THE
Picktree Lane, Rickleton, Washington, Tyne and Wear, NE38 9JZ. Tel:(0191) 415 1272, Fax:(0191) 415 5541

Warwickshire

BLACKDOWN CLINIC
Old Milverton Lane, Blackdown, Leamington Spa, Warwickshire, CV32 6RW. Tel:(01926) 334664, Fax:(01926) 425291

NUNEATON PRIVATE HOSPITAL
132 Coventry Road, Nuneaton, Warwickshire, CV10 7AD. Tel:(01203) 353000, Fax:(01203) 346645

WARWICKSHIRE NUFFIEID HOSPITAL
The Chase, Old Milverton Lane, Leamington Spa, Warwickshire, CV32 6RW. Tel:(01926) 427971, Fax:(01926) 428791

West Midlands

BMI MERIDEN WING
Walsgrave Hospital, Clifford Bridge Road, Coventry, West Midlands, CV2 2DX.
Tel:(01203) 602772, Fax:(01203) 602329

BUPA HOSPITAL LITTLE ASTON
Little Aston Hall Drive, Little Aston, Sutton Coldfield, West Midlands, B74 3UP.
Tel:(0121) 353 2444, Fax:(0121) 353 1592

BUPA PARKWAY HOSPITAL
1 Damson Parkway, Solihull, West Midlands, B91 2PP. Tel:(0121) 704 1451, Fax:(0121) 711 1080

CHG WEST MIDLANDS HOSPITAL
Colman Hill, Halesowen, West Midlands, B63 2AH. Tel:(01384) 560123, Fax:(01384) 411103

WOLVERHAMPTON NUFFIELD HOSPITAL
Wood Road, Tettenhall, Wolverhampton, West Midlands, WV6 8LE. Tel:(01902) 754177, Fax:(01902) 741379

Wiltshire

CLOUDS
Clouds House, East Knoyle, Salisbury, Wiltshire, SP3 6BE. Tel:(01747) 830 733, Fax:(01747) 830 783

NEW HALL HOSPITAL
Bodenham, Salisbury, Wiltshire, SP5 4EY.
Tel:(01722) 422333, Fax:(01722) 435158

RIDGEWAY HOSPITAL
Moormead Road, Wroughton, Swindon, Wiltshire, SN4 9DD. Tel:(01793) 814848, Fax:(01793) 814852

Worcestershire

BUPA SOUTH BANK HOSPITAL
139 Bath Road, Worcester, Worcestershire, WR5 3YB. Tel:(01905) 350003, Fax:(01905) 350856

DROITWICH PRIVATE HOSPITAL
St Andrew's Road, Droitwich, Worcestershire, WR9 8DN. Tel:(01905) 794793, Fax:(01905) 779095

Yorkshire

PUREY CUST NUFFIELD HOSPITAL
Precentors Court, York, Yorkshire, YO1 2EL.
Tel:(01904) 641571, Fax:(01904) 643115

RETREAT, THE
107 Heslington Road, York, Yorkshire, YO1 5BN.
Tel:(01904) 412 551, Fax:(01904) 430 828

STOCKTON HALL HOSPITAL
The Village, Stockton-on-the-Forest, York, Yorkshire, YO3 9UN. Tel:(01904) 400500, Fax:(01904) 400354

Yorkshire (East)

BUPA HOSPITAL HULL & EAST RIDING
Lowfield Road, Anlaby, Hull, Yorkshire (East), HU10 7AZ. Tel:(01482) 659471, Fax:(01482) 654033

HULL NUFFIELD HOSPITAL
81 Westbourne Avenue, Hull, Yorkshire (East), HU5 3HP. Tel:(01482) 342327, Fax:(01482) 470133

Yorkshire (North)

BUPA BELVEDERE HOSPITAL
Belvedere Road, Scarborough, Yorkshire (North), YO11 2UT. Tel:(01723) 365363, Fax:(01723) 377513

HARROGATE CLINIC
23 Ripon Road, Harrogate, Yorkshire (North), HG1 2JL. Tel:(01423) 500599, Fax:(01423) 531074

ST JOHN OF GOD HOSPITAL
Scorton, Richmond, Yorkshire (North), DL10 6EB. Tel:(01748) 811535, Fax:(01748) 812345

Yorkshire (South)

BMI THORNBURY HOSPITAL
312 Fulwood Road, Sheffield, Yorkshire (South), S10 3BR. Tel:(0114) 266 1133, Fax:(0114) 268 6913

Private Hospitals

Yorkshire (South) *continued*

CHG DONCASTER HOSPITAL
51 Bawtry Rd, Bessacarr, Doncaster, Yorkshire (South), DN4 7AA. Tel:(01302) 370219, Fax:(01302) 536990

CHG PARK HILL HOSPITAL
Thorne Road, Doncaster, Yorkshire (South), DN2 5JH. Tel:(01302) 730300, Fax:(01302) 322499

CLAREMONT HOSPITAL
401 Sandygate Road, Sheffield, Yorkshire (South), S10 5UB. Tel:(0114) 263 0330, Fax:(0114) 230 9388

DANUM LODGE CLINIC
123 Thorne Road, Doncaster, Yorkshire (South), DN2 5BQ. Tel:(01302) 325508, Fax:(01302) 768206

PARKFIELD HOSPITAL (ROTHERAM) LTD
Parkfield Road, Rotherham, Yorkshire (South), S65 2AJ. Tel:(01709) 828928, Fax:(01709) 828372

Yorkshire (West)

ALLERTON HOSPITAL
18 Allerton Park, Leeds, Yorkshire (West), LS7 4ND. Tel:(0113) 2683758,

BUPA HOSPITAL ELLAND
Elland Lane, Elland, Yorkshire (West), HX5 9EB. Tel:(01422) 375577, Fax:(01422) 377501

BUPA HOSPITAL LEEDS
Roundhay Hall, Jackson Avenue, Leeds, Yorkshire (West), LS8 1NT.
Tel:(0113) 2693939, Fax:(0113) 2681340

HUDDERSFIELD NUFFIELD HOSPITAL
Birkby Hall Road, Birkby, Huddersfield, Yorkshire (West), HD2 2BL.
Tel:(01484) 533131, Fax:(01484) 428396

MARIE STOPES CENTRE
10 Queen Square, Leeds, Yorkshire (West), LS2 8AJ. Tel:(0113) 244 0685, Fax:(0113) 244 8865

Yorkshire (West) *continued*

METHLEY PARK HOSPITAL
Methley Lane, Methley, Leeds, Yorkshire (West), LS26 9HG. Tel:(01977) 518518,

MID YORKSHIRE NUFFIELD HOSPITAL
Outwood Lane, Horsforth, Leeds, Yorkshire (West), LS18 4HP. Tel:(0113) 2588756, Fax:(0113) 2583108

PRIORY GRANGE
Micklefield Lane, Rawdon, Leeds, Yorkshire (West), LS19 6BA. Tel:(0113) 239 1999,

THE LEEDS PRIVATE HOSPITAL
The Fallodon Private Surgical Hospital, 4 Allerton Park, Leeds, Yorkshire (West), LS7 4ND. Tel:(0113) 2692231,

THE YORKSHIRE CLINIC
Bradford Road, Bingley, Yorkshire (West), BD16 1TW. Tel:(01274) 560311, Fax:(01274) 551247

NOTES

NOTES

NOTES

NOTES